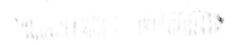

HIV and AIDS

HIV and AIDS

A GLOBAL VIEW

Edited by Karen McElrath

A World View of Social Issues
Andrew L. Cherry, Series Adviser

Greenwood Press
Westport, Connecticut • London

278274

MAY 2 9 2003

Library of Congress Cataloging-in-Publication Data

HIV and AIDS : a global view / edited by Karen McElrath.
   p. cm.—(A world view of social issues, ISSN 1526–9442)
   Includes bibliographical references and index.
   ISBN 0–313–31403–9 (alk. paper)
   1. AIDS (Disease)—Cross-cultural studies. I. McElrath, Karen, 1959– II. Series.
   RA643.8 .H58   2002
   362.1'969792—dc21   2001023886

British Library Cataloguing in Publication Data is available.

Library of Congress Catalog Card Number: 2001023886
ISBN: 0–313–31403–9
ISSN: 1526–9442

First published in 2002

Greenwood Press, 88 Post Road West, Westport, CT 06881
An imprint of Greenwood Publishing Group, Inc.
www.greenwood.com

Printed in the United States of America

The paper used in this book complies with the
Permanent Paper Standard issued by the National
Information Standards Organization (Z39.48–1984).

10 9 8 7 6 5 4 3 2 1

CONTENTS

SERIES FOREWORD

Why are child abuse in the family and homelessness social conditions to be endured or at least tolerated in some countries while in other countries they are viewed as social problems that must be reduced or eliminated? What social institutions and other factors affect these behaviors? What historical, political, and social forces influence a society's response to a social condition? In many cases, individuals around the world have the same or similar hopes and problems. However, in most cases we deal with the same social conditions in very dissimilar ways.

The volumes in the Greenwood series A World View of Social Issues examine different social issues and problems that are being faced by individuals and societies around the world. These volumes examine problems of poverty and homelessness, drugs and alcohol addiction, HIV/AIDS, teen pregnancy, crime, women's rights, and a myriad of other issues that affect all of us in one way or another.

Each volume is devoted to one social issue or problem. All volumes follow the same general format. Each volume has up to fifteen chapters that describe how people in different countries perceive and try to cope with a given problem or social issue. The countries chosen represent as many world regions as possible, making it possible to explore how each issue has been recognized and what actions have been taken to alleviate it in a variety of settings.

Each chapter begins with a profile of the country being highlighted and an overview of the impact of the social issue or problem there. Basic policies, legislation, and demographic information related to the social issue are covered. A brief history of the problem helps the reader better understand the political and social responses. Political initiatives and policies are also discussed, as well as social views, customs, and practices related to the problem or social issue. Discussions about how the countries plan to deal with these social problems are also included.

These volumes present a comprehensive and engaging approach for the study of international social conditions and problems. The goal is to provide a convenient framework for readers to examine specific social problems, how they are viewed, and what actions are being taken by different countries around the world.

For example, how is a problem like crime and crime control handled in Third World countries? How is substance abuse controlled in industrialized countries? How are poverty and homelessness handled in the poorest countries? How does culture influence the definition and response to domestic violence in different countries? What part does economics play in shaping both the issue of and the response to women's rights? How does a national philosophy impact the definition and response to child abuse? These questions and more will be answered by the volumes in this series.

As we learn more about our counterparts in other countries, they become real to us, and our worldview cannot help but change. We will think of others as we think of those we know. They will be people who get up in the morning and go to work. We will see people who are struggling with relationships, attending religious services, being born, growing old, and dying.

This series will cover issues that will add to your knowledge about contemporary social society. These volumes will help you to better understand social conditions and social issues in a broader sense, giving you a view of what various problems mean to different people and how these perspectives impact a society's response. You will be able to see how specific social problems are managed by governments and individuals confronting the consequences of these social dilemmas. By studying one problem from various angles, you will be better able to grasp the totality of the situation, while at the same time speculating as to how solutions used in one country could be incorporated in another. Finally, this series will allow you to compare and contrast how these social issues impact individuals in different countries and how the effect is dissimilar or similar to your own experiences.

As series adviser, it is my hope that these volumes, which are unique in the history of publishing, will increase your understanding and appreciation of your counterparts around the world.

Andrew L. Cherry
Series Adviser

INTRODUCTION

Within a span of two decades, AIDS (Acquired Immunodeficiency Syndrome) has become one of the most important public health concerns in contemporary society. Recent data suggest that an estimated 36.1 million persons (adults and children) are living with HIV (Human Immunodeficiency Virus) or AIDS (UNAIDS/WHO 2000). Approximately 21.8 million persons have died from AIDS-related illnesses by year-end 2000 (UNAIDS/WHO 2000). To date, several projections about future estimates have been unreliable—underestimated for some countries and overestimated for others. The pandemic requires considerable political commitment if we are to prevent the spread of HIV—the virus that causes AIDS. This volume addresses HIV and AIDS and the related social health challenges that we face as a result of the pandemic. Included within this volume are 14 chapters, representing 15 different countries or regions of the world. Each chapter addresses various issues relating to HIV and AIDS within the respective country. These issues include the history of HIV and AIDS, including prevalence, incidence, and modes of transmission; the stigma faced by persons living with HIV and AIDS; available treatment; government responses to HIV and AIDS; and the role of nongovernmental organizations (NGOs).

Vast regional differences exist both across and within continents and countries in terms of prevalence, incidence, service provision, and cultural perceptions about HIV and AIDS. The developing and most impoverished countries of the world have been most affected by the disease. For example, HIV and AIDS have led to catastrophic conditions in Africa. Recent figures suggest that 70% of all persons living with HIV reside in sub-Saharan Africa

(UNAIDS/WHO 2000). In Botswana, one-third of all adults are living with HIV (Schwartländer et al. 2000). Shortened life expectancies have led some scholars to predict an average life span of 30 years by the year 2010 in several countries within southern Africa (Stephenson 2000). Within this volume, Helen Jackson and Tim Lee address these issues with respect to sub-Saharan Africa, and Elizabeth Pisani uses two countries—Kenya and Uganda—to illustrate the impact of and response to the disease.

Other countries have been disproportionately affected as well. Haiti, discussed in this volume by Mary Comerford, has been described as the "worst affected country outside Africa" with an adult HIV prevalence rate estimated to be 5% (Schwartländer et al. 2000). Huge increases in the number of persons living with HIV have been observed in recent years within Central and Eastern Europe. In this volume, Jean-Paul Grund describes these changes and discusses the effects of the political and social conditions within this region.

Probable modes of HIV transmission differ by world region (UNAIDS/WHO 2000), and the chapters herein illustrate these differences. Some contributors note that the primary mode of transmission is men having sex with men (e.g., Australia, Switzerland, United States), whereas in other regions behaviors associated with injecting drug use are believed to be the primary exposure category for HIV or AIDS (e.g., Central and Eastern Europe, China, Spain, Ireland). Other scholars have warned that we have become so concerned about HIV infection spread through sexual means that "we are in danger of missing a great opportunity to stop some of the most explosive AIDS outbreaks now occurring in many developing countries—huge outbreaks of HIV associated with injection drug use" (Drucker 2000: 776). Modes of transmission can differ greatly between countries despite close geographic proximity. Within this volume, Kathryn Higgins and Sally Haw note that men having sex with men represents the most common method of HIV transmission in the United Kingdom. Ireland lies across the Irish sea to the west, yet despite the geographic proximity of the two countries, Karen McElrath notes that injecting drug use represents the most common exposure category in the south of Ireland.

In some countries, the distribution of cases across transmission categories is changing. For example, some countries are experiencing increases in HIV infection among heterosexuals, and chapters within this volume highlight those changes (e.g., Ireland, Switzerland, United Kingdom). Other contributors have noted that increases in heterosexual transmission has resulted from non–injecting drug users (non-IDUs) becoming infected from their IDU partners (e.g., Spain). In their chapter on China, Clyde McCoy and his colleagues cite evidence that suggests the emergence of a similar pattern within areas in that country. Nearly all of the chapters highlight regional differences in the prevalence and incidence of HIV and AIDS *within* countries.

In the early stages of the epidemic, scholars and practitioners referred to "risk groups," that is, groups at greater risk for HIV infection. However, the term *risk group* is in many ways inappropriate because "risk groups" can effectively alter their behavior over time. For example, although collectively gay males have been proactive in their efforts to change individual behavior to prevent the spread of HIV, recent data suggest that in some regions risk behaviors have increased among men who have sex with men, leading some researchers to conclude that "safer sex messages, common in the 1980s and early 1990s, have lost their impact" (Rani, Woolley, and Chandiok 2000: 1531). Equally important is that any one group can contain diverse cohorts, composed of individuals whose behaviors can vary in degree and context from those within other cohorts of the same group (Weniger and Berkley 1996). For example, Susan Goode and Toni Makkai note in this volume that HIV infections have increased among *young* gay males in Australia.

Globally, most persons who are living with HIV are men. However, regional differences are noteworthy. In sub-Saharan Africa, women account for 55% of persons living with HIV (UNAIDS/WHO 2000). Further, life expectancies among females living with HIV and AIDS in this region are approximately 10 years lower compared to their male counterparts (Stephenson 2000). Within this volume, Elizabeth Pisani discusses the implications of the high prevalence of HIV among *young* women in Kenya. In her chapter on Haiti, Mary Comerford notes that heterosexual transmission is the primary route of infection within that country and suggests that this mode of transmission is most common in developing nations. Several chapters within this volume serve to highlight this important point, because the mode of transmission often differs between developing and developed countries. A related issue concerns the changing gender proportion of HIV cases. For example, some countries (e.g., United States) have experienced an increase in females infected with HIV and AIDS. Indeed, Karen Giffin and Letícia Legay Vermelho in their chapter on Brazil refer to this change as the "feminization" of the epidemic. Other contributors have reported that gender role expectations within the dominant culture affect women's sexual health. For example, in their chapter on Mexico, Roberto Castro and René Leyva report that males in that country are resistant to wearing condoms. Although some chapters describe programs that are specifically designed for women who test positive for HIV antibodies (e.g., Ireland), Castro and Leyva present evidence that suggests that these programs tend to target "specific populations" of women, for example, sex workers, while neglecting other groups of women.

Prevention of HIV can occur through what appear to be very simple methods—for example, cleaning injection equipment, avoiding the lending and borrowing of injection equipment, and using condoms consistently and appropriately. However, strong cultural beliefs can impede prevention efforts. The extent of condom use, for example, can be low in cultures dominated by masculine ideologies. Yet, research has demonstrated the effectiveness of prevention efforts in this regard. For example, following a widespread national effort in Thailand to promote the use of condoms during commercial sex encounters, research has shown that the number of sexually transmitted disease (STD) cases declined considerably among sex workers, as did HIV prevalence among army personnel (Celentano et al. 1998; Rojanapithayakorn and Hanenberg 1996). Within this volume, contributors have noted that attitudes and use of condoms can improve (e.g., Switzerland) and that this change can contribute to lower HIV prevalence rates (e.g., Uganda). Some contributors report data drawn from studies conducted within the respective countries that show infrequent or inconsistent use of condoms (e.g., Brazil, Ireland), and other contributors (e.g., Jager and Limburg) cite evidence that supports these findings. Several of the chapters within this volume highlight those factors that impede prevention within the respective countries and also demonstrate the importance of cultural practices when implementing prevention programs.

Antiretroviral therapies have represented one of the most important medical advances in recent years. Known as highly active antiretroviral therapy (HAART), this intervention is not a cure for HIV or AIDS but has contributed greatly to the quality of life for persons living with HIV. In the United States and in several Western European countries, these interventions have increased survival rates among persons living with HIV and have delayed the onset of AIDS. Additionally, a few chapters demonstrate that cases of vertical transmission of HIV from mother to child have declined among women who have received zidovudine during pregnancy (e.g., Spain, United States).

One drawback of antiretroviral therapies is that intervention must be introduced shortly after an individual has become infected with HIV, and the intervention must be used for long periods of time. In some countries described in this volume, antiretroviral therapy is accessible free of charge to persons designated as in need of the intervention (e.g., Brazil, Ireland, the Netherlands); however, some developing countries do not have the type of "health system infrastructure needed to adequately administer complex drug regimes" (Stephenson 2000: 557). Such is the case in Haiti, where Mary Comerford cites evidence that indicates that approximately half of the Haitian population do not have access to primary care. Further, even when the treatment is freely available, some individuals do not utilize the treatment. Other forms of medical care for persons living with HIV and AIDS also are not distributed equally across and within countries. For example, Castro and Leyva note within this volume that many physicians and dentists in Mexico have refused to treat persons living with HIV or AIDS in that country.

In the early stages of the AIDS epidemic, several governments were either slow to respond or responded inappropriately. For example, some contributors to this volume note that early government efforts designed to educate the public about HIV and AIDS were misguided (e.g., the Netherlands) or alarmist in context (e.g., Australia, Brazil). Other contributors note that the Catholic Church (e.g., in Ireland, Mexico, and Spain) and other Christian-based religious groups (e.g., in Kenya) have impeded HIV and AIDS policy regarding condom use and other reproductive issues.

Government denial no doubt worked to delay the introduction of effective interventions, and in some countries this denial may have contributed to the epidemic (Ainsworth and Teokul 2000). For example, research in France has shown that failure to implement harm reduction efforts in a timely manner contributed to a "health catastrophe" among injecting drug users in that country (Moatti and Souteyrand 2000). Within this volume, Jesús Castilla and his colleagues note the early resistance to harm reduction policies in Spain. Jean-Paul Grund describes the resistance to harm reduction practices in some countries within Central and Eastern Europe, despite the large proportion of injectors in that region who are living with HIV. He also notes the often contradictory objectives between international efforts to address HIV and AIDS and international efforts to reduce the use of illicit drugs (i.e., the latter are often based on abstinence-only policies). In contrast to the current situation in Central and Eastern Europe, Johannes Jager and Wien Limburg note within this volume that harm reduction policies—for example, needle exchange, methadone—were introduced prior to or during the early stages of the AIDS epidemic in the Netherlands. These efforts might have contributed to the low proportion of injecting drug users as represented in the cumulative total of AIDS cases within that country. Jesús Castilla and his colleagues describe the innovative harm reduction programs that have been implemented in several prisons in Spain. In another chapter, Elizabeth Pisani uses the examples from Kenya and Uganda to show how differences in the type and extent of government and community responses can affect HIV prevalence.

People who were directly affected by HIV and AIDS were among the first to raise awareness about the disease and to highlight the stigma faced by people living with HIV and AIDS (O'Malley, Kim, and Lee 1996). Indeed, within this volume several contributors have noted that gay activists were among the first to draw attention to the disease within the respective country (e.g., Brazil, Ireland, United Kingdom). NGOs also have played important roles in that they often are able to reach "marginalised groups who may actually fear contact with government" (Ainsworth and Teokul 2000). NGOs vary in terms of goals and objectives, service provision and delivery, persons for whom services are available, size, accountability, and a host of other factors (O'Malley, Kim, and Lee 1996). In many countries, government recognition of and involvement with NGOs developed slowly and was much more apparent in Europe than in the United States (O'Malley, Kim, and Lee 1996). Most of the chapters within this volume describe various

NGOs within the respective countries or regions and note their contributions in addressing HIV and AIDS.

One theme that emerges from several chapters concerns the disproportionate effect of HIV and AIDS within marginalized groups. Moreover, individuals within these groups who become infected with HIV often become even more marginalized (Moatti and Souteyrand 2000). Persons so stigmatized risk further damage to health when they fail to obtain treatment and support (Herek and Glunt 1995). Within this volume, Dale Chitwood describes the stigma attached to persons with AIDS in the United States. Stigma emerged despite differences in the profiles of persons living with AIDS. At times, stigma surrounding HIV and AIDS is firmly embedded in the discriminatory views about certain types of people infected with HIV. Several chapters within this volume highlight this stigma. For example, Castro and Leyva note that in Mexico gay males who are living with HIV and AIDS are subject to discrimination from both the heterosexual community and other gay males. Cultural discrimination against injecting drug users is noted by several contributors to this volume, for example, Giffin and Vermelho (Brazil), McElrath (Ireland), and Castilla and his colleagues (Spain). In contrast, Jean-Paul Grund notes that drug injecting carries less social stigma within Central and Eastern Europe compared to the United States and Western Europe. Some chapters highlight the special challenges that countries face with respect to HIV and ethnic minorities (e.g., Australia, Central and Eastern Europe, China). Contributors describe that patterns of exposure may differ greatly between ethnic minorities or indigenous populations and the dominant group (e.g., Australia, Kenya, United Kingdom).

We now know that HIV is usually spread within social networks, but we know less about how to effectively encourage *consistent* risk reduction within various groups and in the general population. In their chapter on the Netherlands, Johannes Jager and Wien Limburg correctly note the importance of "local circumstances" in understanding the epidemic. In the chapters that follow, we demonstrate the importance of cultural values with respect to individual knowledge about HIV and AIDS, prevention and treatment efforts, and government and community response to the epidemic. We describe progress and setbacks as well as future challenges.

The country case studies in this volume have all been chosen to represent the different regions of the world as well as those places where the epidemic has been particularly severe and/or the problem has been recognized and/or addressed. The goal is to provide chapters in which students can easily compare and contrast all the different aspects of the disease and what has been done to stop its spread. Due to the fact that the vast majority of persons living with HIV or AIDS reside in Africa and that the continent has been devastated by the epidemic, two chapters address this region of the world (one chapter on sub-Saharan Africa and one on Uganda and Kenya).

Uganda is the only country within Africa that can claim to have implemented a successful prevention program to fight AIDS. It is the only African country that has demonstrated that HIV is actually declining among youth. For these reasons, even though it is located within sub-Saharan Africa (as are most countries on the continent), Uganda is addressed in a separate chapter, along with Kenya, because a detailed contrast between Uganda and Kenya helps to highlight the important differences in health policy between them and to show how these differences have affected HIV prevalence in the respective countries. The chapter on sub-Saharan Africa deals only briefly with these two countries, providing a broader overview, so students can understand the effects of the disease in other countries in Africa.

BIBLIOGRAPHY

Ainsworth, Martha, and Waranya Teokul. 2000. "Breaking the Silence: Setting Realistic Priorities for AIDS Control in Less-Developed Countries." *Lancet* 356: 55–60.

Celentano, David D., Kenrad E. Nelson, Cynthia M. Lyles, Chris Beyrer, Sakol Eiumtrakul, Vivian F.L. Go, Surinda Kuntolbutra, and Chirasak Khamboonruang. 1998. "Decreasing Incidence of HIV and Sexually Transmitted Diseases in Young Thai Men: Evidence for Success of HIV/AIDS Control and Prevention Program." *AIDS* 12: F29–F36.

Drucker, Ernest. 2000. *Stopping AIDS in Asia: An Operating Manual.* Book Review. *Lancet* 356: 776.

Herek, Gregory M., and Eric K. Glunt. 1995. "An Epidemic of Stigma: Public Reaction to AIDS." In *AIDS: Readings on a Global Crisis*, Elizabeth Rauh Bethel, ed., pp. 25–36. Boston: Allyn and Bacon.

Moatti, Jean-Paul, and Yves Souteyrand. 2000. "Editorial: HIV/AIDS Social and Behavioural Research: Past Advances and Thoughts about the Future." *Social Science and Medicine* 50: 1519–1532.

O'Malley, Jeffrey, Nguyen Vinh Kim, and Sarah Lee. 1996. "Nongovernmental Organizations." In *AIDS in the World II: Global Dimensions, Social Roots, and Responses*, Jonathan M. Mann and Daniel J.M. Tarantola, eds., pp. 341–361. New York: Oxford University Press.

Rani, Ranjana, Paul D. Woolley, and Swatantrata Chandiok. 2000. "Increased High Risk Sexual Behaviour in Homosexual Men; Findings Are Similar in Manchester." Letter. *British Medical Journal* 321: 1531.

Rojanapithayakorn, Wiwat, and Robert Hanenberg. 1996. "The 100% Condom Program in Thailand." *AIDS* 10: 1–7.

Schwartländer, Bernhard, Geoff Garnett, Neff Walker, and Roy Anderson. 2000. "AIDS in a New Millennium." *Science* 289: 64–67.

Stephenson, Joan. 2000. "Apocalypse Now: HIV/AIDS in Africa Exceeds the Experts' Worst Predictions." *JAMA* 284: 556–557.

UNAIDS/WHO. 2000. *AIDS Epidemic Update: December 2000.* Geneva: Joint United Nations Programme on HIV/AIDS (UNAIDS) and World Health Organization.

Weniger, Bruce G., and Seth Berkley. 1996. "The Evolving HIV/AIDS Pandemic." In *AIDS in the World II: Global Dimensions, Social Roots, and Responses*, Jonathan M. Mann and Daniel J.M. Tarantola, eds., pp. 57–70. New York: Oxford University Press.

1

AUSTRALIA

Susan Goode and Toni Makkai

INTRODUCTION

Australia responded to the threat of HIV/AIDS quickly and effectively when it first appeared in the early 1980s. This period reflected significant policy shifts within the then Federal Department of Health and Aged Care, the agency responsible for national policy and program development for both HIV/AIDS and illicit drug use. These shifts were greatly facilitated by a newly elected federal Labor health minister who was acutely aware of the need to deal quickly with the issue of HIV/AIDS (Blewett 1987). This response occurred at a time when illicit drug use was becoming a major political issue, and the two coalesced, enabling policymakers to institute major treatment, education, and rehabilitation interventions that could deal with HIV/AIDS.

AIDS was first diagnosed in Australia in late 1982, and a further six cases were diagnosed in 1983. The need to monitor HIV/AIDS on a national basis was recognized at an early stage, and a national register of AIDS cases was established in 1984 (Crofts 1992: 35–36). The major risk group identified at this time were homosexual men. The majority of the earliest cases were among men in Sydney who had reported sexual contact with men on the West Coast of the United States (Crofts 1992: 35). Even today, when the route of infection is known, the majority of diagnosed cases of HIV infection are among men as a result of sexual contact between men (Federal Department of Health and Family Services 1996: 9).

This chapter will outline policy responses to HIV/AIDS since the early

1980s and discuss the various special interest groups and policy initiatives that have been undertaken over the past 15 years. We begin with a brief overview, move on to discuss policy development, and conclude with a discussion of the various special interest groups.

ISSUES RELATING TO HIV AND AIDS

Direct evidence of the history of the spread of HIV infection in Australia is scarce, as much of the spread among homosexual men had taken place before antibody testing became widely available in mid-1985. It is believed that AIDS cases had occurred in the 1970s, but it was not until the early 1980s that the first case was officially diagnosed. There was a rapid increase in the number of reported cases during the early to mid-1980s, but by the late 1980s, the rate had begun to slow. The bulk of HIV transmission among gay men in Australia occurred prior to 1986 (Crofts 1992). Consistent with the geographic location of high-risk groups in Australia, HIV/AIDS rates of infection have been, and are, higher in the capital cities than in rural and regional Australia. In fact, the highest per capita rates are reported in New South Wales, particularly "those parts of Sydney that are recognized as focal points for the gay community" (Federal Department of Health and Family Services 1996: 9).

Various attempts have been made to estimate the incidence of the disease over time. "Using the method of back projection, based on AIDS cases and the known rate of progression from HIV infections to AIDS, it is estimated that the annual incidence of new HIV infection peaked at about 3,000 in 1984 and then declined sharply to around 500 in 1990. As a consequence, the number of people progressing to AIDS increased for the 10 years following the 1984 peak in HIV transmission but is now approaching a plateau" (Federal Department of Health and Family Services 1996: 8).

Table 1.1 shows an overall decline in the number of new AIDS diagnoses since 1990 in Australia. In 1991 there were 804 new AIDS diagnoses, declining to 196 in 1999. The table shows the various exposure categories, and male homosexual contact accounts for the vast majority of new diagnoses. In the early 1990s the next highest group involved injecting drug users (IDUs); however, over time the number of new diagnoses through heterosexual contact have exceeded the IDU exposure category. In 1999, 62.7% of the new cases were found among males with homosexual contact, 20.9% through heterosexual contact, and 4.6% among those who had a history of injecting drug use.

In 1999, the total number of persons with HIV infection was estimated to be 12,160, of whom 2,520 were estimated to be living with AIDS. New diagnoses of HIV were just over 679 in 1999, with new AIDS diagnoses being around 196 cases for that year. The rate of new AIDS diagnoses is expected to remain steady at around 190 cases until 2003 (National Centre

Table 1.1
Number of AIDS Diagnoses Adjusted for Reporting Delay by HIV Exposure Category, Pre-1990–1999

HIV exposure category	Pre-90	91	92	93	94	95	96	97*	98*	99*	(Total)
Male homosexual contact	2,256	650	627	659	768	626	496	265	199	123	(6,669)
Male homosexual contact and injecting drug use	80	31	38	56	46	42	37	12	9	8	(359)
Injecting drug use**	46	30	16	27	29	28	24	20	24	9	(253)
Heterosexual contact	45	38	50	51	53	50	52	50	54	41	(484)
Hemophilia/ coagulation disorder	47	11	13	11	10	15	7	4	1	0	(119)
Receipt of blood/tissue	88	16	15	8	9	5	6	1	4	1	(153)
Health care setting	0	0	1	1	1	1	0	0	0	0	(4)
Mother with/at risk for HIV infection	6	3	4	0	6	4	0	1	2	0	(26)
Other/undetermined	55	25	24	31	33	34	35	22	22	14	(295)
Total	(2,623)	(804)	(788)	(844)	(955)	(805)	(657)	(375)	(315)	(196)	(8,362)

*Adjusted for reporting delay; AIDS cases diagnosed in previous years were assumed to be completely reported.
**Excludes males who also reported a history of homosexual contact.

Source: National Centre in HIV Epidemiology and Clinical Research 2000: 290.

in HIV Epidemiology and Clinical Research 2000). Between 1990 and 1999 approximately 5,850 Australians had died from AIDS (National Centre in HIV Epidemiology and Clinical Research 2000).

In comparative terms, Australia has been very successful in its HIV/AIDS policy. Figure 1.1 shows the AIDS incidence per 100,000 population in seven countries. The data show that in all but one country the incidence of AIDS peaked in the early 1990s. The exception is Thailand, where the rate of infection continued to increase through the 1990s. In terms of Australia, the rate of infection has been lower than all other countries except for the United Kingdom. Most noticeably, the difference in the rate of infection between Australia and the United States disproportionately increased throughout the 1990s.

Special Interest Groups

Indigenous Australians

By the mid-1990s the data showed that the rate of diagnosis of HIV/AIDS among Indigenous Australians was increasing (Federal Department of Health and Family Services 1996: 10–11). Between 1992 and 1994 new diagnoses of HIV represented only 17% of cumulative HIV notifications. However, over that same period among Aboriginal and Torres Strait Islander people new diagnoses represented 50% of the cumulative diagnoses. Not only was the rate increasing, but the patterns of infection among Indigenous Australians appeared to be different. For Indigenous Australians the cumulative proportion of HIV cases attributed to heterosexual contact (24%) was much higher than in the non-Indigenous HIV-infected population (7%). The implication was that there were a growing number of Indigenous women at risk. The limited available data and the growing anecdotal evidence led authorities to question the effectiveness of HIV/AIDS and sexually transmitted disease (STD) education and prevention strategies among Australia's Indigenous population (Federal Department of Health and Family Services 1996: 11).

Following the recommendations of Feachem's (1995) evaluation of the second National HIV/AIDS Strategy (discussed in the next section), the Australian National Council on AIDS and Related Diseases (ANCARD) undertook a consultation process that resulted in the establishment of the Australian National Council on AIDS (ANCA) Working Party on Indigenous Australians' Sexual Health. This working party produced the first National Indigenous Australians' Sexual Health Strategy (NIASHS) in 1997 (Australian National Council on AIDS and Related Diseases Working Party 1997). The discussion document on the fourth National HIV/AIDS Strategy identifies seven priorities for health promotion that include Indigenous Australians. The discussion document argues that NIASHS should be an integral

Figure 1.1
AIDS Incidence in Selected Countries by Year

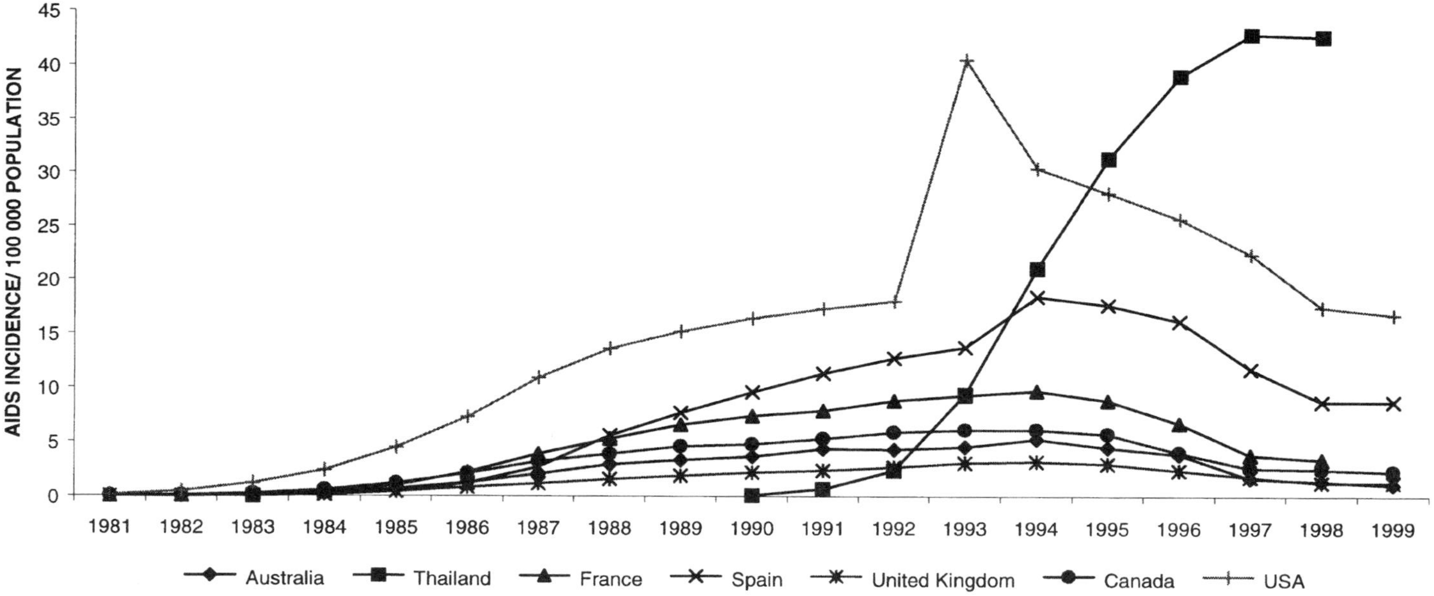

U.S. AIDS case definition changed in 1993 to include people with a CD4+ count of <2000.

Source: National Centre in HIV Epidemiology and Clinical Research 2000.

part of the fourth National HIV/AIDS Strategy. Contained within this strategy were health promotion priorities for homosexually active men and IDUs within the Indigenous community. The discussion document also calls for greater self-determination over models of best practice.

Homosexually Active Men

Consistently throughout the national HIV/AIDS strategies, gay and homosexually active men have been a priority area. As Table 1.1 shows, homosexual males account for the bulk of HIV and AIDS cases. "Although the proportion of new diagnoses of HIV/AIDS occurring in homosexually active men has remained high the overall number of new HIV diagnoses in this group has seen a considerable decrease from 2284 in 1987 to 567 in 1995" (Federal Department of Health and Family Services 1996: 10).

Studies of members of the homosexual community in Australia have shown that the percentage of homosexuals having intercourse without protection has decreased from 1984 to present. However, there are still an unacceptably high percentage of homosexuals engaging in unsafe sexual practices, and this continues to be the primary method of HIV transmission in Australia (Crawford, Bermingham, and Kippax 1996).

Case Study: "Project Male-Call"

In 1994 "Project Male-Call" was conducted by the Federal Department of Human Services and Health. The project involved a national telephone survey of men who have sex with men. The sample consisted of 2,583 men from metropolitan and regional areas in Australia. The aims of the survey were: "(1) to describe homosexually active men's knowledge of HIV and AIDS and their sexual practices with special focus on the adoption of 'safe' sexual strategies; and (2) to examine the ways in which knowledge and safe sexual practice are related to a number of demographic and contextual variables" (Kippax Crawford, Rodden, and Benton 1994: 1).

Of the gay men surveyed, over one-third reported having more than 100 partners in their lifetime, and a further quarter reported having between 11 and 50 partners in their lifetime. This finding has important implications for prevention of the HIV/AIDS epidemic in the gay community, and it reinforces the need for these men to use safe sex practices (Kippax et al. 1994). This study also examined the knowledge that homosexual men had of HIV and AIDS. Levels of knowledge on the whole were high; however, men who had been tested for HIV and those with high levels of gay community attachment were more knowledgeable than those who had not been tested for HIV and those with low levels of gay community attachment (Kippax et al. 1994).

Prison Inmates and AIDS

Throughout the world the prevalence of HIV among prison inmates is higher than that of the wider community (Shewan and Davies 2000). HIV prevalence in Australian prisons remains low by international standards. The first reported case of an inmate becoming infected in prison was in 1994 (Dolan and Crofts 2000). Since 1991 the prevalence of HIV among inmates in Australian prisons has been about 0.5% (approximately eight times higher than that in the nonprison population) (National Centre in HIV Epidemiology and Clinical Research 2000). From 11 different studies carried out between 1988 and 1994, it has consistently been shown that there is a high level (average of 72%) of sharing of injecting equipment among IDUs in prison (Crofts, Webb-Pullman, and Dolan 1996). Given the risks associated with sharing of needles the potential threat of HIV/AIDS in prisons remains very real.

In Australia the number of prison inmates has continued to rise over the last 15 years, and there is a very high turnover rate of inmates. This trend, together with the increasing mobility of inmates within the prison system, makes it difficult to estimate the prevalence of and effectively prevent and manage HIV/AIDS in prisons (Dolan and Crofts 2000). The primary responsibility for determining HIV/AIDS policy in relation to prisons lies with states and territories. As a result, different jurisdictions have responded with a variety of strategies. For example, condoms and bleach are available to inmates in three jurisdictions, whereas methadone maintenance is available in one jurisdiction. Dolan and Crofts (2000) report that HIV/AIDS interventions in prisons have been minimal in the past four years.

The evaluation of the third National HIV/AIDS Strategy noted the specific problems associated with HIV/AIDS in prisons and argued that health promotion within this environment should be expanded and "based on the principle of harm minimisation" (Australian National Council on AIDS and Related Diseases 1999: 58). The ongoing concern about HIV/AIDS in prisons is also reflected in the discussion document for the fourth National HIV/AIDS Strategy, which argues for a national perspective aimed at reducing the spread of HIV in prisons (Federal Department of Health and Aged Care 1999).

Injecting Drug Users and AIDS

Most surveys show that the prevalence of HIV infection among IDUs in Australia is low, at about 2% (excluding male IDUs who also have a history of homosexual contact). The rates of "needle sharing in the last month" reported by IDUs in Australia have declined greatly over the last decade, from 90% to less than 20%. However, the continued high prevalence and incidence of hepatitis C infection among IDUs suggests that the existing strategy is yet to bring this epidemic under control (Federal Department of Health and Family Services 1996: 11). Table 1.1 shows that approximately 4.6% of AIDS cases in 1999 are found among people who have been injecting drug users.

Between 1992 and 1997 the prevalence of HIV was very low (less than 0.6%) for males and females who attended metropolitan health centers and identified themselves as IDUs. HIV prevalence among IDUs who attended needle and syringe exchange between 1995 and 1997 was also low (less than 2%), except among those men who identified themselves as homosexual, for whom the mean HIV prevalence was 27.3%. In contrast to the very low prevalence of HIV in IDUs, the prevalence of hepatitis C continues to remain high (Australian National Council on AIDS and Related Diseases 1999: 9).

The number of IDUs continues to rise in Australia (McAllister and Makkai 2001) and is associated with high rates of opiate use among particular groups (Makkai 2000), with injecting being the preferred mode of administration. Harm minimization strategies in Australia are aimed at reducing the risk of transmission of bloodborne viruses. As a result methadone maintenance is widely available in Australia, and needle and syringe programs exist in all states and territories. There are currently under way proposals for injecting rooms in two jurisdictions. In addition, programs to divert drug-dependent offenders out of the criminal justice system into education and treatment programs are also being implemented.

RESPONSES TO HIV/AIDS

In the early 1980s there was little consensus on the overall policy direction for AIDS in Australia. Surveys of the Australian population at that time indicated that many believed HIV/AIDS would not affect them—that it was a disease confined to a number of marginal groups in the community. Lack of awareness and concern for the issue resulted in a variety of policy directives that ranged from calls for the compulsory testing of high-risk groups to published guidelines on confidentiality and education programs. At its simplest level, state and territory governments have the major responsibility for the provision of health care within Australia. The federal government's role is to coordinate and provide sufficient resources.

State governments had established their own programs on AIDS, but the epidemic was attracting increasing attention, particularly in the media. With the news of the first case of AIDS being diagnosed in Australia, the Working Party on AIDS was established in 1983 (Altman 1992; Penington 1987). This was quickly followed in 1984 by a national reporting mechanism for all cases of AIDS in Australia and special funding by the National Health and Medical Research Council for AIDS research. However, the report of a case of AIDS caused by blood transfusion in July 1984, followed by the deaths of three babies through blood transfusion, heightened awareness and concern within the broader Australian community.

A special meeting of Health ministers was convened in November 1984, and two major policy decisions were undertaken (Penington 1987):

• The voluntary exclusion of donors at high risk of contracting the disease was to be replaced with state and territory legislation requiring all donors to sign a declaration

form indicating their exposure status; severe penalties were attached for false dec-
larations.

• A new committee structure was to be established that would include a working
  committee called the National AIDS Task Force and a National Advisory Committee on AIDS (NACAIDS) to liaise between government and the general community. The latter included community representatives.

By mid-1983 the Australian Red Cross, which is responsible for almost all
the blood banks in Australia, had issued a statement recommending that
blood should not be collected from "sexually active homosexual or bisexual
men with multiple partners, from intravenous drug users or from their partners" (Altman 1992: 56). However, blood transfusion remained a source of
infection. The introduction of the new legislation requiring declaration of
exposure status resulted in a dramatic decline in contaminated blood so that
by 1985 only 3 out of 800,000 donations were found to be positive. By
1985 a national screening of all blood donations for HIV antibodies had
been instituted and remains to this day. Table 1.1 shows the steady decline
in the number of people who have contracted AIDS from blood transfusions
in the 1990s.

The new committee structure sought to move toward a more managed
response to HIV/AIDS in Australia. It was in this setting that the Intergovernmental Committee on AIDS (IGCA) was established in June 1987
with the aim of coordinating and strengthening public health policy and
financial arrangements between the federal and state governments (Altman
1992: 57–58). In the complex political structure of a federal system, this
model was used to develop consistent policy approaches endorsed by all
governments in Australia. It also enabled strategic alliances to be struck
between policymakers, treatment providers, and "at risk" groups in the community.

The decision was made to undertake a major media campaign of a type
not seen in Australia before. The "Grim Reaper" campaign, with images of
death mowing down a wide range of victims in a bowling alley, was launched
in April 1987. These advertisements were widely criticized as they implied
that all people were equally at risk of contracting AIDS. However, Buttrose
(1987), who was chair of NACAIDS at the time, said that the purpose of
the campaign was to raise awareness of AIDS and to encourage Australians
to talk about issues such as safe sex and sexually transmitted diseases. Monitoring data showed that six weeks after the campaign was launched, 95%
of Australians were aware of AIDS.

Community-based responses to AIDS developed prior to the implementation of formal government committees. Most states and territories had
established community AIDS councils or action committees. In 1984 the
federal government had allocated funds for AIDS activities and education
programs run by the newly established community AIDS councils. In 1985

the federal Health minister had indicated that it was only by harnessing and enhancing community-based programs with community involvement would the HIV/AIDS epidemic be successfully controlled. In 1985 community-based education programs were fostered and funded by government, particularly among people with hemophilia, the gay community, injecting drug users, and prostitutes.

In 1985 the Australian Federation of AIDS Organisations (AFAO) was established and funded by the federal government to be the peak organization for HIV/AIDS–related community organizations. The Haemophilia Foundation has retained a separate status from the AFAD and was also funded by the federal government (Altman 1992). The strong commitment to community-based organizations was later confirmed in the first national HIV/AIDS strategy through formal consultative mechanisms. The involvement of the community sector at the highest levels of government policy-making has remained an important feature of Australia's national HIV/AIDS strategy.

The First National HIV/AIDS Strategy

In 1988 the Australian National Council on AIDS replaced NACAIDS, and the federal government decided to develop a national strategy on AIDS. This required the production of a Green Paper[1] that was to be the basis of widespread national discussion on the AIDS epidemic and strategies to deal with it (Altman 1992: 58). Six panels of experts were convened to seek views of the public on Aboriginals, Islanders, and HIV; discrimination and other legal issues; education and prevention; IDU and HIV; testing and treatment; and services and care (Federal Department of Community Services and Health 1989: 4).

The Green Paper was presented to the federal and state Parliaments in late 1988 and became the basis for a White Paper on HIV/AIDS. The White Paper was tabled in federal Parliament almost a year later and committed the federal government to a four-year planning and funding program. The process had taken four years and involved extensive policy development and consultation. The White Paper outlined a national HIV/AIDS strategy that had two key goals:

• to eliminate transmission of the virus; and
• to minimise the personal and social impact of HIV infection. (Federal Department of Community Services and Health 1989: 23)

The strategy sought to emphasize that the HIV epidemic had the potential to impact on all Australians and that specific groups should not be targeted for fear of stigmatization. Instead, the focus of the strategy was that HIV transmission could only be contained if all Australians understood and utilized the educational and preventive measures available (Federal Department of Community Services and Health 1989). "The Strategy was welcomed by a wide audience including state government, federal opposition parties, health care professions, community organisations and people living with HIV/AIDS" (Australian Federation of AIDS Organisations 1992: 2).

Altman (1992) reports that it was hoped that the White Paper would be accompanied by a period of consensus and consolidation. However, the government was somewhat concerned over AIDS organizations that were competing for control of the AIDS agenda. This period had seen a new militancy among AIDS activists and new issues emerging as emphasis shifted from prevention to treatment. A new chapter in AIDS policy emerged, as there was the growing possibility of medical intervention to help prolong the lives of HIV suffers (Altman 1992: 59).

The first National HIV/AIDS Strategy incorporated a number of concepts that were derived from the *OTTOWA Charter for Health Promotion* (Australian National Council on AIDS and Related Diseases 1999). The strategy had also stipulated that a national evaluation be undertaken in 1992 for consideration in the 1993–1994 budget context. Under the direction of the National Evaluation Steering Committee (NESC) the evaluation report was completed in December 1992. The report was favorable, indicating that Australia had been successful in containing the spread of HIV and that "considerable progress had been made in minimising the personal impact of HIV in Australia" (National Evaluation Steering Committee 1992). The report highlighted that unlike many other countries the Australian government had provided extensive funding for HIV/AIDS treatment services, and the Australian system of universal health care had provided reasonable health care for those infected with AIDS (National Evaluation Steering Committee 1992).

The evaluation concluded that a major achievement of the strategy had been the development of a tripartite partnership that involved:

- Government at all levels
- Scientific, medical and health care professionals and
- The communities and social groups particularly affected by HIV/AIDS, including people with HIV infection. (National Evaluation Steering Committee 1992: 120–121)

The Second National HIV/AIDS Strategy

The second National HIV/AIDS Strategy was guided by a major evaluation of existing policies and programs that was completed in January 1993. The goals of the first National HIV/AIDS Strategy were adopted for the second strategy with the primary goal being supported by a national target "[t]o reduce the incidence of new HIV infection in Australia to an annual rate of no more than 2 persons per 100,000 by the year 2000" (Federal Government of Australia 1993: 9). The Australian Health Ministers Council (AHMC) endorsed the second National HIV/AIDS Strategy in July 1993.

The two guiding principles of the second strategy were the following:

• Transmission of HIV is preventable through changes in individual behaviour. Education and prevention programs are necessary to bring about such changes.
• Each person must accept responsibility for preventing themselves becoming infected and for preventing further transmission of the virus. (Federal Government of Australia 1993: 9)

The Australian Federation of AIDS Organisations had supported the first National HIV/AIDS Strategy, but at the same time they recommended some major changes for the second National Strategy. These changes included:

• Change in the order of priorities for education programs;
• A more humane approach in regard to prisoners;
• Significant changes to the arrangements for trial, availability, and funding of treatments; and
• Increased commitment to international and regional partnerships.

This period was characterized by a strong push from AIDS activists to speed up the testing and approval of new drugs from the United States and Britain. However, the government was not very responsive to this push, and it remained a slow and cumbersome process to have these drugs approved for use in Australia (Altman 1992: 60). Overall, this period was characterized by dissatisfaction from those affected by AIDS, and there were a number of attacks by powerful forces on the preventative education messages, particularly the language they used and the way in which specific groups were targeted.

As required by federal cabinet, an evaluation of the second National HIV/ AIDS Strategy was conducted during 1995. An independent overseas evaluator, Richard Feachem of the London School of Hygiene and Tropical Medicine, was appointed, with support being provided by the Surveillance and Evaluation Unit in the AIDS/Communicable Diseases Branch of the Federal Department of Human Services and Health. Feachem referred to Australia's response as "prompt and creative," and he noted two important features of the approach:

• Nonpartisan political support and
• Partnerships between governments, researchers, and health professionals and the community groups affected by HIV. (Feachem 1995)

He concluded that the epidemic had been contained among IDUs, sex workers, and heterosexuals. However, he pointed to the continuing high rates of infection among gay men and the emerging epidemic among Indigneous Australians as two important areas that needed to be confronted. He concluded that the goals of the national strategy were "still clear and valid" and that the strategy was "more than the sum of its parts" (1995: 8). In total, Feachem made 79 recommendations including the necessity for a third National HIV/AIDS Strategy that would run for five rather than three years. He also saw the need to mainstream HIV/AIDS policy with the development of a "national communicable diseases and/or sexual health policy" (1995: 204).

The Third National HIV/AIDS Strategy

As recommended, the third National HIV/AIDS Strategy saw a focus on lowering the rates of infection among homosexually active men and preventing an epidemic emerging in the Indigenous communities. This strategy called for efforts to be made to decrease the disturbingly high rate of HIV infections in younger homosexually active men through the development of new revitalized education and prevention strategies. In the strategy it was stated that the gap between the HIV response for Indigenous and non-Indigenous Australians must be bridged and that the government must move quickly to develop more effective programs to prevent the emerging HIV epidemic and ongoing high rates of sexually transmissible diseases in the Indigenous communities (Federal Department of Health and Family Services 1996).

In response to many of Feachem's recommendations, a number of factors distinguish the third National HIV/AIDS Strategy from the first two strategies. Thus the third strategy was framed in the context of related communicable diseases including hepatitis C and sexually transmissible diseases. However, the implementation of the third strategy occurred at a time of far-reaching reform in the health sector, especially in the public health funding arrangements. In particular, the federal government was seeking to concentrate on its core business of national policy development and coordination and leaving the implementation of policy to state governments. During this period there were important advances in the treatment of HIV/AIDS with combination therapies. The result was to greatly improve the prognosis for people living with HIV/AIDS, but the implications for health care provision were enormous. Rather than managing people who face a terminal disease, the new treatments meant that people now faced ongoing chronic pain management. The third strategy sought to confront the problem of HIV/AIDS among Indigenous Australians with the development of the National Indigenous Australians' Sexual Health Strategy (Australian National Council on AIDS and Related Diseases 1999: vii).

The Fourth National HIV/AIDS Strategy

The terms of the third National HIV/AIDS Strategy for 1996–1997 to 1998–1999 (*Partnerships in Practice*) expired on 30 June 1999. National consultations on the directions for a fourth National HIV/AIDS Strategy were undertaken between late April and July 1999. A draft of the fourth National HIV/AIDS Strategy was developed in light of the outcomes from the national consultation forums, the recommendations contained in the Australian National Council on AIDS and Related Diseases document *Proving Partnership: Review of the National HIV/AIDS Strategy 1996–97 to 1998–99*, and a national one-day forum for peak national HIV/AIDS, state, and territory health departments and key scientific, medical, and social research organizations. The draft was also developed in close consultation with the state and territory Health Department representatives on the Intergovernmental Committee on AIDS and Related Diseases (IGCARD). The fourth evaluation report is due out at the end of 2000.

CONCLUSION

Using a national strategy as a way of responding to the epidemic has been a constant feature of the Australian response. Evaluations of the first three National HIV/AIDS Strategies concluded that a single strategic document was a very effective way of generating a coordinated response. In terms of both HIV and AIDS, Australia has been highly successful in reducing and controlling the rates of infection to this date. As a result, the rate of infection in Australia is considerably less than in comparable countries like the United States, and the forward projections are that this rate will remain low. How do we explain this success? It is impossible to pinpoint any one factor, as many factors have come together at the correct time. Some of the more important include:

1. Strong bipartisan commitment to HIV/AIDS policy.
2. An articulate and active community sector.
3. A welfare state that has provided comprehensive medical cover to all in need.
4. A strong emphasis on education and prevention.
5. A national HIV/AIDS strategy.

There are still major areas of concern, and some researchers have argued that the high rates of infection of hepatitis may not bode well for the future, especially within the prison environment. From 1990 to 1999, 140,000 cases of hepatitis C have been reported.

In addition, major shifts are occurring in the funding and provision of both welfare and health. The provision of antiretroviral therapy in Australia has had a major impact on AIDS diagnoses since 1996. The implications for health care provision are enormous. Whereas before AIDS victims were facing terminal illnesses, they now have a greater chance of facing ongoing chronic illnesses. Ultimately the latter will require greater resources and support. This is occurring at a time when the federal government is continuing its major reform of both welfare and health provision in order to reduce costs. The long-term implications of these reforms and their impact on HIV/AIDS sufferers remain unknown at this time.

NOTE

1. A Green Paper is usually the discussion document that precedes the White Paper that outlines the government's formal policy position.

BIBLIOGRAPHY

Altman, Dennis. 1992. "The Most Political of Disease." In *AIDS in Australia*, Eric Timewell, Victor Minichello, and David Plummer, eds., pp. 55–72. Sydney: Prentice-Hall of Australia.

Australian Federation of AIDS Organisations. 1992. *National HIV/AIDS Strategy: Beyond 1993*. Sorry Hills, NSW, Australia: Australian Federation of AIDS Organisations.

———. 2000. *Strategic Plan*. Available on the World Wide Web at: http://www.afao.org.au

Australian National Council on AIDS and Related Diseases. 1999. *Proving Partnership: Review of the National HIV/AIDS Strategy 1996–97 to 1998–99*. Canberra: Federal Department of Health and Family Services.

Australian National Council on AIDS and Related Diseases Working Party. 1997. *The National Indigenous Australians' Sexual Health Strategy 1996–97 to 1998–99*. Canberra: Federal Department of Health and Family Services.

Blewett, Neal. 1987. "Some Reflections on the Australian Experience." In *WHO/Australian Inter-regional Ministerial Meeting on AIDS*, Elizabeth Reid, ed., pp. 25–33. Canberra: Australian Government Publishing Service.

Buttrose, Ita. 1987. "The National Advisory Committee on AIDS: Education and Prevention Programs in Australia." In *WHO/Australian Inter-regional Ministerial Meeting on AIDS*, Elizabeth Reid, ed., pp. 215–222. Canberra: Australian Government Publishing Service.

Crawford, June, Suzanne Bermingham, and Susan Kippax. 1996. *An Analysis of Trends over Time in Social and Behavioural Factors Related to the Transmission of HIV in Men Who Have Sex with Men*. Technical Appendix 3. Canberra: Australian Government Publishing Service.

Crofts, Nick. 1992. "Patterns of Infection." In *AIDS in Australia*, Eric Timewell, Victor Minichello, and David Plummer, eds., pp. 24–54. Sydney: Prentice-Hall of Australia.

Crofts, Nick, J. Webb-Pullman, and Kate Dolan. 1996. *An Analysis of Trends over Time in Social and Behavioural Factors Related to the Transmission of HIV among Injecting Drug Users and Prison Inmates.* Technical Appendix 4. Canberra: Australian Government Publishing Service.

Dolan, Kate, and Nick Crofts. 2000. "A Review of Risk Behaviours. Transmission and Prevention of Blood Borne Viral Infections in Australian Prisons." In *Drug Use and Prisons: An International Perspective*, David Shewan and John Davies, eds., pp. 215–232. Australia: Harwood Academic Publishers.

Feachem, Richard. 1995. *Valuing the Past . . . Investing in the Future: Evaluation of the National HIV/AIDS Strategy 1993–94 to 1995–96.* Canberra: Federal Department of Human Services and Health.

Federal Department of Community Services and Health. 1989. *National HIV/AIDS Strategy: A Policy Information Paper.* Canberra: Australian Government Publishing Service.

Federal Department of Health and Aged Care. 1999. *Discussion Document towards the Fourth National HIV/AIDS Strategy.* Canberra: Australian Government Publishing Service.

Federal Department of Health and Family Services. 1996. *Partnerships in Practice: National HIV/AIDS Strategy 1996–97 to 1998–99.* Canberra: Australian Government Publishing Service.

Federal Government of Australia. 1993. *National HIV/AIDS Strategy 1993–94 to 1995–96.* Canberra: Australian Government Publishing Service.

Kippax, Susan, June Crawford, Pamela Rodder, and Kim Benton. 1994. *Report on Project Male-Call: National Telephone Survey of Men Who Have Sex with Men.* Canberra: Australian Government Publishing Service.

Makkai, Toni. 2000. "Drug Use Monitoring in Australia: 1999 Annual Report on Drug Use among Adult Detainees." *Research and Public Policy Series No. 26.* Canberra: Australian Institute of Criminology.

McAllister, Ian, and Toni Makkai. 2001. "The Prevalence and Characteristics of Injecting Drug Users in Australia." *Drug and Alcohol Review* 20:29–36.

National Centre in HIV Epidemiology and Clinical Research. 2000. *2000 HIV/ AIDS, Hepatitis C & Sexually Transmissible Infections in Australia Annual Surveillance Report.* Sydney: National Centre in HIV Epidemiology and Clinical Research.

National Evaluation Steering Committee. 1992. *Report of the Evaluation of the National HIV/AIDS Strategy.* Canberra: Author.

Penington, David. 1987. "The National AIDS Task Force." In *WHO/Australian Inter-regional Ministerial Meeting on AIDS*, Elizabeth Reid, ed., pp. 209–214. Canberra: Australian Government Publishing Service.

Shewan, David, and John Davies, eds. 2000. *Drug Use and Prisons: An International Perspective.* Australia: Harwood Academic Publishers.

2

BRAZIL

Karen Giffin and Letícia Legay Vermelho

INTRODUCTION

Brazil is a huge country with immense natural resources, the world's eighth
largest economy, a population of 164 million, and one of the world's most
unequal income distributions: In the 1960s, the richest 10% received 34
times what the poorest 10% received; in 1990, they received 78 times more
(Cohn 1997). Brazil has the highest school dropout rate in the world, with
40% of children leaving school before grade eight (Brasil 1999a; Monteiro
1995). The majority of the population depends on public health services,
which are free of charge.

Formally a democracy, the first elected president following the 25-year
military regime resigned in 1992 as a result of widespread corruption and
misuse of public funds, in a process that also revealed entrenched interests
of the international drug trade in political and military structures.[1] The use
of public policy to generate private wealth is, however, a long-standing political tradition in Brazil, and in this tradition social policies have acted as
an obstacle to democratic institution building, rather than contributing to
the consolidation of citizen's rights and social well-being (W. Santos 1987).
In such an exclusionary model, the existence of socially advanced laws is no
guarantee that they will be put into effect, a fact that is often difficult for
international observers to fully appreciate.[2]

The current government has been enthusiastically carrying out the "structural adjustments" demanded by the International Monetary Fund, including privatization and denationalization of essential service industries, mineral

resources, and heavy industry. While this process has been generating massive unemployment and increasing impoverishment, spending on social services has been cut, and immense public resources have been spent in shoring up private and public financial institutions. The national Congress has recently approved a constitutional amendment that will allow the executive exclusive control over 20% of Brazil's annual budget. This change represents, for the year 2000, about U.S.$18 billion that the government can spend as it wishes, without "interference" from either Congress or civil society. This amendment may be seen as the latest example of the "administration of exclusion," which characterizes many of Latin America's formally democratic political cultures (Alvarez, Dagnino, and Escobar 1998: 10). In the case of present-day Brazil, however, this tendency is accompanied by a drive to achieve a stronger position in the new global economic order.

The Brazilian Health Ministry's (BHM) National AIDS Programme (PN-DST/AIDS), an impressive example of technical prowess and political agility, has from its inception been highly articulated with international organizations.[3] Brazil currently participates in the Joint United Nations Programme on HIV/AIDS (UNAIDS) program-coordinating committee and coordinates the horizontal technical collaboration group. PN-DST/AIDS is heavily financed by one of the World Bank's largest loan programs: U.S.$160 million for AIDS I (1994–1998) plus U.S.$165 million for AIDS II (1999–2002). The national counterpart totaled U.S.$225 million for 1994–2002 (Brasil 1999a).

PN-DST/AIDS is distinguished by universal free provision of antiretroviral drugs and extensive participation of nongovernmental organizations (NGOs) whose activities, coordinated by the Health Ministry, are also financed by the World Bank. Opening the XII International AIDS Congress, attended by Brazil's first lady, the director of UNAIDS affirmed that this is a model to be internationally emulated (Galvão 1999).

PN-DST/AIDS exists as "a Swiss island in a sea of misery," an expression Brazilians use to refer to privileged enclaves in a context of generalized need: in this case, an elaborate, internationally financed, and highly publicized program, implanted in a public health system subject to political neglect and progressive degradation in which basic materials, infrastructure, drugs, hygienic conditions, and so on, are lacking.

ISSUES RELATING TO HIV AND AIDS

History of HIV/AIDS

The first cases of AIDS were notified in 1983 in Rio de Janeiro and São Paulo, Brazil's largest cities, both located in the southeast. By November 1999, 179,541 cases had been registered: 132,213 in men, 41,160 in women, and 6,168 in children under 13.[4]

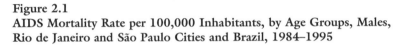

Figure 2.1
AIDS Mortality Rate per 100,000 Inhabitants, by Age Groups, Males,
Rio de Janeiro and São Paulo Cities and Brazil, 1984–1995

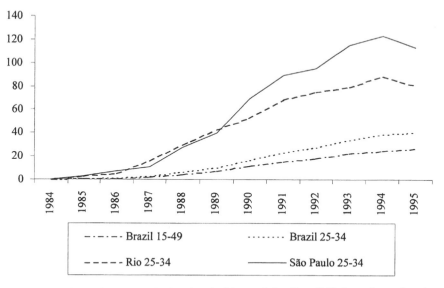

Source: Lowndes et al. 2000: 1271. Reprinted with permission from C.M. Lowndes et al. and
 Lippincott, Williams, & Wilkens.

Analysis of AIDS mortality from 1984 to 1995 (Lowndes et al. 2000)
showed a total of 68,270 deaths for age 13 and over, with women representing 3.4% of the total in 1985 and 22.6% in 1995. In 1995, AIDS accounted for 11.3% of total deaths of men, and 9.9% of women, in the age
group 25–34. The evolution of male and female mortality is shown in Figures 2.1 and 2.2.

The rate of incidence increased from .9/100,000 in 1986 to 14.2/
100,000 in 1997 (Figure 2.3). During the last three years, approximately
21,000 cases have been reported annually. Current estimates show around
536,920 people between ages 15 and 49 infected by HIV.

Estimates indicate that only 15% of cases are *not* notified. Given delays in
notification, however, data from 1998 and 1999 are currently less reliable,
as they may be altered in the future. From 1995, case classification was
amplified, which also makes comparison more difficult.

The greatest incidence occurs in the age group 20–39, in both sexes (Figures 2.4 and 2.5). From 1994 to 1999, however, a reduction occurred in
the age group 15–29 (Figure 2.6), which may be the result of increasing
condom use.

For those over 18, comparison over time reveals the *impoverishment* of
the epidemic, with 27% of cases in the 1980s and 57% in the 1990s having

Figure 2.2
AIDS Mortality Rate per 100,000 Inhabitants, by Age Groups, Females, Rio de Janeiro and São Paulo Cities and Brazil, 1984–1995

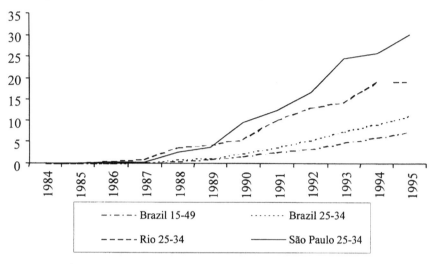

Source: Lowndes et al. 2000: 1271. Reprinted with permission from C.M. Lowndes et al. and Lippincott, Williams, & Wilkens.

Figure 2.3
AIDS Incidence Rate per 100,000 Inhabitants, by Year of Diagnostics, According to Sex,* Brazil, 1985–1996

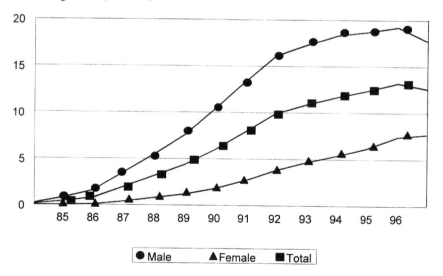

*Cases notified through August 1999.

Source: Brasil 1999c.

Figure 2.4
AIDS Incidence Rate per 100,000 Inhabitants, Males, by Age Groups,*
Brazil, 1985–1996

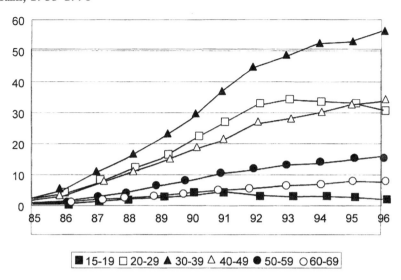

*Cases notified through August 1999.

Source: Brasil 1999c.

Figure 2.5
AIDS Incidence Rate per 100,000 Inhabitants, Females, by Age Groups,*
Brazil, 1985–1996

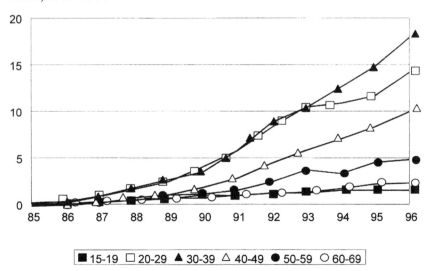

*Cases notified through August 1999.

Source: Brasil 1999c.

Figure 2.6
Proportional Distribution of AIDS Cases, by Age Group and Period of
Diagnosis,* Brazil, 1984–1999

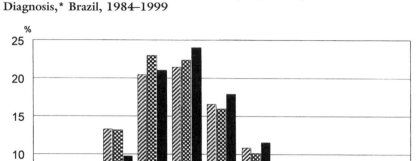

*Cases notified through August 1999.

Source: Brasil 1999c.

primary-level education. (Figure 2.7). Although around 75% of reported cases are men, the sex ratio of new cases has changed rapidly, from 16/1 in 1986 to 2/1 in 1997, indicating the epidemic's feminization or hetero-sexualization.

Although the vast majority of cases are concentrated in the Southeast region, the tendency is to stabilization of the rate of incidence in that area. All other regions show increases, with certain municipalities in the Southern region showing the most rapid increases. While 80% of existing cases are concentrated in 100 municipalities and 22 state capitals, more than one-half of all 5,500 Brazilian cities and towns now have at least one one case (Figure 2.8).

Sexual transmission accounts for 54% of all accumulated cases, with sig-nificant variation occurring through time. During 1984–1988, 56% of new cases were related to homo/bisexual exposure and only 6% to heterosexual exposure. From 1989 to 1993, exposure through injecting drug use (IDU) showed the greatest increase, accounting for 24% of new cases. From 1994 to 1999, heterosexual transmission accounted for the greatest proportion (29.3%) of reported cases, and 26.7% of all cases were considered as "un-defined" (Figures 2.9 and 2.10).

Figure 2.7
Proportional Distribution of AIDS Cases in 20+ Age Group, by Sex and Educational Level,* Brazil, 1984–1999

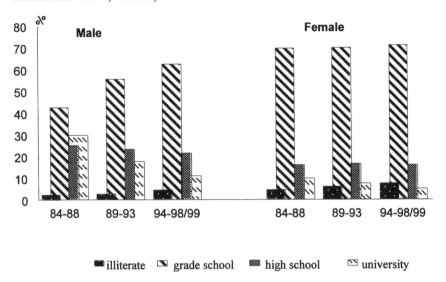

illiterate ☒ grade school ☷ high school ☒ university

*Cases notified through August 1999.

Source: Brasil 1999c.

Figure 2.8
AIDS Incidence Rate per 100,000 Inhabitants, by Region of Residence,* Brazil, 1984–1997

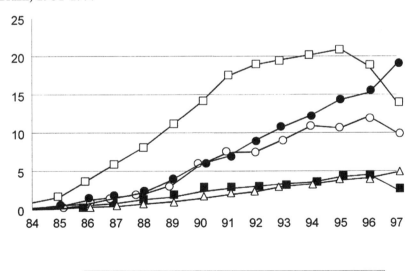

△ North ■ Northeast □ Southeast ● South ○ Center-west

*Cases notified through August 1999.

Source: Brasil 1999c.

Figure 2.9
**AIDS Cases in Males Aged 12+ Years, by Exposure Categories,* Brazil,
1984–1999**

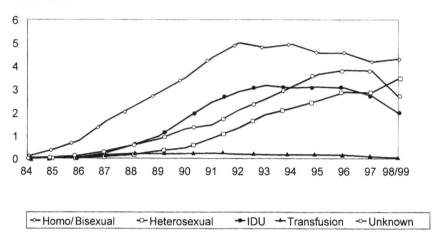

*Cases notified through May 1999.

Source: Brasil 1999b.

Figure 2.10
**AIDS Cases in Females Aged 12+ Years, by Exposure Categories,* Brazil,
1985–1999**

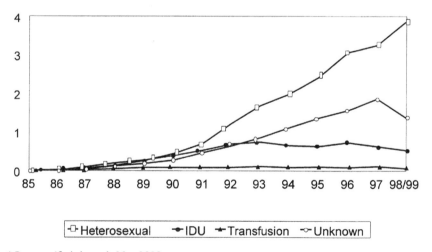

*Cases notified through May 1999.

Source: Brazil 1999b.

Figure 2.11
AIDS Incidence Rate per 100,000 Population in Women and Children and
by Perinatal Transmission,* Brazil, 1985–1999

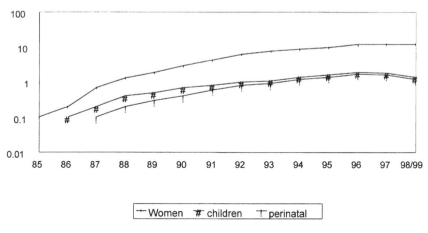

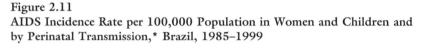

*Cases notified through May 1999.

Source: Brasil 1999b.

IDU transmission was responsible for 26.5% of new cases in 1991 and 16.9% in 1997. Despite this decrease in the relative weight of IDU, transmission to their sexual partners and children is now having a major impact on the epidemic, as the data on vertical transmission indicate.

Mother-child vertical transmission (VT) has been responsible for 90% of all cases in children under 13, or 2.8% of all cases. The first case was reported in 1985; and by November 1999, 4,974 cases had been reported, with 40% mortality. In the 1990s, the growth rate of VT, and of cases in all children, accompanies the rate of AIDS in women (Figure 2.11).

Average age at the time of diagnosis is shown in Figure 2.12, with the poorest North and Northeast regions showing later diagnoses. This pattern certainly reflects both greater prevalence of other childhood illnesses (and malnutrition) as well as more deficient health services in these regions.

Transmitting mothers are infected through heterosexual transmission in 47% of cases; 16% are IDUs; and 34% of cases are undefined (Figure 2.13). Heterosexual transmission is more prevalent in the poor North and Northeast regions, compared with the importance of IDU in the South and Southwest, where the drug traffic routes have been established. This is true for both the mothers and their partners (Figure 2.14). Thus, more than one-half of VT in Brazil, and 63% in the Southeast, is related to IDU.

Injecting drug use is a relatively recent habit in Brazil, where new international drug routes, established in the last 20 years, represent an important source of income in a context of increasing unemployment and impoverish-

Figure 2.12
AIDS in Children Infected through Vertical Transmission, Average Age Distribution at Diagnosis by Region of Residence,* Brazil, 1993–1999

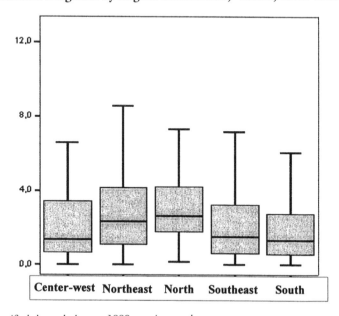

*Cases notified through August 1999; age in months.

Source: Brasil 1999c.

Figure 2.13
Proportion of Cases of Vertical Transmission, by Category of Mother's Infection,* Brazil, 1983–1999

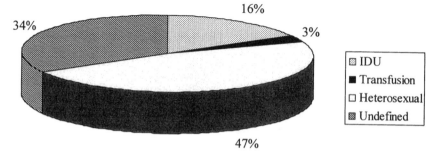

*Cases notified through May 1999.

Source: Brasil 1999b.

Figure 2.14
Proportion of Cases of Vertical Transmission, Mother Infected Through Heterosexual Transmission, by Mother's Partner's Transmission Category,* Brazil, 1993–1999

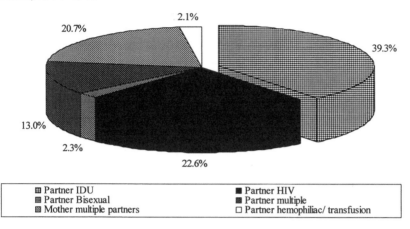

Partner IDU	Partner HIV
Partner Bisexual	Partner multiple
Mother multiple partners	Partner hemophiliac/ transfusion

*Cases notified through May 1999.

Source: Brasil 1999b.

ment (Mesquita 1995). In these geographical areas, in the early 1990s, seroprevalence in IDUs reached world highs (60% in Santos, 38% in Rio de Janeiro, according to the World Health Organization in 1993; in Bucher 1995). Researchers have noted that such IDUs are the most stigmatized and least powerful segment of the high-risk categories, whose members have no associations and no role in discussing HIV/AIDS in Brazil (Bastos 1995). Cocaine is the predominant injectable drug, and these users have been shown to be active sexually, with consequent effects on both heterosexual transmission and VT.

The epidemic in Brazil is not under control, despite generous international financing, political support, partnerships with NGOs and other institutions, and diversified strategies, which have been undertaken by PN-DST/AIDS.

Representations of Seropositivity

Mass media, NGOs, and public health personnel have all been important actors in constructing and changing representations of the epidemic and of those infected by HIV. In Brazil, AIDS has been a mass media topic since 1981, about two years before the first national cases were identified. As in other countries, this strange disease was originally presented as being exclusive to gay men. In Brazil, however, those affected were first perceived to be an elite group of gay intellectuals, activists, or artists, participants in in-

ternational gay circles and accustomed to world travel. In 1983, the death
of a well-known fashion designer consolidated this view (Parker et al. 1994).

In this same year, gay activist groups (whose members often tended to
be well-educated members of the middle class, including university teachers
and researchers committed to gay identity politics) began distributing educational material and pressuring public health authorities in São Paulo,
where the first AIDS program was initiated. Gay activists were also important in creating the first AIDS/NGO in 1985, with the objectives of influ-
encing and monitoring public policy, disseminating information, and
providing legal services to seropositive persons, with an emphasis on civil
rights (Galvão 1999). The term *civil death*, used to denounce discriminatory
and exclusionary practices, became a watchword of AIDS activism in Brazil.
Perversely, the extent and visibility of elite gay activism from the earliest
days of the epidemic may itself have acted to reinforce the general public's
notion of AIDS as restricted to gay men.

Church groups and religious institutions began carrying out support projects to provide food and shelter to people with AIDS (Galvão 1999), although conservative members of the Catholic hierarchy also linked infection
to "immoral behavior."

In Rio, two former political exiles, both seropositive, created an AIDS/
NGO (Associação Brasileira Interdisciplinar de AIDS [ABIA]) whose members were health professionals involved with research in AIDS and other
concerned academics and social activists (Parker 1994). ABIA was instrumental in organizing the AIDS VI International Congress in Montreal in
1989, where seropositive activism and the notion of "living with AIDS"
were consolidated internationally (Galvão 1999).

One of ABIA's founders was director of a large, well-established NGO,
which carried out research on social problems and would later lead a nationwide campaign against hunger. He was a heterosexual hemophiliac who
had contracted HIV through blood transfusion, as had his two brothers.
One of them was a famous cartoonist, also well known and highly esteemed
throughout the country. In 1987, the year preceding promulgation of the
new national Constitution, ABIA helped make commercial blood banks an
important political issue.[5] Compulsory testing of blood for transfusions became required by law, and the following year selling blood was prohibited
by the Constitution, which also defined health care as a basic social right.

While the issue of blood transfusions may have contributed to broadening
the definition of HIV carriers to include recognized and respected citizens
with heterosexual preferences, the BHM's first prevention project targeted
high-risk groups such as gay men, prostitutes, prison inmates, and injecting
drug users. If these categories also extended the original representation of
AIDS as a problem exclusive to gays, together they reinforced the association of AIDS with illegal and/or socially stigmatized activities.

According to a recent document of the BHM, in the early years of the epidemic AIDS was not perceived as a public health priority, and mass media sensationalism generated reactions of panic, fear, and discrimination in the general public (Brasil 1998). NGOs, on the other hand, pointed out that some of the BHM's early mass media campaigns were themselves stigmatizing, threatening, and counterproductive, as they offered little in the way of useful information and disseminated frightening images combined with slogans such as "I have AIDS and I'm going to die" and "If you don't look after yourself, AIDS will get you" (Parker et al. 1994: 56).

If the gay activists were faced with the dilemma of drawing attention to their needs and demanding resources for combatting AIDS, while at the same time resisting the stigmatizing definitions of "high risk," an opposite problem may be said to have occurred with the general female population. As in other countries, the predominant risk stereotypes made identification of female cases difficult, and such "invisibility" increased their vulnerability. By 1985, 15 cases of AIDS in women had been diagnosed (Koifman et al. 1991), and to the extent that prostitution was identified as a transmission route, both heterosexual men and women would, in principle, also be exposed. The "invisibility" of women in the epidemic may have been reinforced in the Brazilian case by a group of front-line medical researchers in Rio whose widely publicized early data on "stable" couples seemed to indicate that men were not being infected by seropositive female partners. Both heterosexual risk and IDU were devalued in notification of female cases (Bastos 1996; N. Santos 1996).

Despite the difficulty of recognizing AIDS in women in the early years, a 1991 publication demonstrated that the male/female ratio of reported cases had narrowed from 73/1 in 1980–1984 to 10/1 in 1989. Sexual transmission accounted for 34% of the female cases diagnosed in this period, and IDU for 38% (Koifman et al. 1991). Yet interviews with leading AIDS infectologists in Rio in the early 1990s revealed that those male cases in which it was not possible to detect homosexual practices or IDU were still being considered by some as "undefined" in terms of transmission. A female doctor interviewed in that study, on the other hand, suggested that this inability to recognize heterosexual transmission was a result of her male colleagues' need to feel safe themselves, particularly in their own clandestine heterosexual relations (Camargo 1994).

Only in 1991 did the feminist movement begin to concern itself with AIDS in women (Barbosa 1996). Primary data from a community study of low-income married women in Rio from the same period revealed that they themselves were aware of their risk and concerned about the possibility of infection, mainly because they could not be sure that their partners were monogamous (Simões Barbosa 1993). This finding is coherent with an international Gallup study from 1987–1988 that showed that 67% of Brazilians interviewed considered the general population to be vulnerable, apparently sometime before many specialists and activists recognized this fact (Webb 1988, in Parker 1994).

Up until recently, AIDS has been an urban phenomenon in Brazil, in both epidemiological and representational terms, and much of the research, activism, and reporting have taken place in the Rio–São Paulo region. While PN-DST/AIDS mass media campaigns have now been aimed at the "general population" for some time, images used are consistently urban. Representations of seropositivity have reflected this fact, even as the epidemic spreads to interior regions.

RESPONSE TO HIV/AIDS

Government Efforts

In Brazil, most public health service units are under the jurisdiction of state and municipal authorities and are only partially financed by BHM.[6] BHM's responsibilities include formulation of public policies, definition of technical norms, and in this case, coordination of actions involving AIDS. While the BHM established HIV tests and directives for control of AIDS in 1985, and a national AIDS commission including representatives of civil society and scientists was created in 1987, only in the early 1990s did AIDS become a public health priority.

PN-DST/AIDS's three Internet homepage sites have 5,296 internal pages with many national and international links, including access to the quarterly epidemiological bulletin in Portuguese and English, and may be seen to symbolize the technical sophistication with which this program has been conceived.

With 12 internal committees, PN-DST/AIDS's network includes 17 BHM service instances (councils, research institutions, national health programs, etc.), 14 other types of ministerial or state-level health programs, 9 types of civil and private initiative entities, and 19 international organizations (including foreign universities). A special sector for articulation with NGOs was created in 1992–1993, in preparation for the AIDS I project.

Diagnosis and Treatment

Testing is, in principle, voluntary. A network of laboratories carries out diagnostic procedures, and 139 centers offer free and anonymous testing and counseling and stimulate partner testing, as well as referring for treatment, when necessary.

Three hundred and fifty hospitals care for patients with AIDS; and 159 maternity units attend seropositive clients. Additionally 150 special service units, 60 outpatient clinics, and 40 home-care units give care to patients on antiretroviral therapy.

Universal free access to AZT (azidothymidine) began in 1991, and highly active antiretroviral therapy (HAART) was included in 1996, but drugs necessary for control and treatment of AIDS-associated health problems are considered to be the responsibility of state and municipal services. Approximately 70,000 patients are receiving HAART, 65% of whom are in double therapy. Three hundred and seventy-eight services offer antiretroviral drugs, and 100 of these use a sophisticated control system designed to reduce costs and guarantee adequate control of stock. A network of approximately 60 laboratories measure viral load, and 70 monitor CD4+ cell counts. Monitoring of resistance to antiretroviral drugs is also conducted.

Epidemiological Surveillance

Special programs have been established at 150 sites for monitoring of specific categories, including sexually transmitted disease (STD) and emergency service users, antenatal clients, army recruits, and IDUs. These studies also monitor the evolution of viral subtypes, as well as incorporating prevention measures.

Studies of seroprevalence, sexual behavior, and drug use are carried out every 2 years on a sample of 750,000 18-years-olds who are obliged to present to the armed forces annually, and ongoing prevention programs are developed (Brasil 1999a).

Fourteen IDU harm reduction programs, including 9 treatment and recuperation centers, have been established in health posts and community settings, despite a legal situation in which needle distribution may be interpreted as a crime. These studies are monitoring serostatus in the field, collecting qualitative data, and attempting to map social networks and estimate specific populations of IDUs.

Educational and Prevention Measures

A recent BHM document, produced with the collaboration of many academics/AIDS activists, stresses the creativity, diversity, and innovative nature of the PN-DST/AIDS approach to prevention, which combines national mass media campaigns and extensive intersectorial distribution of educational material, with support of NGOs in community-level peer education and outreach projects.[7] Other authors have noted, however, that this model is an example of the World Health Organization's most recent general approach to health promotion (Rocha 1999).

PN-DST/AIDS supports a national human rights network, disseminating information and promoting advocacy on human rights issues in the form of bulletins, workshops, seminars, and so on, including national meetings of persons living with AIDS. This network currently has 1,382 members, including individuals, institutions, libraries, hospitals, NGOs, and government organizations (Brasil 1998).

Sixteen national television campaigns were carried out between 1993 and 1998, at an average cost of $U.S.1.5 million each, making PN-DST/AIDS a preferred client for advertising agencies in the country. These campaigns adopt a 30-second "commercial" format, in which basic information is presented. Each national campaign also distributes pamphlets, posters, manuals for multipliers, and videos to local health posts and prevention projects.

Specific information campaigns are directed at truck drivers, indigenous groups, miners, and prostitutes. A bulletin designed for children and teenagers is distributed monthly to 100,000 grade-school students, a population of approximately 38 million children and youth who are in school.

BHM notes that problems with delivery of antiretroviral drugs and condoms have occurred, integration of university centers has been problematic, training has been deficient, and laboratory capacity is still insufficient, but authorities are confident that these problems will be overcome. Many professionals involved in what BHM considers "exemplary experiences" point to the need for more adequate evaluation of numerous aspects of this program (Brasil 1999a).

Independent of the problems that have, inevitably, occurred, the Health minister estimated a savings of about $U.S.3 million in hospitalization costs for 1997–1999 (O Globo 2000). This result reflects the abrupt interruption of mortality and morbidity trends achieved by initiation of widespread distribution of antiretroviral drugs. It must be remembered, however, that consistent reduction in these trends will depend on reducing the incidence of disease—that is, on effective prevention measures.

Epidemiological surveillance is perhaps the least criticized of all aspects of PN-DST/AIDS and represents a major tool for control of the epidemic if results are adequately used. Data from the survey of army recruits in 1996 showed that rural residence and low education levels were related to less accurate information on HIV/AIDS (Brasil 1998). This finding is compatible with current tendencies to pauperization and "interiorization" of the epidemic, which demonstrate that wider segments of the population are being directly affected.

While many segments of the Brazilian population appear to be reasonably informed about transmission and prevention, behavioral changes are more difficult to detect (Brasil 1999a). The limits of an individual/rational/informational approach, especially in a context of increasing impoverishment, are now being raised.

National data demonstrate that men have many sexual partners, and girls are becoming sexually active at earlier ages (Brasil 1999a). The demographic and health study from 1996, based on a large national sample, showed that only 14% of men reported using condoms, while 24% of the women interviewed reported having had an STD in the preceding year (BEMFAM 1996).

According to BHM, the sale of condoms increased 466% between 1992 and 1998, to an average of 6 condoms per year for the male population between the ages of 15 and 69 (Brasil 1999a). A major distortion of the

PN-DST/AIDS model is expressed in the fact that, given the high cost of condoms relative to income, antiretroviral drugs are in fact more accessible than condoms in Brazil (Rocha 1999).

Compared to the investment in education and prevention in NGOs, there has been no systematic attempt to develop these actions with existing human resources in public health services, a fact that will become more crucial when external funding for NGOs ceases (Rocha 1999).

Nongovernmental Organizations

As has been noted, gay activist groups were the first to react to the epidemic, carrying out peer education, giving legal advice, and pressuring public authorities. The first specific AIDS/NGO dates from 1985, and in 1986, hemophiliacs and other seropositive actors began organizing. Their emphasis on citizenship and civil rights resonated with the preconstitutional debates that were occurring at that time.

Since 1987, AIDS/NGOs have been included in official AIDS committees that define many aspects of the operationalization of public policy and participate in officially sponsored seminars, meetings, and so forth. With official support, the number of AIDS/NGOs grew rapidly, and 600 entities are currently listed on the BHM mailing list. At least 350 of these organizations are concerned primarily with AIDS (Brasil 1999a). Many academic activists have acted as consultants to BHM and/or have been absorbed as coordinators in PN-DST/AIDS (Galvão 1999).

During 1994–1998, U.S.$18 million of the AIDS I World Bank loan was invested in 444 community projects, including those developed and carried out by 175 NGOs. The first stage of AIDS II (1999–2002) has approved 250 projects, with women, children, adolescents, and "the poor" as priority groups (Brasil 1999a).

Selected through public competition coordinated by PN-DST/AIDS, AIDS I projects included support to people living with AIDS; information, education, and communication; behavior modification; and institutional development. While specific target groups and approaches varied, the BHM offered training in planning, supervision, and evaluation to participating NGOs. Educational material was distributed, and seminars held for exchange of experiences (Brasil 1998). In general, the KAP (knowledge, attitudes, practices) approach to education was promoted, often through multipliers trained in international programs.

Given the diversity of organizations, goals, time frames, target groups, and social contexts, assessment of this strategy for AIDS prevention is an almost impossible task. In fact, some critics characterize this strategy as fragmentation of educational efforts, in which evaluation is reduced to quantitative measures, example, number of multipliers trained or number of pamphlets distributed (Brasil 1999a).

AIDS I is also criticized for importation of behavioristic educational models based on the idea of a "free" individual who "chooses behaviors" with no social constraints (Fee and Kreiger 1993, in Galvão 1999). Others note that Brazil's long tradition in popular education, which aimed at promoting critical consciousness in disadvantaged social groups, has been totally ignored by PN-DST/AIDS (Rocha 1999).

Grassroots prevention programs are notoriously difficult to evaluate, and lessons learned in developing primary health care for poor communities have also not been taken into account. As one of the international NGOs involved in AIDS I has pointed out, this omission has led to repetition of problems that typically confront such projects: Even where community participants are remunerated, their prevention efforts are demoralized when their own communities' priorities are ignored; demoralization and demotivation also occur when provision of basic inputs such as condoms, which depend on official sources, is irregular (Brasil 1999a).

This points to a classic barrier to success of community-based projects: the difficulty of guaranteeing the support of official health services for supplies and for systematic supervision and recycling of community agents. On another plane, some activists who have been key integrants of this process are now questioning the transformation of NGOs from political and cultural actors to increasingly specialized and depoliticized professionals, dependent on external financing and divided by competition for project funds (Galvão 1999).

CONCLUSION

Institutionalization: The Recognized Challenge

Achieving institutionalization and sustainability at the state and municipal level is now a major objective of PN-DST/AIDS, as World Bank financing will not be repeated (Brasil 1999a). This means, in effect, involving a huge service network that has been marginal to the development of PN-DST/ AIDS, especially in terms of the huge investment made in prevention and education. The major challenges identified by BHM are political instability of coordinating teams; lack of priority for STD/AIDS; inadequate management structures; and scarcity of trained managers (Brasil 1999a).

These problems are directly related to the neglect of public health, a chronic condition that is itself aggravated by accumulated national debt (including World Bank loans) and regressive social policy. Beyond this, cost factors will certainly weigh heavily on services currently subject to diminishing financial support.

Epidemiological Tendencies and Prevention Possibilities

It has been noted that current tendencies to pauperization and interiorization of the epidemic will demand more complexity in action (Brasil

1999a), while deficiencies in public policy and services have more serious consequences for these populations (Bastos 1995).

Extensive vulnerability that results from poverty, lack of employment opportunities, and social exclusion is a clear sign of the weakness of citizenship in Brazil. In such a situation, involvement with drugs and prostitution represents a survival strategy for otherwise unemployed youth. These activities are difficult to measure, but studies show that drug use is increasing in school-age children, and age of first use is diminishing; despite efforts so far, systematic drug prevention programs are not in place even though the law "guarantees" them (Bastos and Carlini-Cotrim 1998). Studies with IDUs have demonstrated the limits of information and the dependence of effective prevention on contextual factors: Users' attempts to clean their used needles have been ineffective because of the low quality of available cleaning substances (Bastos 1995).

Despite the now undeniable feminization/heterosexualization of the epidemic in Brazil, prevention and educational measures have tended to adopt the "condom literacy" approach developed from the point of view of the masculine/gay aesthetic, in which the eroticization of condoms and the right to multiple partners are dominant themes. Ignoring both gender power relations and female sexual/affective preferences in intimate relationships, this approach tends to reproduce gender hierarchy and reinforce male-oriented sexuality (Giffin 1998; Goldstein 1994).

While the idea of promoting "empowerment" for women is now common in prevention discourse, few researchers and activists have as yet attempted to confront an even more difficult question that arises in reproductive relations: the fact that practicing "safe sex," defined as condom use, assumes that no more babies will be born (Treichler 1988). Within these conceptual limits, reproduction is opposed to survival, an obviously untenable stance for prevention, which has yet to be dealt with in Brazil and elsewhere.

Final Considerations

The decreases in morbidity-mortality that have been achieved with universal antiretroviral therapy are evidence of improvement in the quality of life of those who are seropositive, which must be defended without losing sight of the need to improve the quality of life of the majority of Brazilians. This challenge requires us to consider the significance of the Brazilian experience, the huge Brazilian market, and the influence of the World Bank for the profit-making international "AIDS industry" (Galvão 1999).

PN-DST/AIDS has invested huge sums in expensive drugs that demand expensive, elaborate support and delivery systems and yet has not assured an adequate supply of condoms, which are both much easier and cheaper to distribute as well as being essential to decreasing future need for drugs. From the point of view of public health, this policy is irrational and unacceptable, especially where people with HIV are living longer and in better health, which increases the need for partner protection.

From an economic point of view, a patent law that prohibits national production of antiretroviral drugs also signifies dependence on international suppliers, thus assuring captive markets and high profits for producers and high costs to users. High costs of essential supplies are a detriment to public health services in general and to citizens' well-being. Chronification of AIDS is, however, the most lucrative of possibilities for the drug industry. Could this state of affairs diminish investments in a vaccine or a final cure? How is the ethic of such patent laws to be defended (Galvão 1999)?

Perhaps more important, how is it to be questioned? In an exclusionary political system, the struggle for rights and citizenship demands strong civil organizations with a combative stance. PN-DST/AIDS support and professionalization of AIDS/NGOs have assured their political authority, at the same time as it tends to reduce their original demands for "rights" and "citizenship" to that which PN-DST/AIDS offers: salaries and resources for direct immediate action.

From the perspective of a political stance that seeks privatization of health and education services, and their transformation into profit-making endeavors, the professionalization of AIDS/NGOs in Brazil may be seen as a halfway measure, in which both potential activists and ordinary citizens become accustomed to the idea that such services be provided by such private entities (Galvão 1999). Unlike organic social movements, AIDS/NGOs are heterogeneous, self-constituted, and not representative of, or answerable to, wider social constituencies in any formal sense. Who controls them? Once World Bank funds cease, who will pay for them?

The new coordinator of PN-DST/AIDS, opening the Third International Conference on HIV in Women and Children, announced that despite the financial and technical investment in AIDS in Brazil, vertical transmission cannot be reduced because of the low quality of antenatal and labor care in the country (*Jornal do Brasil* 2000). This acknowledgment can be seen as recognition that there is no technical solution to the epidemic that is capable of bypassing the absence of basic social rights or the right to citizenship.

NOTES

The authors of this chapter are grateful to Catherine M. Lowndes and Willer Baumgarten for comments and suggestions.

1. These interests are currently becoming more visible on the level of states and municipalities across the country, and their presence is also clearly reflected both in the fact that violence is the leading cause of death in Brazilian youth (Vermelho and Mello Jorge 1996) and in the spread of HIV, as will be shown.

2. For one of many examples, see Giffin (1994) on the question of basic health care for women and children.

3. The founding director of PN-DST/AIDS is a qualified public health specialist and the sister of a long-standing director of the PAHO/WHO (Pan-American Health Organization/World Health Organization). When her first term of office was interrupted in 1990, she spent two years at WHO, returning in 1992 to resume the post. In her 11 years as director, she survived five health ministers, a rare occurence in a country where technical staff and program priorities tend to change with each new minister.

4. Unless otherwise specified, data in this section are from Brasil (1999b, 1999c).

5. One of the questions that became clear in this debate was that those who regularly sell their blood are often needy, marginalized, and in ill health. Beyond HIV, hepatitis and Chagas disease have also been commonly transmitted through transfusions in Brazil (Santos, Moraes, and Coelho 1994).

6. Unless otherwise specified, data in this section are from Brasil (1998).

7. Unless otherwise specified, data in this section are from Brasil (1999a).

BIBLIOGRAPHY

Alvarez, Sonia E., Evelina Dagnino, and Arturo Escobar, eds. 1998. *Cultures of Politics, Politics of Cultures*. Boulder and Oxford: Westview Press.

Barbosa, Regina. 1996. "Feminismo e AIDS." In *Quebrando o silencio: Mulheres e AIDS no Brasil*, Richard Parker and Jane Galvão, eds., pp. 153–168. Rio de Janeiro: ABIA/Relume-Dumará/IMS-UERJ.

Bastos, Francisco I. 1995. "Limitações estruturais à implementação de estratégias preventivas relativas à disseminação do HIV entre usuários de drogas injetáveis no Brasil." In *AIDS: Pesquisa social e educação*, Dina Czeresnia, Elizabeth M. dos Santos, Regina H. Simões Barbosa, and Simone Monteiro, eds., pp. 167–192. Rio de Janeiro: HUCITEC/ABRASCO.

———. 1996. "Cenas nubladas: A usuária de drogas injetáveis e a epidemia da AIDS." In *Quebrando o silencio: Mulheres e AIDS no Brasil*, Richard Parker and Jane Galvão, eds., pp. 61–78. Rio de Janeiro: ABIA/Relume-Dumará/IMS-UERJ.

Bastos, Francisco I., and Beatriz Carlini-Cotrim. 1998. "O consumo de substâncias psicoativas entre os jovens Brasileiros: Dados, danos, e algumas propostas." In *Jovens acontecendo nas trilhas das politicas públicas*, Vol. 2, pp. 645–670. Brasília: Commissão Nacional de População e Desenvolvimento.

BEMFAM. 1996. *Pesquisa nacional de demografia e saúde*. Rio de Janeiro: Author.

Brasil. 1998. Ministério da Saúde, PN DST/AIDS. *AIDS no Brasil: Um esforço conjunto governo-sociedade*. Brasília: Author.

———. 1999a. Ministério da Saúde, PN DST/AIDS. *A resposta Brasileira ao HIV/AIDS: Experiências exemplares*. Brasília: Author.

———. 1999b. Ministério da Saúde, PN DST/AIDS. *Boletim Epidemiológico AIDS*, Ano XII (4): 35–47.

———. 1999c. Ministério da Saúde, PN DST/AIDS. *Boletim Epidemiológico AIDS*, Ano XII (2): 9–21.

Bucher, Richard. 1995. "O usuário de drogas injetáveis na política preventiva ao HIV/AIDS." In *AIDS: Pesquisa social e educação*, Dina Czeresnia, Elizabeth M. dos Santos, Regina H. Simões Barbosa, and Simone Monteiro, eds., pp. 147–166. Rio de Janeiro: HUCITEC/ABRASCO.

Camargo, Kenneth R. 1994. *A ciência da AIDS e a AIDS da ciência: O discurso médico e a construção da AIDS.* Rio de Janeiro: ABIA/Relume-Dumará/IMS-UERJ.
Cohn, Amélia. 1997. "Considerações acerca da dimensão social da epidemia de HIV/AIDS no Brasil." In *A epidemia de AIDS no Brasil: Situação e tendências,* Brasil, Ministério da Saúde, pp. 45–53. Brasília: M.S. PN DST/AIDS.
Fee, Elizabeth, and Nancy Kreiger. 1993. "Understanding AIDS: Historical Roots of the Limits of Biomedical Individualism." *American Journal of Public Health* 83 (10): 1477–1486.
Galvão, Jane. 1999. *AIDS no Brasil: A agenda de construção de uma epidemia.* Ph.D. diss., Universidade Estadual do Rio de Janeiro.
Giffin, Karen. 1994. "Women's Health and the Privatization of Fertility Control in Brazil." *Social Science and Medicine* 39 (3): 355–360.
———. 1998. "Beyond Empowerment: Heterosexualities and the Prevention of AIDS." *Social Science and Medicine* 46 (2): 151–156.
Goldstein, Donna. 1994. "AIDS and Women in Brazil: The Emerging Problem." *Social Science and Medicine* 39 (7): 919–929.
Jornal do Brasil. 2000. "Recursos para evitar contágio de AIDS são mal utilizados no Brasil." 7 April, p. 5.
Koifman, Rosalina, Eleonora P. Quinhões, Gina T. Monteiro, Regina Rodrigues, and Sergio Koifman. 1991. "AIDS em mulheres adultas no município do Rio de Janeiro." *Cadernos de Saúde Pública* 7 (2): 232–250.
Lowndes, Catherine M., Francisco I. Bastos, Karen Giffin, Ana C.G. Vaz dos Reis, Eleonora D'Orsi, and Michel Alary. 2000. "Differential Trends in Mortality from AIDS in Men and Women in Brazil (1984–95)." *AIDS* 14 (9): 1269–1273.
Mesquita, Fábio C. 1995. "HIV/AIDS entre usuários de drogas injetáveis: A experiência do Brasil." In *AIDS: Pesquisa social e educação,* Dina Czeresnia, Elizabeth M. dos Santos, Regina H. Simões Barbosa, and Simone Monteiro, eds., pp. 137–146. Rio de Janeiro: HUCITEC/ABRASCO.
Monteiro, Simone. 1995. "Projeto vivendo a vida: Prevenindo AIDS na escola." In *AIDS: Pesquisa social e educação,* Dina Czeresnia, Elizabeth M. dos Santos, Regina H. Simões Barbosa, and Simone Monteiro, eds., pp. 122–136. Rio de Janeiro: HUCITEC/ABRASCO.
O Globo. 2000. "AIDS contamina mais adultos que jovens." 15 March, pp. 1, 4.
Parker, Richard. 1994. *A construção da solidariedade: AIDS, sexualidade e política no Brasil.* Rio de Janeiro: ABIA/Relume-Dumará/IMS-UERJ.
Parker, Richard, Cristiana Bastos, Jane Galvão, and José S. Pedrosa, eds. 1994. *A AIDS no Brasil (1982–1992).* Rio de Janeiro: ABIA/Relume/Dumará/IMS-UERJ.
Rocha, Maria Fátima G. 1999. *Política de controle ao HIV/AIDS no Brasil: O lugar da Prevenção Nessa Trajetória.* Master's thesis, Escola Nacional de Saúde Pública ENSP/FIOCRUZ, Rio de Janeiro.
Santos, Luiz A.C., Cláudia Moraes, and Vera S. Coelho. 1994. "Sangue, AIDS e constituinte: Senso e contra senso." In *A AIDS no Brasil (1982–1992),* Richard Parker, Cristiana Bastos, Jane Galvão, and José S. Pedrosa, eds., pp. 307–324. Rio de Janeiro: ABIA/Relume/Dumará/IMS-UERJ.
Santos, Naila J.S. 1996. "A AIDS entre as mulheres no estado de São Paulo." In

Quebrando o silencio: Mulheres e AIDS no Brasil, Richard Parker and Jane Galvão, eds., pp. 33–60. Rio de Janeiro: ABIA/Relume-Dumará/IMS-UERJ.

Santos, Wanderley G. 1987. "Gênese e apocalipse: Elementos para uma teoria da crise institucional Latino-Americana." Paper presented at the International Conference Identidad Latinoamericana, Modernidad e Postmodernidad, Buenos Aires.

Simões Barbosa, Regina. 1993. *Gênero e AIDS: As mulheres de uma comunidade favelada do Rio de Janeiro*. Master's thesis, Escola Nacional de Saúde Pública, ENSP/FIOCRUZ, Rio de Janeiro.

Treichler, Paula. 1988. "Gender and Biomedical Discourse: Current Contests for Meaning." In *AIDS: The Burden of History*, Elizabeth Fee and David Fox, eds., pp. 190–246. Berkeley: University of California Press.

Vermelho, Letícia Legay, and M.H. Mello Jorge. 1996. "Mortalidade de Jovens: Análise do Período 1930–1991." *Revista de Saúde Pública* 30 (4): 319–331.

Webb, N.L. 1988. "Gallup International Survey on Attitudes towards AIDS." In *The Global Impact of AIDS*, A. Fleming, ed. New York: Alan R. Liss.

WHO. 1993. "An International Comparative Study on HIV Prevalence and Risk Behavior among Drug Injectors in 13 Cities." *Bulletin of Narcotics* 45 (1): 19–46.

3

CENTRAL AND EASTERN EUROPE

Jean-Paul C. Grund

INTRODUCTION

Until 1995 Central and Eastern Europe as well as the Asian republics of the former Soviet Union have been more or less devoid of epidemic outbreaks of HIV infection. In this region with more than 450 million inhabitants (United Nations 1997), the total number of HIV infections was estimated lower than 30,000 (UNAIDS 1996; WHO 1995). Most of these infections resulted from sexual and nosocomial (originating or taking place in a hospital) transmission. In 1995 this epidemiologically soporific picture started changing drastically in two ways. First, reports on rapid HIV outbreaks in various parts of the former Soviet Union started to surface; second, these new infections were almost exclusively associated with another major public health crisis that until then had gone largely unnoticed: the rapid diffusion of drug injecting. Indeed, the social networks of drug injectors have provided an almost custom-tailored infrastructure for the virus to spread through the former Soviet Union, and most HIV cases are reportedly related to illicit drug injecting. Except for Poland and Yugoslavia, the countries in Central and Southeast Europe have not yet experienced epidemic HIV spread, although in many of these countries drug injecting has become a major public health concern as well.

At the end of the year 2000, there were an estimated 700,000 people living with HIV in this region; 250,000 of them acquired the virus in the new millennium. Most of these infections are among injecting drug users (IDUs) (UNAIDS/WHO 2000f). This chapter will provide an overview of

the development of the epidemic in the region and discuss some of its epidemiological and social peculiarities. Subsequently, it will bring to the
reader's attention some of the social and political impediments to developing
appropriate responses, which are rooted in its recent totalitarian past and
exacerbated by the "backdrop of social-economic turmoil" (UNAIDS/
WHO 2000h) that characterizes the postcommunist transition process.
Next, it will discuss the human rights aspects of the drugs-AIDS nexus, as
well as its link to another historically unsettling feature of this region: its
traditionally abysmal treatment of ethnic minorities, in particular the stateless Roma. To counter some of the pessimism these issues may have elicited
in the reader, the chapter ends with a—given the immensity of the region,
inevitably partial—description of interventions that nevertheless have developed.

ISSUES RELATING TO HIV AND AIDS

History of HIV/AIDS

It was in 1995 that the first reports appeared on outbreaks of HIV in
different parts of the former Soviet Union, including the Black Sea ports
Odessa and Nikolayev, the northwestern Russian enclave of Kaliningrad (a
seaport as well), and Svetlogorsk in southern Belarus. Only separated by
months, epidemics developed in these three countries with highly similar
features.

In Ukraine less than 100 HIV infections were registered between 1988
and 1994, which concerned mainly foreigners. However, in March and April
1995 more than 1,000 cases were detected among drug injectors in Odessa
and Nikolayev, after the militia was instructed to round up registered drug
users for testing. HIV prevalence among drug injectors arrested by the militia or in contact with narcology centers[1] grew rapidly from virtually zero
to 30% in Odessa and 57% in Nikolayev (Khodakevich 1997). Within a year
HIV infections were reported among drug injectors from all 25 regional
capitals, and more recent reports suggest continued spread into rural areas
and cities in the eastern and central parts of the country (UNAIDS 2000f).
Countrywide, the registered number of new HIV infections rose to 1,490
in 1995, up from 31 in the year before. An additional 5,400 new cases were
registered in 1996, and this number peaked at 8,913 in the following year.
A total of 8,575 new infections were registered in 1998 and 5,827 in 1999,
resulting in a cumulative total of 30,388 reported cases at the end of 1999
(WHO-EURO 2000). At the end of 1999, UNAIDS estimated the number
of HIV-positive people in Ukraine at 240,000, and between 50% and 80%
are associated with injecting drug use (UNAIDS 2000f).

Fewer than 1,100 HIV cases were registered in the Russian Federation
between the start of registration in 1987 and the end of 1995. Among these

cases were very few IDUs (Pokrovskyi, Savtchenko, and Ladnaia 1997). Kaliningrad first reported a rapidly escalating number of infections among drug injectors, but the outbreak was not contained to this East Sea enclave. In 1996 and 1997 cities all over the Russian map, including Krasnodar, Nizhnyi Novgorod, Rostov Na Donu, Saratov, Tula, Tumen, and Tver, reported epidemic spread among IDUs as well (Burrows et al. 1998; Pokrovskyi et al.). In early 1999 the epidemic hit the federal capital. One year later (June 2000 data), Moscow has officially registered 6,670 HIV infections and an additional 8,904 infections in the surrounding Moscow oblast (administrative region). With 782 and 222 officially registered HIV cases, St. Petersburg and its surrounding oblast Leningrad still seem to lag behind (Ministry of Health of the Russian Federation 2000). However, a 1999 survey among IDUs in St. Petersburg found that HIV prevalence rates rose in six months from 12% to 19% (UNAIDS 2000h). To appreciate the epidemic's geographical dimension, the remote city of Irkutsk has already registered 5,773 cases (Ministry of Health of the Russian Federation 2000). At the end of 2000 the epidemic has spread to over 30 cities across Russia, and 82 out of 89 oblasts had reported HIV cases (UNAIDS/WHO 2000a).

Overall, the number of registered new cases in Russia increased from 196 in 1995 to 1,546 in 1996 and 4,399 in 1997. During 1998 new cases decreased to 3,947, but the following year they jumped to 19,661. More than 90% of new cases in 1998 and 1999 were registered among injecting drug users. The average age of HIV-infected individuals was 18 to 25 years. Nine HIV-positive cases concerned 11- to 14-year-olds who became infected through injecting drug use. With 15,696 new cases in the first half year, the 2000 incidence is projected to supercede the total prevalence of 1999 (30,624 cases) (Ministry of Health of the Russian Federation 2000) and to climb to 50,000 by year's end (UNAIDS/WHO 2000b). At the start of 2000, UNAIDS estimated the number of HIV-positive people in the Russian Federation at 130,000 (UNAIDS 2000e). At the end of the year this figure will have climbed to 300,000 (UNAIDS/WHO 2000a). Close to 90% of cases are associated with injecting drug use.

In the beginning of 1996 the first case of HIV in an IDU since 1992 was established in Minsk, the capital of Belarus. This case concerned a resident of Svetlogorsk, a town of 72,000 in the southern Gomel oblast. Subsequent mass screening (targeting known drug users) revealed 1,125 HIV infections, 88% among drug injectors (Bezruchenko-Novachuk and Romantsov 1998). In 1997 an HIV prevalence of 67% was found in blood samples drawn from the syringes of participants of the Svetlogorsk needle exchange (Bezruchenko-Novachuk and Romantsov 1998). That same year, HIV was detected among IDUs in all oblasts of Belarus. The number of registered new cases in Belarus increased from 8 in 1995 to 1,021 in 1996 but fell to 653 in 1997 and continued to decrease to 554 and 411 in the subsequent two years (WHO-EURO 2000). At the end of 1999, there were 2,752 cases of HIV infection registered in Belarus (WHO-EURO 2000), but UNAIDS estimated the number of HIV-positive people at 14,000 at the end of 1999, and more than 80% are associated with injecting drug use (UNAIDS 2000b).

Moldova experienced an outbreak of HIV soon after Ukraine, Belarus, and Russia, but hitherto the number of cases remained lower. Registered new cases rose from 7 in 1995 to 48 in 1996, and further to 404 and 408 in the subsequent two years, but fell to 155 in 1999 (WHO-EURO 2000). A total of 1,034 cases of HIV infection were registered in Moldova at the end of 1999 (WHO-EURO 2000), but according to UNAIDS the number of HIV-positive people was 4,500. Most infections have been detected in the two major cities Chisinau and Baltsi, and more than 80% are associated with injecting drug use (UNAIDS 2000a).

More recently HIV has diffused into populations of IDUs in the Baltic states as well, most notably in Latvia where in 1998 the number of new cases jumped to 163, up from 25 in the previous year, while 241 new cases were registered in 1999. At the end of 1998, 122 cases were registered among IDUs (WHO-EURO 2000). These numbers may not seem dramatic, but they put Latvia among the three countries in the entire (World Health Organization [WHO]) European region with incidence rates (per million population) over 100 in 1999, the other two being Russia and Ukraine. After initial reports on outbreaks among IDUs in its port city Klaipeda, Lithuania seems to have been able to contain epidemic spread. At the end of 1998, 66 cases had been registered among IDUs (WHO-EURO 2000). But in 2000, a new epidemic emerged among drug injectors in Narva, Estonia, with the result that the country reported far more HIV cases than in any previous year (UNAIDS/WHO 2000b). In the three Caucasus republics Armenia, Azerbaijan, and Georgia the number of infections is also on the rise. Although in a large number of registered HIV cases in this subregion the transmission category was unknown (e.g., prisoners or military personnel who may have injected drugs), most of these infections are associated with injecting drug use as well (WHO-EURO 2000). Central Asia has remained largely untouched by the global AIDS pandemic, but in 1999 HIV infections were reported among IDUs in four of the five countries. Furthermore, the detention-related outbreak of HIV among IDUs in Temirtau, in the Karaganda oblast of Kazakhstan, demonstrates that this subregion is not immune to rapid epidemic spread. Prior to the detection of HIV among drug users imprisoned in the local prison, there were just 69 registered cases of HIV in Kazakhstan. Since then, testing of drug users has been intensified. As a result, 736 new cases were reported between 1997 and 1998, 88% among injecting drug users (UNAIDS 2000c).

Most former communist countries in Central Europe have thus far not reported epidemic spread of HIV, except for Poland. While homosexual and bisexual men in the region are the most affected population group, overall reported prevalence remained relatively low. Nonetheless, Poland was hit by an outbreak among drug injectors in the late 1980s. The numbers of reported infections among IDUs jumped from 1 in 1988 to 411 in 1989, and since 1995 between 539 and 638 new infections are registered yearly (WHO-EURO 2000). The majority of those are associated with injecting drug use (UNAIDS 2000d). At the end of 1999 the cumulative total reported cases in Poland was 6,118 (WHO-EURO 2000), but UNAIDS estimates the total number of HIV-positive people at 13,000 (UNAIDS 2000d). As in Central Europe, HIV infections among injecting drug users in the Balkan countries have remained low, except in Yugoslavia (Serbia and Montenegro), which experienced an early IDU-driven epidemic similar to Poland. Most other countries in this subregion primarily reported heterosexual transmission, but transmission between men who have sex with men (MSM) is likely to be underreported because of strong stigmatization. Assessment of the levels of HIV and injecting drug use in Southeastern Europe are severely hampered by the recent political events in the region.

All in all, both in Central and Southeastern Europe the preconditions exist for epidemic outbreaks of HIV infection among IDUs. While IDU populations are perhaps still smaller than in several of the newly independent states (NIS), a growing number of authors have suggested that drug injecting is on the increase throughout both subregions (Grund and Nolimal 1995; Honti and Zelenai 1999; Khodakevich and Dehne 1998; Nolimal and Jerman 1996; Polanecky, Sijda, and Studnickova 1996). Likewise, anecdotal reports suggest high prevalence of hepatitis C among IDUs in many parts of these two subregions.

Data Collection Issues

In most countries in this large region—almost 30 countries between Germany's eastern border and the Pacific Ocean, stretching 11 time zones—HIV reporting is based on mandatory mass screening and a two-stage registration process, introduced in 1987. Reporting of HIV/AIDS cases is required by law and Ministry of Health (MoH) regulations. Screening targets include both low-risk (e.g., pregnant women, blood donors, occupational groups) and vulnerable populations (drug users, prisoners, sexually transmitted disease [STD] patients). For years millions of dollars have been invested in this costly but inefficient pursuit—in 1995 approximately 95% of the Ukrainian HIV/AIDS budget was spent on testing kits: That same year the epidemic struck the country's IDU networks.

Testing policies for low-risk populations have become less stringent since the early 1990s. Officially, most HIV tests are now voluntary, except for blood donors and foreigners (e.g., in Russia). Yet routine mandatory screening without informed consent and pre- and posttest counseling of high-risk populations, including identified drug users, prisoners, and STD patients, remains a routine exercise throughout the region. Since 1999–2000, innovative methods of HIV surveillance (e.g., sentinel surveillance, which collects HIV data from selected sites or from particular subgroups within the population) are being slowly implemented in a few countries, but officially these are not yet included in the national guidelines on HIV monitoring (Y. Kobyshcha, personal communication). Voluntary, confidential, or anonymous testing accounts for only a fraction of both tests and positive results registered. This pattern is perhaps associated with the fact that the anonymity of people testing HIV-positive is often not upheld.

Registration includes the recording of all test results and the referral of positive results to an AIDS Center for confirmation, history taking, official registration, and treatment (when available). Classification (and reclassification of, for example, prisoners) into transmission category is based on the clinic interview. In most countries, reporting is based on the registration of the AIDS Centers. Because of intense stigmatization and potentially serious consequences (from losing one's employment or driver's license to imprisonment and ongoing police harassment, including unlawful entry of the home) many people are unwilling to disclose a history of drug use.

Furthermore, incomplete referrals between the initial test site and the health institution responsible for registration have resulted both in underreporting and biased distributions over transmission categories. For example, in Ukraine, each person with a confirmed HIV-positive test result is obliged to attend an AIDS Center or other specialized infectious diseases clinic for extensive clinical and biological examinations, which must be completed before official registration. But in practice a large number of people found HIV-positive after laboratory testing (mainly drug users) do not show up for further examination at these clinics, resulting in delays in reporting and considerable underreporting. Thus, during the first years of the epidemic (1996–1997), only 50% of people with HIV-positive test results were officially registered (Y. Kobyshcha, personal communication). Likewise, Russian data for 1996 and 1997 included more than 2,000 cases for which the transmission mode was unknown. The HIV data presented in this section are therefore in all likelihood an underestimate of the true dimensions of the HIV epidemic in this region.

Colliding Epidemics: HIV and Injecting Drug Use

Research in diverse regions of the world has established rapid HIV spread associated with transmission among IDUs (Angarano, Pastore, and Monno 1985; Ball, Rana, and Dehne 1998; Hamers et al. 1997; Ismail 1998; Rebagliato, Avino, and Hernandez–Aguado 1995; Stimson 1994; Zheng et al. 1994), sometimes resulting in increases of HIV prevalence among drug injectors from less than 5% to 30% to 50% in one to three years (Burns, Brettle, and Gore, 1996; Crofts, Reid, and Deany 1998; Des Jarlais et al. 1994;

Htoon et al. 1994; Stimson 1994; Weniger et al. 1991). Khodakevich (1997) reported equally rapid HIV spread in Svetlogorsk, Belarus, and Odessa and Nikolayev in Ukraine. By mid-1999 HIV transmission among IDUs was reported from 114 countries, and in many countries, injecting drug use has been the main mode of transmission (UNAIDS 2000g). However, in no other region is the overall proportion of reported cases associated with drug injecting as high as in Eastern Europe, in particular in the NIS. In this section we will discuss some of the factors that may be associated with this issue. This discussion will concentrate on the countries of the former Soviet Union, as those are hit hardest by the HIV epidemic.

While certainly not unknown before the breakdown of communism, drug use seems to have rapidly increased in the 1990s. Officially registered injecting drug users in Ukraine rose from around 20,000 in the early 1990s to 80,000 in 1997 (Dehne et al. 1999). According to the Russian Ministry of Internal Affairs the number of people undergoing drug treatment was 249,000 in 1996, up from 91,000 two years earlier (Khodakevich and Dehne 1998). The country's Ministry of Health reported a more modest increase: from 25,000 in 1990 to 85,000 in 1996 (Khodakevich and Dehne 1998). Such a discrepancy illustrates the unreliability of these statistics. Before the political changes in the Soviet Union drug use was officially nonexistent and consequently not enumerated. In reality drug users were persecuted indiscriminately by militia, sentenced to many years in prison, and committed to inhumane mandatory treatment and other repressive measures. Nowadays these practices still prevail in many parts of the region, with the result that people who use drugs avoid contact with drug treatment and other health institutions as much as possible. As a consequence, the official number of registered drug users is only a small proportion of the real size of the drug user population.

In 1997 the Ukrainian Ministry of Internal Affairs estimated the total number of drug users between 600,000 and 700,000, and IDUs represented 75% to 80% of these cases (Khodakevich and Dehne 1998). Estimates in Russia range from 600,000 to 1 to 2.5 million (Brunet 1996; USAID and Centers for Disease Control and Prevention 1998). While their reliability is difficult to assess, these estimates suggest that in both countries more than 1% of the population is involved in drug use. "Rapid Situation Assessments" (WHO 1998) in a number of Russian cities estimate the number of IDUs at 35,000 for Nizhniy Novgorod, 9,500 to 10,000 in Rostov Na Donu, 70,000 in St. Petersburg, and 18,000 in Volgograd. The author's fieldwork in these cities during 1999 suggests that the use of injectable opiates in particular has become a regular feature of the social ecology of many neighborhoods in these cities. As one outreach worker in Volgograd explained, "People drink or inject in this place." Likewise, an epidemiologist in Rostov Na Donu thought that "it [was] difficult to find a building in this town that is not affected by drug use."

While more recently the use of (imported) heroin has increased drastically in many cities, drug use patterns throughout the NIS are characterized by two rather specific observations, which add dramatically to the potential for drug-related harm. First, the tradition of kitchen production of alcoholic beverages seems to have been extended to a number of other psychoactive substances. Simple "bathtub chemistry" is used to process opium poppies into a strong injectable opioid cocktail, and ephedrine-based medications into methamphetamine and methcathinone, both powerful psychostimulants. Second, there seems to be a prevailing perception among a majority of drug users that, perhaps apart from cannabis, drugs are to be injected. Thus, while in the United States snorting Ketamine (a dissociative anesthetic primarily used in veterinary medicine) has gained considerable popularity in gay dance clubs, in Russia this drug is primarily injected among straight middle-class youth. The self-produced opioids and amphetamines are generally prepared for injection as well.

Many risk behaviors identified in drug injecting–related HIV epidemics elsewhere are relevant to the reported rapid spread. For example, sequential use (sharing) of syringes and needles has been reported from many cities throughout the region, including Moscow, St. Petersburg, Kaliningrad, Nizhniy Novgorod, Rostov Na Donu, Volgograd, and Pskov in Russia, Poltava and Odessa in Ukraine, Svetlogorsk in Belarus, Almaty and other cities in Kazakhstan, and Tblisi in Georgia. In a recent study of syringe exchange participants in five Russian cities, 38% (N = 1076) of the participants admitted that in the 30 days before they joined the program they had injected with a syringe that was previously used by someone else (Grund, Kobzev, et al. 2001).

However, a number of region-specific risk factors can be identified, associated to the home preparation of injectable drugs, in particular opiates. Using water and common household chemicals, including ethyl acetate, soda, vinegar, and acetic anhydride, IDUs boil opium poppies or opium gum into a strong injectable cocktail of opioid alkaloids (containing, codeine, morphine, and heroin in varying proportions). The resulting cocktail is known under a number of different names in the region, including Cheornaya (black), Chemia or Himya (chemistry), Mak, Shirka, and Hanka.

A number of authors have wondered whether HIV might be introduced into the mixture during the production process through the use of contaminated mixing containers. Others hypothesized that the (nowadays rare) practice of using blood to filter solid particles from the solution might have caused rapid outbreaks of HIV in several Russian and Ukrainian cities (Bolekham and Zmushko 1998; Liitsola et al. 1998; Lukashov et al. 1998). However, recent ethnographic observations of the production process in Russia (Grund, unpublished data; Dehne et al. 1999) and laboratory simulations of the process (Heimer, personal communication) show that contamination of the drug solution during the production process is extremely unlikely. Even when contaminated blood is used, the solution is subsequently repeatedly boiled for extended periods, and at the end of the process, acetic anhydride (a highly caustic chemical) is added. (For a description of the process and its potential for HIV transmission, see Dehne et al. 1999.)

A perhaps more plausible hypothesis is related to how the practice of self-production has shaped the drug culture (Grund 1998b) in this region. A typical feature of the self-production and use of opiates is that it is mostly conducted within groups of two or more people, and when the drugs are ready for consumption, they are divided by squirting them from one (large) syringe into those of the group members. This technique—termed "front-loading" or "syringe-mediated drug sharing" (SMDS)—has been described in many other parts of the world and is associated with HIV seroconversion (Grund et al. 1991, 1996; Jose et al. 1993). The regular practice of preparing and using in groups is also likely to result in higher frequencies of needle sharing than in more individualistic cultures of drug injecting. Nevertheless, a recent study of syringe exchange participants in five Russian cities indicated that while syringe sharing decreased substantially (from 38% to 11%) after respondents joined the exchange program, several behaviors associated with the context of group drug use decreased to a much lesser degree. The practice of injecting with friends itself was hardly affected by participation in the needle exchange program, going from 91% before to only 86% after joining the program. Likewise, sharing drug paraphernalia other than needles and syringes only went down from 82% to 73%, whereas SMDS decreased only from 58% to 48% (Grund, unpublished data).

Thus, the social context of drug injecting, especially the seemingly ubiquitous practice of preparing and using drugs in groups, may well be responsible to a large extent for the rapid diffusion of HIV among the IDU populations in the region. Many questions arise from this hypothesis—for example, concerning the density and connectivity of IDU networks. Nevertheless, home production and its communal aspects in particular may well produce considerably higher rates of established risk behaviors than in more individualistic drug injecting cultures where (imported) powder drugs are used.

In summary, the circumstances under which HIV is transmitted among IDUs in the region is at present insufficiently understood. This situation is in urgent need of thorough ethnographic and epidemiological study. Not only is it essential to gain a better understanding of transmission among IDUs themselves, but research should also address the questions of the potential and mechanisms of secondary spread into non-IDU populations. At the presentation of the December 2000 AIDS epidemic update, WHO's director general, Dr. Gro Harlem Brundtland, warned that "in just three to four years, Russia may well have a generalized epidemic" (UNAIDS/WHO 2000a). Elsewhere, Dehne and colleagues (1999) reviewed this hazard and hypothesized that the overlap between drug injecting and sex work could well become the critical link in the epidemiological chain between the current HIV epidemics among IDUs and a generalized epidemic. Another scenario might be based on the sheer magnitude of the fast-paced, postcommunist epidemic of drug injecting in Central and Eastern Europe and the former Soviet Union and its apparent normalcy in many communities.

Although reliable statistics are lacking, injecting drug use appears to have touched a significant proportion of the population in the region. Drug injectors may be subject to intense state repression, but they appear to remain fairly well integrated in family structures and social networks that are not necessarily built around drug-related activities (Grund, unpublished data). Likewise, self-injection does not always seem to invoke the same level of stigmatization known in Western Europe or the United States and is reportedly a commonly accepted method of taking both medical and recreational drugs in parts of the region (Jong, Tsagarelli, and Schouten 1999). When the stigma against drug injecting is limited, and when IDUs spend relatively more time in "nondrug" networks, they are likely to meet more sexual partners who do not inject drugs than when they only socialize with other drug users. Ergo, the widespread practice of drug injecting may provide for many links in the epidemiological chain toward a generalized epidemic that will be unprecedented in the Northern Hemisphere.

RESPONSES TO HIV/AIDS

Obstacles to Controlling the HIV/AIDS Epidemics in the Region

The common denominator of this region is that all countries are undergoing a transition process from closed societies with state-controlled economies toward more democratic, open societies with free market economies—until now, with various results. For most people the transition includes a significant drop in the quality of life, set against a background of profound social and political change. For many citizens, unemployment and decreased access to housing, health care, and social services have been the price for economic and political liberalization. Where formal economies stagnate, informal economies have mushroomed, and organized crime is growing rapidly. Increasingly, illicit drugs are becoming a prime commodity within this "shadow economy." The region's transition process, its communist legacy, and the associated economic crises in many parts of the region can be seen to hamper the response to the HIV epidemic in many ways.

In most, if not all, of the NIS countries that experienced significant HIV outbreaks among IDUs, appropriate governmental responses only developed after these outbreaks were firmly established, despite the writings on the wall. Instead of timely introducing public health–based HIV prevention programs targeting IDUs, governments relied on outmoded and ineffective mass screening procedures and police repression of drug users. What's more, most of the (Central European) countries that have been spared epidemic HIV spread so far seem bound to repeat this mistake, as funding levels for needle exchange and other HIV prevention activities targeting IDUs are, generally speaking, grossly inadequate. In fact, most needle exchange programs in the region exist on foreign funding.

One of the most important lessons in this epidemic is that successful responses require "multisectoral and multilevel" approaches (UNAIDS 2000g). However, such thinking does not tie in well with the bureaucratic legacy of the communist era we find in many, if not most, countries in the region. The Soviet approach to management was strictly hierarchical and multilayered, and in many places few structural changes have taken place in the bureaucracy. Governmental health structures are extremely complex, and frequently the number of local, state, and federal institutions involved in HIV prevention planning runs into the double digits. Furthermore, in establishing a training program to assist Russian health professionals and others involved in HIV prevention among IDUs, Burrows and colleagues (1999) observed a highly competitive atmosphere among (government) health agencies involved in this area. Absence of interagency collaborations and of information sharing within and between agencies seemed to be the usual modus operandi. They linked this situation to the scarcity of funds, but such a culture of secrecy and competition is of course a remnant of the communist past as well. As one Lithuanian narcologist explained: "Why would you share information or your ideas about a certain matter? It could only be used against you."

Absence of sufficient funding is nonetheless a genuine issue. Salaries of health and other government workers (e.g., militia) are often months behind, buildings are in poor shape, and funds for equipment, medications, and professional literature are often lacking. In one regional AIDS Center in the south of Russia, the library was filled with the dust-covered complete works of Lenin and Stalin. Russian or international professional literature was nearly absent.

Another serious problem is the absence of a positive nongovernmental organization (NGO) climate, in particular in the NIS but, for example, in Slovakia as well. Not only are NGO legislation and regulation often unnecessarily complicated, but many state health workers consider NGOs with Argus's eyes, that is, as a new set of competitors in a shrinking market. To make matters more complex, while "real NGOs" certainly exist in the HIV/ AIDS field, many are closely linked to government institutions. In the previously mentioned evaluation study of Russian needle exchange programs, three out of five of the programs were administered by NGOs that were run by the head physician and core staff of the AIDS Center, and all three were located at the premises of the AIDS Center. The primary function of this type of NGO seems to be attracting and channeling nongovernmental and foreign funding. It also provides AIDS Center staff a chance to be innovative and operate outside the rigid structures that determine their usual work (Burrows et al. 1999). And last but not least, it offers a possibility to boost their regular (devaluated ruble) salaries with hard currencies, such as U.S. dollars. Some of these initiatives have built impressive (peer/outreach-based) needle exchange projects, but elsewhere middle-aged epidemiologists and laboratory workers in white coats have taken up the outreach profession.

A problem of a different order is that in most countries in the region policymakers and professionals alike seem to believe that the situation in their country is not comparable to any other place in the world. "My country is different" is a mantra that many foreign consultants have heard over and over again, where "my country" can be substituted by "our mind-set," "our drug users' mentality," and other variants. Burrows and colleagues (1999) refer to this phenomenon as "Russianness," but this author has been exposed to it in at least 10 countries in the region and elsewhere as well. The upshot of such remarks is generally that pragmatic interventions for IDUs tried successfully elsewhere will not work in the country. Perhaps associated with the Cold War, such beliefs go hand in hand with a mistrust of "Western" research and approaches, and with this comes a moral dismissal of many aspects of what UNAIDS terms "Best Practice" (UNAIDS 1999). The explicit ban on the use of methadone in the new Russian drug law serves as an apt example.

Particularly strong are misconceptions of drug users and their ability to adjust their behaviors, which are embedded in obsolete and unscientific ideas on the dynamics of drug use, addiction, and the careers of drug users. Many narcologists and psychiatrists were trained to believe that, after their first injection, IDUs have on average three to four years to live and that drug users are "hopeless" cases who do not care whether they live or die (Burrows et al. 1999). When the prevailing sense is that drug users are not interested in protecting themselves and their family and friends against HIV, pragmatic, unmoralistic prevention becomes a hard sell. Along with these ideas comes an unwarranted belief in repressive approaches and mandatory treatment—hence the emphasis on mass screening, contact tracing, and regular mandatory reporting.

In areas such as drugs, prostitution, and infectious diseases, the health and law enforcement structures (Internal Affairs) have traditionally maintained fairly cooperative relationships in the Soviet Union and its successor states. As the director of the AIDS Center in a large city east of Moscow explained, "The police have some same points of interest and same directions of work." In particular, "Narcology" maintained close ties with law enforcement—according to Burrows and colleagues (1999), Narcology in Russia was until the 1990s largely an instrument of Internal Affairs. A psychologist of a narcological center in the south of Russia put it in plain terms: "The relations with the police are good. They do a lot of mutual work."

Indeed, in the early stages of the epidemics in many cities in Russia, Ukraine, Belarus, and other countries in the region, drug users (and prostitutes) have been rounded up by militia and mandatorily tested at the nearest AIDS Center.

One can certainly find "enlightened" police officials in the region, who have more thoughtful ideas on drug use and HIV, especially outside of the capitals (and political spotlight)—in Ukraine, one of the first needle exchanges was initiated by (among others) a militia major. But overall the position of Internal Affairs toward innovative HIV prevention programs, such as needle exchange, has been highly censorious (Medecins Sans Frontieres-Holland 1999). The first two needle exchange programs in Russia (St. Petersburg and Yaroslavl) were closely monitored and frequently hassled by Internal Affairs (Medecins Sans Frontieres-Holland 1999; Sergeyev et al. 1999). Sergeyev and colleagues (1999) quoted a Russian national newspaper to illustrate the activities of Internal Affairs in the city of Yaroslavl:

For two weeks Drug Enforcement Officers have been watching closely the gray van running around Yaroslavl and attracting local drug users. The attention of police officers is focused on the needle exchange facility inside the van. The police are taking notice of every client attending the needle exchange so that their officers can report about the victories in the fight against drugs later on. (795)

Perhaps because the St. Petersburg and Yaroslavl programs took a lot of the political heat, most of the more recently initiated needle exchange programs in Russia have some sort of agreement in place with the locally active branches of Internal Affairs. Outside of the political spotlight, at the oblast and city levels, the authorities have more autonomy, and they seem simply less dogmatic and sensitive to pragmatic considerations. However, while police officials in the region are politically less dependent on Moscow and have some room for creative interpretation, they cannot totally ignore the federal (drug) laws or the views of the Ministry of Internal Affairs. As the head physician of an AIDS Center that started needle exchange in the south of Russia explained:

The city and oblast police departments . . . approve of the program activities. But the drug legislation is repressive. It is necessary to change it. Now the attitude of the Ministry of Internal Affairs toward such programs is negative. That's why it is difficult to work with police at the exchange sites.

Thus, agreements with one (of the several) police department(s) do not preclude the negative influence of Internal Affairs on IDUs' participation in needle exchange and other HIV prevention programs.

Furthermore, street militia is not always aware of these agreements and continues to hassle drug users around needle exchange programs. In the previously mentioned multicity evaluation of needle exchange, 44% of respondents mentioned being harassed by the police or militia because they were suspected of carrying needles. Of those, 74% mentioned that they were verbally abused or threatened, whereas 59% said they were physically abused or pushed and shoved around. Another 59% said they were detained; 67% mentioned that the police had confiscated their injecting equipment, whereas 44% were forced to destroy or dispose of injecting equipment in front of the officer. That such treatment negatively influences program participation seems self-evident, as 40% of the respondents said that they normally do not carry injection equipment at all. Of those, 58% explained that they feared discovery by the police as the reason for not doing so.

Thus, IDUs may run serious immediate risks (police hassling and brutality, arrest, and subsequent withdrawal) by participating in an intervention, which helps them avert risks, which only matter in the long term. Under such conditions, visiting the needle exchange may score higher on the IDUs' "Hierarchy of Risk" (Connors 1992) than averting some unclear infection (note that at present only a few infected drug users in Central and Eastern Europe have developed clinical manifestations).

A related matter seriously troubling the development of adequate responses to the HIV epidemic in the region is the recent passing of increasingly repressive drug legislation. In April 1998 the Russian Duma passed a new, very repressive drug law, under which substitution treatment of opiate addiction with methadone is forbidden, while syringe exchange and other HIV prevention activities might be interpreted as abetting to drug use. Soon after President Boris Yeltsin signed the law, police harassment of the St. Petersburg and Yaroslavl needle exchange programs increased. In Yaroslavl the needle exchange operation closed its doors for two months for fear it was in violation of the new law, and in June 1998 the police tried to close down the St. Petersburg project. In the following excerpt from an email, the program's codirector from Medecins Du Monde described the situation:

News from the front. The bus has trouble with the police again. They are trying to stop it and for a while the bus is staying day and night in Pravoberejniy Rynok. The threat is that if the bus moves the police will take away all the driver's licenses. For several days now, the bus has stayed put and the staff is sleeping in it to avoid problems. (B. Stambul, email, 29 June 1998)

Several other countries in the region have recently introduced more repressive drug legislation as well, among them the Czech Republic (1998), Poland (1997), and Hungary (1999). The Slovak Republic stiffened up drug laws as early as 1993. The most important difference with previous legislation is that all these new laws make possession of drugs a criminal act, although both the Polish and Czech laws made exceptions for possession of small quantities, treating those as a misdemeanor (Grund 1998a).

While human rights concerns—the proposed legislation punishes the victims rather than the perpetrator—prompted Czech President Václav Havel to veto these legislative proposals, this veto was overturned by an ad hoc majority in Parliament, which included Communists and Christian Democrats (Jakl 1998). What's more, on 17 November 2000 Polish President Aleksander Kwasniewski approved an even tougher antinarcotics bill, which banned the possession of even small amounts of drugs and introduced compulsory treatment. Two days later, a senior official from the Country Planning and Programme Development section of UNAIDS sent the following reaction to the email listserver of the Central and Eastern Europe (CEE) Harm Reduction Network:

If [this new law] is properly reinforced it may isolate drug users from the service providers, with the well known consequences. We had such an example in one city of the region in 1996. At the end of that year the police made intensive raids on the apartments where traditionally built small groups of drug users/friends met to prepare and inject drugs. Following these raids, the groups reshuffled, mixing the members of different groups and the demand for ready solution prepared elsewhere grew up. This was considered at least one of the reasons that at the beginning of the next year the HIV epidemic blew up among IDUs in that city. (L. Khodakevich, email, 19 November 2000)

UNAIDS has played an important role in developing a response to the HIV epidemics in this region. However, it has had great difficulties convincing another—for this effort crucial—UN agency, the United Nations Drug Control Program (UNDCP), of the necessity of harm reduction approaches to HIV prevention among IDUs, and, until very recently, this UN agency has not been involved in the "Joint United Nations Program." For years UNDCP has been promoting repressive drug legislation in the region, opposing methadone, needle exchange, and other harm reduction interventions. With the recent establishment of a new UNAIDS office in Vienna, next to the UNDCP headquarters, this will hopefully change. Nevertheless, this contradiction within the UN system illustrates perhaps the most essential problem in policymaking for HIV prevention among IDUs: the fundamentally different goals and interests of the international struggle against HIV/AIDS and the globalized war on drugs.

Colliding International Concerns: Drugs, AIDS, and Human Rights

Because such measures counter marginalization, and thus vulnerability to HIV, UNAIDS stresses that "[p]romoting human rights and tolerance is

. . . important in fighting AIDS as well as in its own right" (UNAIDS 2000g). Its June 2000 *Report on the Global HIV/AIDS Epidemic* reads that "[m]any factors in vulnerability—the root causes of the epidemic—can best be understood within the universal principles of human rights." The report continues with pointing toward a number of factors that engender vulnerability to HIV/AIDS. These include lack of respect for "freedom of expression and association," "the rights to liberty and security," "freedom from inhuman or degrading treatment," and "the right to privacy and confidentiality" (UNAIDS 2000g). When it comes to drug users, just about all of these rights are severely compromised in most countries in this region. Participants of focus groups of drug users in the previously mentioned multisite needle exchange evaluation in Russia told many stories of police abuse. They maintained that the police persecute drug users with HIV/AIDS. They thought that the police still have the idea that the only way to stop the epidemic is by isolation of all infected people. One of the respondents told his story:

On April 30 I came out of the prison for HIV positives and was stopped 3 times by the police in the following 9 days. I have to report 2 times a month to the police. Three different police departments can come into my home whenever they want. I think the police hounds us because we are HIV positive.

Historically, this region does not have a good reputation for championing human rights, and focus group participants were well aware of their marginalized situation. They felt that civil rights are meaningless to them: "What human rights?" said one of them, while rubbing his fingers. "No money; no human rights! Ta ta!"

UNAIDS insists that successful interventions can only develop when partnerships are created, and communities—including the drug user community—are taken into trust and not confronted (UNAIDS 1999). Nonetheless, the dominant approach toward the community hit hardest by the HIV epidemic in this region (and elsewhere) is rooted in a mixture of repression and grave disrespect for human rights.

The combustible properties of this mixture are likely to be exacerbated by yet another volatile ingredient: the treatment of ethnic minority communities. For example, the recent HIV outbreak (and drug injecting in general) in Narva, Estonia mainly concerns IDUs from the Russian minority in the city. However, in particular the stateless Roma, which are present in almost every corner of the region, may be hit hard by the epidemic in the near future. A recent study reported a number of unsettling findings. In many cities across the region a substantial proportion of the Roma community is involved in drug injecting. The overall prevalence of injection drug use in these cities equals or greatly exceeds those known in Western Europe and other established market economies. However, proportionally, injection drug use seems to have touched the Roma community in these cities to a much greater (2 to 20 times) extent. Thus, in Vilnius, the capital of Lithuania, reportedly 0.3 to 0.5% of the overall population are drug injectors, while the prevalence of drug injecting in the local Roma community is estimated at 6 to 10% (Grund Öfner, and Verbraeck 2001). The problems seem to concentrate in one Roma tabor (settlement) on the edge of town, where some 50 out of approximately 250 residents are drug injectors (Subata and Tsukanov 1999), whereas Roma living in the city—who are more "integrated" and economically better off—seem less affected. Likewise, in Szeged in southern Hungary, the overall prevalence is reportedly slightly less than 1%, but among the local Roma it is 5% to 7%. In all, 80 out of 200 participants of the local peer outreach–based syringe exchange are Roma IDUs (Grund, Öfner, and Verbraeck 2001).

Heroin use is rapidly gaining popularity among Roma youth, and reportedly they start injecting at a very early age. The study points toward many factors that suggest an increased vulnerability of the Roma for HIV infection. These include increased levels of HIV risk behaviors among Roma IDUs, barriers to clean needles and other HIV prevention services (HIV testing and education; drug treatment), as well as socioeconomic matters, such as the community's structural exclusion from the mainstream economy. HIV prevention and drug treatment projects targeting drug users in this minority community are virtually absent.

Throughout the region, Roma are considered to be an undesirable underclass, and they are still heavily discriminated on the labor market, in the educational system, in health care, and in many other services. Given their structural exclusion from the mainstream economy and historical reliance on the "shadow economy" for their sustenance, it should not come as a surprise that Roma communities in many parts of the region are reportedly involved in supplying heroin and other drugs. Thus, Subata and Tsukanov (1999) reported that about 70% of the production of opiates from poppy straw in the region takes place in the mentioned Roma tabor. In all five cities in the Russian needle exchange evaluation study, the local Roma population was reportedly the main source of opiates and other drugs, whereas in Bratislava consumption-level heroin dealing is dominated by Roma as well.

Against the background of a mounting drug war atmosphere in the region, their involvement in drugs is likely to pose a genuine threat to both their already compromised health status and the historically delicate human rights situation of the Roma communities in the region at large. It is not undue to expect that the police will increasingly target the Roma community under the pretext of the fight against drug dealers, in particular under the new repressive drug legislation. Furthermore, law enforcement targeting Roma drug users and dealers may implicitly or explicitly, and perhaps even deliberately, foster the impression that the drug problem and Roma are synonymous and that Roma are to blame as perpetrators rather than victims. Both the World Bank and UNAIDS have warned that the more marginalized and oppressed minority populations are, the more vulnerable they become to HIV epidemics. Hopefully, the sketched scenario will not become a case study of this important observation.

Glimmers of Hope?

The picture sketched in this chapter does not evoke a lot of confidence in the possibilities of developing appropriate and timely responses to HIV in the region. Reading the December 2000 AIDS epidemic update, jointly issued by UNAIDS and WHO and providing a global summary of the HIV/ AIDS epidemic up to that moment (UNAIDS/WHO 2000a), one gets the impression that the epidemiologists at UNAIDS and WHO share much of this pessimism (UNAIDS/WHO 2000a).

Despite this grim picture, there are signs that a response is developing in the region. Because of the large number of countries in this region it is nearly impossible to outline country-specific responses in this chapter. Therefore, the following section does not pretend to provide a comprehensive overview of policy and project development in Central and Eastern Europe but merely discusses some interesting developments.

At the level of policy development, UNAIDS, WHO, and other UN agencies, as well as international organizations, such as Medecins Sans Frontieres (MSF), Medecins Du Monde (MDM), and the Lindesmith Center, a project of financier George Soros' Open Society Institute (OSI), have played a leading role in developing the initial response. UNAIDS, WHO, and other UN agencies have invested much time and energy in supporting national governments' efforts to develop integrated "multisectoral and multilevel" approaches (UNAIDS 2000g). It seems that this onerous exercise is starting to yield rewards in some countries. For example, despite its Soviet bureaucratic tradition, in Belarus practically all ministries and state committees are involved in the response to HIV, which includes harm reduction interventions for IDUs and awareness-raising campaigns conducted by the national railways (UNAIDS/WHO 2000b). Reliance on obsolete mass screening techniques is reportedly decreasing in many countries and substituted by more intelligent HIV sentinel surveillance and education of the population. In 1998, Ukraine passed legislation embracing a modern public health–based philosophy toward controlling its HIV epidemic. Among other positive changes, the country stopped compulsory screening of inmates and isolating those found HIV-positive and, instead, started prevention programs in the prisons. Voluntary drug treatment is also developing in the country, and steps have been taken toward the introduction of methadone maintenance treatment for opiate addicts.

In Russia, Medecins Sans Frontieres–Holland has developed an intensive training project on HIV prevention among IDUs for health care providers and others working on HIV prevention. Between January 1998 and February 2000, the project trained 200 people from 61 Russian cities (U. Weber, personal communication; Burrows et al. 1999). The program is developed in consultation with the Ministry of Health and is part of a strategic alliance with Medecins Du Monde and the International Harm Reduction Development (IHRD) program of the Lindesmith Center/Open Society Institute. This alliance, the Russian AIDS Prevention Initiative—Drugs (RAPID), is unique in the world in the sense that following the training, successful trainees are supported in applying for funding at a grants program funded by IHRD and OSI Russia. Thus, it includes intensive initial training, support with project formulation and budget development (which are new concepts), and project funding, including further technical assistance. Until today, IHRD has funded more than 150 harm reduction programs, including needle exchanges and methadone maintenance programs. These projects are not only in Russia but throughout the region, both in areas that reported significant outbreaks of HIV in IDUs and in low-prevalence areas.

With its growing magnitude, a realization grows that drastic, unconventional, and innovative measures are required to counter and control the HIV epidemic. Research from around the world has built a strong scientific case for harm reduction approaches (Des Jarlais 1995; Drucker 1995), and after initial—largely ideological—resistance, support for this comprehensive approach is rapidly growing in Central and Eastern Europe, as well as in the central Asian countries. Strengthened by the support of fortunately an increasing number of other international (donor) organizations, researchers, activists, and professionals in the region have started to develop a wide range of harm reduction projects. An equally important development is the formation of networks in the region, such as the Central Eastern European Harm Reduction Network, the South East European Harm Reduction Coalition, and the recently established Central Asian Harm Reduction Network. These, often Internet-based, networks are a definitive departure from the old culture of secrecy and competition, and they connect scientists, professionals, and activists not only within the region but also to the international drugs and AIDS community.

While the HIV epidemic is getting out of control in Russia, the overall number of new infections in Ukraine and Belarus seems to have decreased. While these results received both UNAIDS praise and extensive media coverage, another, possibly more significant, result just across the border in Lithuania caught less attention—perhaps because until now a large outbreak has not yet occurred in the country. According to the Lithuanian AIDS Center, early prevention programs have helped Lithuania—which shares borders with HIV epicenters Poland, Belarus, and Russia's Kaliningrad region—keep its HIV infection rate the lowest in Central Europe, at 6.8 cases per 100,000 people. In 2000 a total of 257 HIV cases had been recorded in Lithuania, including 56 new infections reported through November of that year (Anonymous 2000). Lithuania belongs to the few countries where before rapid HIV spread among IDUs was reported, concerned clinicians, activists (e.g., parents of drug users), and policymakers worked together in implementing "best practice" or proven harm reduction interventions. The country largely abandoned the Soviet narcology system and has developed perhaps the most pragmatic government guidelines on methadone (maintenance) treatment in the region. Likewise, needle exchange, outreach, and peer strategies were timely introduced, giving the country, compared to its neighbors, a headstart in contacting and educating out-of-treatment drug users about HIV.

It remains to be seen whether the country can maintain its low infection rate, as harm reduction services for IDUs are not present in all cities, and such services must compete for scarce funds with primary drug prevention programs and low-volume, high-threshold drug treatment programs. As the director of the Vilnius Substance Abuse Treatment Center contended:

Definitely, the low HIV prevalence is not due to primary drug prevention or the twelve treatment slots in [the country's] therapeutic community. On the other hand I am not sure that there is no potential "Narva" in one of the industrial cities in Lithuania, which have no methadone maintenance treatment and needle exchange programs for IDUs. No services, no IDUs reached, no HIV positives. Just as three months ago in the Estonian city of Narva. (E. Subata, personal communication)

CONCLUSION

This chapter described the HIV epidemic in Central and Eastern Europe. Based on a review of the epidemiological evidence, we can conclude that more than anywhere else the rapid pace of HIV spread is fueled by illicit drug injection. Examination of the injecting drug use patterns prevalent in the region suggested that the characteristic social setting of drug injecting (group use) might have facilitated rapid spread within this population. Likewise, the widespread nature and relatively high level of community tolerance of drug injecting may set the stage for a rapid secondary diffusion into the general population by way of sexual transmission.

In some parts of the region the responsiveness of politicians and bureaucrats to the epidemic seems to have improved, and a number of innovative HIV prevention projects have been established. Nevertheless, the overall conclusion must be that the response to the epidemic has developed at a pace too slow to control further spread. The chapter described several (sociocultural and political) obstacles from which this slow development resulted. Many of these are associated with the slow transition away from totalitarianism.

How the response to HIV in the region further progresses may depend very much on the developments in Russia. Having been educated within the Soviet system, policymakers and professionals in leading positions throughout the region are confused about how to address the drug inject-ing–driven HIV epidemic and many, in particular in the central Asian suc-cessor states of the former Soviet Union, are looking toward Moscow for guidance and leadership. Russia's emphasis on the allegedly unique features of its culture and the resulting dismissal of "best practice" is in this context an important impediment to controlling the epidemic in the whole region. Of course, the design of appropriate interventions must include a cultural sensitivity to the particularities of each culture facing the epidemic. How-ever, the international experience teaches that certain best practice interven-tions can transcend such cultural specificity. A lackluster response of archaic bureaucratic structures can therefore not be hidden behind a front of "Rus-sianness" or its regional variations.

In particular, the vulnerable position of drug users is of great concern: Intense repression of drug users has alienated them from the public health system to a great extent. This outcome is associated with the dominant influence of Internal Affairs in matters of public health. Not only are Min-istries of internal affairs vocal opponents of needle exchange, methadone treatment, and other examples of "best practice," but their repressive ap-proach to drug users is a main obstacle to the region's struggle against HIV/ AIDS and brings about serious human rights concerns. While the experience elsewhere shows that good collaborative relationships between public health and law enforcement structures are important for developing successful in-terventions, such collaborations ought not to be determined by a law en-forcement agenda but by the requirements of an efficient public health–based response to the virus.

An additional worry is the influx of highly stigmatized ethnic minorities into the drug injecting population, such as the Roma. This trend is expected to result in rapid HIV spread in these communities and further complicate the human rights aspects of the epidemic, as they may easily become scape-goats for the failures of the authorities in controlling the twin epidemics of drug injecting and HIV.

The recent introduction of more repressive drug laws in several countries suggests that joining the international war on drugs may seem attractive to governments of countries where the legacy of communist bureaucracy is still tangible in many areas of public policymaking. Referring to its negative con-sequences, including HIV/AIDS, George Soros wrote that U.S. drug policy "offers a prime example of adverse, unintended consequences." He argued that "there is perhaps no other field where our public policies have produced an outcome so profoundly at odds with what was intended" (Soros 1997: C1). The U.S. drug war has facilitated the spread of disease (Grund et al. 1992), and its opposition to harm reduction measures, such as needle exchange, has resulted in extensive human and economic loss (Lurie and Drucker 1997). Embarking on an U.S.-style drug war would further compromise the region's response to HIV. One should not forget that from a biological viewpoint the struggle against HIV/AIDS is an interspecies battle, whereas the drug war has become an intraspecies conflict.

It may perhaps nowhere else become more obvious than in Central and Eastern Europe, and in particular in the former Soviet Union, how, from a public health perspective, the HIV epidemic among drug injectors has become a sentinel measurement for assessing the success of our drug policies. With up to 90% of injecting drug users among the region's registered HIV cases, the region can simply not afford for its leaders to jump on the abstinence only bandwagon of the drug war.

NOTES

Some of the work referred to in this chapter was funded by grants from the International Harm Reduction Development Program, Open Society Institute, New York.

1. Narcology is a medical specialization, usually held by psychiatrists, though narcology staff also tends to include psychologists. Prior to 1991, when drug use was decriminalized in Russia (which was undone again in 1998), alcohol and drug treatment was punitive and draconian, involving prison sentences, labor camps, and specialized correctional centers, based on medical, moral, and Pavlovian treatment models. Confidential treatment was nonexistent. Nowadays, narcology staff performs many of the functions of drug and alcohol workers in Western countries, including efforts to prevent drug use, assessment for treatment, and detoxification. Detoxification is provided at narcological hospitals and is normally supported by medication, but this seems to depend on whether the patient can afford those. Medications appear to be mainly Russian-made variations of minor tranquilizers and analgesics. Present detoxification treatment models vary widely and include Western-style (psychological) individual and group counseling but also neural surgery, hyperthermic heating of the blood, aromatherapy, coma therapy, and music therapy. The exact methodology seems to depend on the ideas and beliefs of the most senior local narcologist. While more patient/client-centered treatment approaches are being introduced, in many places treatment assessment continues to be an involuntary practice in many cases, as clients are often brought to the clinic by police or parents. Detoxification is often undergone under pressure from families, and once a detoxification center is entered, clients are usually locked in and cannot leave. Only limited postdetoxification treatment is available, usually involving counseling. Residential rehabilitation is still rare and usually run by NGOs, which contract narcologists as consultants (Burrows, personal communication; Green, Holloway, and Fleming 2000).

BIBLIOGRAPHY

Angarano, G., G. Pastore, and L. Monno. 1985. "Rapid Spread of HTLV III Infection among Drug Addicts in Italy." *Lancet* ii: 1302.

Anonymous. 2000. "Prevention Keeps Lithuania AIDS Rate Lowest in Central Europe." *Agence France Presse*, 21 November. Available on the World Wide Web at: http://www.afp.com.

Ball, A., S. Rana, and K.L. Dehne. 1998. "HIV Prevention among Injecting Drug Users: Responses in Developing and Transitional Countries." *Public Health Reports* 113 (Suppl. 1): 170–181.

Bezruchenko-Novachuk, M., and V. Romantsov. 1998. "Sentinel Surveillance Conducted within the Frame of the Project of HIV Prevention among IDUs in the Town of Svertlogosrk, Gomel Region, Belarus." Paper presented at the Twelfth International Conference on AIDS, Geneva (abstract 43467).

Bolekham, V., and E.L. Zmushko. 1998. "Home-made Drugs as an Active Factor of HIV-Transmission in Russia." Paper presented at the Twelfth International Conference on AIDS, Geneva (abstract A23186).

Brunet, J.B. 1996. *Report on Visit to Russia*. Saint-Maurice, France: European Centre for the Epidemiological Monitoring of AIDS.

Burns, S.M., R.P. Brettle, and S.M. Gore. 1996. "The Epidemiology of HIV Infection in Edinburgh Related to the Injecting of Drugs: A Historical Perspective and New Insight Regarding the Past Incidence of HIV-Infection Derived from Retrospective HIV Antibody Testing of Stored Samples of Serum." *Journal of Infections* 32: 53–62.

Burrows, D., T. Rhodes, F. Trautmann, M. Bijl, G.V. Stimson, Y. Sarankov, A. Ball, and C. Fitch. 1998. "HIV Associated with Drug Injecting in Eastern Europe." *Drug and Alcohol Review* 17: 452–463.

Burrows, Dave, Franz Trautmann, Murdo Bijl, and Yuri Sarankov. 1999. "Training in the Russian Federation on Rapid Assessment and Response to HIV/AIDS among Injecting Drug Users." *Journal of Drug Issues* 29: 805–843.

Connors, M.M. 1992. "Risk Perception, Risk Taking and Risk Management among Intravenous Drug Users: Implications for AIDS Prevention." *Social Science and Medicine* 34: 591–601.

Crofts, N., G. Reid, and P. Deany. 1998. "Injecting Drug Use and HIV Infection in Asia." *AIDS* 12 (Suppl. B1): S69–S78.

Dehne, Karl L., Jean-Paul C. Grund, Lev Khodakevich, and Yuri Kobyshcha. 1999. "The HIV/AIDS Epidemic among Drug Injectors in Eastern Europe: Patterns, Trends and Determinants." *Journal of Drug Issues* 29: 729–776.

Des Jarlais, Don C. 1995. "Harm Reduction—A Framework for Incorporating Science into Drug Policy." *American Journal of Public Health* 85: 10–12.

Des Jarlais, D.C., S.R. Friedman, J.L. Sotherhan, J. Wenston, M. Marmor, and S. Yankovitz. 1994. "Continuity and Change within an HIV Epidemic: Injecting Drug Users in New York City, 1984 through 1992." *Journal of the American Medical Association* 271: 121–127.

Drucker, E. 1995. "Harm Reduction: A Public Health Strategy." *Current Issues in Public Health* 1: 64–70.

Green, Anita J., David G. Holloway, and Philip M. Fleming. 2000. "Substance Misuse in Russia: A Partnership for Policy Change and Service Development." *International Journal of Drug Policy* 11: 393–405.

Grund, Jean-Paul C. 1998a. "Není Všeobjímajících Rešení: Potreba Inovace a Poucené Debaty o Drogové Politice" [No golden bullets: Contextualizing the need for innovation and informed debate in drug policy]. In *Drogy na predpis—lékarská preskripce narkotik. Vedecké podklady a první zkušenosti*, Kolektiv autoru, pp. 356–389. Olomouc, Czech Republic: Votobia, Publishers and Open Society Fund Praha. (Epilogue to the Czech edition of *The Medical Prescription of Narcotics.*)

———. 1998b. "The Subculture of Injecting Drug Use." In *Encyclopedia of AIDS: A Social, Political, Cultural and Scientific Record of the HIV Epidemic*, Ray A. Smith ed., pp. 289–292. Chicago and London: Fitzroy Dearborn Publishers.

Grund, Jean-Paul C., S.R. Friedman, L.S. Stern, B. Jose, A. Neaigus, R. Curtis, and D.C. Des Jarlais. 1996. "Drug Sharing among Injecting Drug Users: Patterns, Social Context, and Implications for Transmission of Blood-borne Pathogens." *Social Science and Medicine* 42: 691–703.

Grund, Jean-Paul C., C.D. Kaplan, N.F.P. Adriaans, and P. Blanken. 1991. "Drug Sharing and HIV Transmission Risks: The Practice of 'Frontloading' in the Dutch Injecting Drug User Population." *Journal of Psychoactive Drugs* 23: 1–10.

Grund, Jean-Paul C., Denis Kobzev, Vitalic Melnikov, Catherine Zadoretsky, Elena Zemlianova, Stephen Titus, Theresa Perlis, Denise Paore, Valentina Bodrova, and Don C. Des Jarlais. 2001. "Drug Use Patterns and HIV Risk Behaviors of Russian Syringe Exchange Participants." Paper presented at the Twelfth International Conference on the Reduction of Drug-Related Harm, April, Delhi, India.

Grund, Jean-Paul C., and D. Nolimal. 1995. *A Heroin Epidemic in Macedonia: Report to the Open Society Institute, New York and the Open Society Institute Macedonia.* New York: Lindesmith Center.

Grund, Jean-Paul C., Paul J. Öfner, and Hans T. Verbraeck. 2001. "Marel o Del, Kas Kamel, le Romes Duvar. (God hits whom he chooses; the Rom gets hit twice.): An Exploration of Drug Use and HIV Risks among the Roma of Central and Eastern Europe." Paper presented at the Twelfth International Conference on the Reduction of Drug-Related Harm, April, Delhi, India.

Grund, Jean-Paul C., L.S. Stern, C.D. Kaplan, N.F.P. Adriaans, and E. Drucker. 1992. "Drug Use Contexts and HIV-Consequences: The Effect of Drug Policy on Patterns of Everyday Drug Use in Rotterdam and the Bronx." *British Journal of Addiction's Special Edition on HIV/AIDS* 87: 381–392.

Hamers, F., V. Batter, A. Downs, J. Alix, F. Cazein, and J.B. Brunet. 1997. "The HIV Epidemic Associated with Injecting Drug Use in Europe: Geographic and Time Trends." *AIDS* 11: 1365–1374.

Honti, J., and K. Zelenai. 1999. "Steps on the Methadone Path in Hungary." Paper presented at the Ninth International Conference on the Reduction of Drug-Related Harm, March, Geneva.

Htoon, M.T., H.H. Lain, K.O. San, E. Zan, and M. Thwe. 1994. "HIV/AIDS in Myanmar." *AIDS* 8 (Suppl. 2): S105–S09.

Ismail, R. 1998. "HIV/AIDS in Malaysia." *AIDS* 12 (Suppl. B): S1–S10.

Jakl, R. 1998. "Deputies Push Through Bill." *The Prague Post*, 20 May.

Jong, Wouter de, Tea Tsagarelli, and Erik Schouten. 1999. "Rapid Assessment of Injection Drug Use and HIV in the Republic of Georgia." *Journal of Drug Issues* 29: 843–860.

Jose, B., S.R. Friedman, A. Neaigus, R. Curtis, J-P.C. Grund, M.F. Goldstein, and D.C. Des Jarlais. 1993. "Syringe-Mediated Drug Sharing (Backloading): A

New Risk Factor for HIV among Injecting Drug Users." *AIDS* 7: 1653–1660.

Khodakevich, Lev. 1997. "Development of HIV Epidemics in Belarus, Moldova and Ukraine and Response to the Epidemics." Paper presented at the Eighth International Conference on the Reduction of Drug-Related Harm, March, Paris.

Khodakevich, Lev, and Karl L. Dehne. 1998. "HIV Epidemics in Drug Using Populations and Increasing Drug Use in Central and Eastern Europe." Paper presented at the Global Research Network on HIV Prevention in Drug Using Populations (Inaugural Meeting), Geneva.

Liitsola, K., I. Tasinova, T. Laukkanen, G. Korovina, T. Smoslkaya, O. Momot, N. Mahkilleyson, S. Chaplinskas, H. Brummer-Korvewnkonito, J. Vanhatalo, P. Leinikki, and M. Salminen. 1998. "HIV-1 Genetic Subtype A/B Recombinant Strain Causing an Explosive Epidemic in Injecting Drug Users in Kaliningrad." *AIDS* 12: 1907–1999.

Lukashov, V.V., E.V. Karamov, V.F. Eremin, L.P. Titov, and J. Goudsmit. 1998. "Extreme Founder Effect in an HIV Subtype A Epidemic among Drug Users in Svetlogorsk, Belarus." *AIDS Research and Human Retroviruses* 14: 1299–1303.

Lurie, P., and E. Drucker. 1997. "An Opportunity Lost: HIV Infections Associated with Lack of a National Needle Exchange Programme in the USA." *Lancet* 349: 604–608.

Medecins Sans Frontieres-Holland. 1999. Unauthorized transcript of a presentation of Mr. Boris Celinsky, Ph.D. (Senior Officer at the Academy of Management of the Ministry of Internal Affairs in Moscow), at the U.S.–Russia Bi-National Workshop Drug Abuse and Infectious Disease Prevention Strategies, St. Petersburg.

Ministry of Health of the Russian Federation. 2000. *Officially Registered HIV Infections in the Russian Federation, 1987–23 June 2000.* (Courtesy of MSF-H Moscow)

Nolimal, D., and T. Jerman. 1996. *Project Extension of the Multi-City Work to Central and Eastern Europe. City Report Ljubljana.* Strasbourg: Pompidou Group/UNDCP.

Pokrovskyi, V.V., I.Y. Savtchenko, and N.N. Ladnaia. 1997. *HIV-Infection Surveillance in Russia in 1987–1996.* Moscow: Russian AIDS Centre. (Statistics)

Pokrovskyi, V.V., I.Y. Savtchenko, N.N. Ladnaia, and A.T. Goliusov. 1998. "A Recent Epidemic of HIV Infection in Russian IVDUs." Paper presented at the Twelfth International Conference on AIDS, July, Geneva (abstract 13191).

Polanecky, V., J. Sijda, and B. Studnickova. 1996. "Prevalence Study of Serious Substance Abuse in the Czech Republic." *Central European Journal of Public Health* 4: 176–184.

Rebagliato, M., M.J. Avino, and I. Hernandez-Aguado. 1995. "Trends in Incidence and Prevalence of HIV-1 Infection in Intravenous Drug Users in Valencia, Spain." *Journal of Acquired Immune Deficiency Syndromes and Human Retrovirology* 8: 297–301.

Sergeyev, Boris, Tatyana Oparina, Tatyana P. Rumyantseva, Valerii L. Volkanevskii, Robert S. Broadhead, Douglas D. Heckathorn, and Heather Madray. 1999.

"HIV Prevention for Drug Injectors in Yaroslavl, Russia: A Peer-Driven Intervention and Needle Exchange." *Journal of Drug Issues* 29: 777–804.

Soros, G. 1997. "The Drug War Cannot Be Won: It's Time to Just Say No to Self-destructive Prohibition." *The Washington Post*, 2 February, C1.

Stimson, G.V. 1994. "Reconstruction of the Subregional Diffusion of HIV-Infection among Injecting Drug Users in Southeast Asia: Implications for Early Intervention." *AIDS* 8(11): 1630–1632.

Subata, Emilis, and Jurij Tsukanov. 1999. "The Work of General Practitioners among Lithuanian Roma in Vilnius: Incorporating Harm Reduction into Primary Medical Practice." *Journal of Drug Issues* 29: 805–810.

UNAIDS. 1996. *Worksheet: Provisional Working Estimates of Adults Living with HIV/AIDS by Subcontinent in 1995*. Geneva: UNAIDS.

———. 1999. "Drug Use and HIV/AIDS." UNAIDS statement presented at the United Nations General Assembly Special Session on Drugs in New York. Geneva: UNAIDS.

———. 2000a. *Epidemic Update June 2000: Table of Country-Specific HIV/AIDS Estimates and Data, June 2000*. Available on the World Wide Web at: http://www.unaids.org/epidemic_update/report/Final_Table_Eng_Xcel.xls

———. 2000b. *Epidemiological Fact Sheet: Belarus, June 2000*. Available on The World Wide Web at: http://www.unaids.org/hivaidsinfo/statistics/june98/fact_sheets

———. 2000c. *Epidemiological Fact Sheet: Kazakhstan, June 2000*. Available on the World Wide Web at: http://www.unaids.org/hivaidsinfo/statistics/june98/fact_sheets

———. 2000d. *Epidemiological Fact Sheet: Poland, June 2000*. Available on the World Wide Web at: http://www.unaids.org/hivaidsinfo/statistics/june98/fact_sheets

———. 2000e. *Epidemiological Fact Sheet: Russian Federation, June 2000*. Available on the World Wide Web at: http://www.unaids.org/hivaidsinfo/statistics/june98/fact_sheets

———. 2000f. *Epidemiological Fact Sheet: Ukraine, June 2000*. Available on the World Wide Web at: http://www.unaids.org/hivaidsinfo/statistics/june98/fact_sheets

———. 2000g. *Report on the Global HIV/AIDS Epidemic, June 2000*. Geneva: UNAIDS.

———. 2000h. "UNAIDS Calls for Intensified Support as Russia's AIDS Epidemic Spreads." Moscow: UNAIDS, 16 November. (Press release)

UNAIDS/WHO. 2000a. "AIDS Epidemic Explodes in Eastern Europe." Berlin: UNAIDS/WHO, 28 November. (Press release)

———. 2000b. *AIDS Epidemic Update: December 2000*. Geneva: UNAIDS/WHO.

United Nations. 1997. *Trends in Europe and North America 1996/1997*. The Statistical Yearbook. Geneva: Economic Commission for Europe.

USAID and Centers for Disease Control and Prevention. 1998. *HIV/AIDS Strategy in Russia, 1998–2000*. Washington, DC: USAID.

Weniger, B.G., K. Limpakarnjanarat, K. Ungchusak, S. Thanprasertsuk, K. Choopanya, S. Vanichseni, T. Uneklabh, P. Thongcharon, and C. Wasi. 1991. "The Epidemiology of HIV Infection and AIDS in Thailand." *AIDS* 5: 571–585.

WHO. 1995. *Weekly Epidemiological Bulletin* 70: 353–360.

————. *The Rapid Assessment and Response Guide on Injecting Drug Use.* G.V. Stimson, C. Fitch, and T. Rhodes, eds. Geneva: World Health Organization, Program on Substance Abuse.

WHO-EURO. 2000. "Table of HIV Infections Newly Diagnosed and Rates per Million Population by Country and Year of Report (1992–1999), and Cumulative Totals, WHO European Region." Available on the World Wide Web at: http:cisid.dk/hiv-aids/table12.htm

Zheng, X.W., C. Tian, J. Zhang, M. Cheng, X. Yang, D. Li, J. Lin, S. Qu, X. Sun, T. Hall, J. Mandel, and N. Hurst. 1994. "Injecting Drug Use and HIV Infection in Southwest China." *AIDS* 8: 1141–1147.

4

CHINA

*Clyde B. McCoy, Douglas Feldman,
Lisa R. Metsch, Robert S. Anwyl,
Shenghan Lai, and Xue-ren Wang*

INTRODUCTION

China represents the world's oldest living civilization, with art, culture, religion, and a language that can be traced as far back as 7,000 years to the beginning of permanent agricultural settlements in the Huang (Yellow) River basin. With a population that has doubled in the last 40 years, from approximately 650 million to 1.3 billion, one of every five of the earth's current population call China home.

China, called "Zhongguo" (or "Middle Country") by the Han Chinese, has undergone major transformations within the past century, including such events as the collapse of its last dynasty, the development of a republic, a brutal Japanese occupation, the instillation of communism, the Great Leap Forward of the 1950s, the Cultural Revolution of the 1960s, and continuing growth of international trade stemming from the opening up of China to a Western market economy beginning in 1978. Accompanying such dramatic changes are changing patterns of social life, including new challenges in the fields of health and criminal justice, such as the new epidemic of drugs, HIV, and AIDS, which has recently entered and begun to spread throughout the country. A more complete understanding of such new challenges are illuminated by tracing older cultural issues such as drug use, the reemergence of which is largely responsible for the recent spread of HIV/AIDS across China's borders.

The British first supplied Indian opium to China as early as the sixteenth century. After the Qing dynasty prohibited opium in 1829, the British began two opium wars that forced the Chinese government to open the door for the importation of the drug. An estimated 200 million Chinese suffered the effects of opium abuse between the sixteenth century and the ascendancy of communism in 1949 (McCoy et al. 1997). While some have argued opium abuse has caused an incredible devastation of Chinese culture (Beeching 1975; Suwanwela and Poshyachinda 1986), Newman (1995) more recently argues opium use in late Imperial China was a normal rather than a deviant activity, and most Chinese were infrequent or nonusers of the drug. While many wealthy Chinese did become addicted, Newman maintains most of the vast Chinese peasantry used opium socially, if at all. Nevertheless, some 5% of the population became addicted to the drug.

In 1950, shortly after the communists seized power in China, the government banned all planting and processing of opium, destroyed all existing opium crops, confiscated all equipment used in making or using opium, and closed all opium dens. While total amnesty was granted to small opium dealers and addicts if they turned over their supplies, long prison terms were given to intermediate-size dealers, and capital punishment was imposed on all major opium dealers. Opium users who stopped using the drug were given government stipends if unemployed or otherwise in need. Local villages throughout China held rallies and public forums to discuss the evils of opium use. Opium and drug paraphernalia were publicly burned, and former users were encouraged to tell of their negative experiences in using the drug.

The government-controlled media successfully linked the antidrug crusade with the collapse of imperialism in China. Young and recent opium users were encouraged to break their addiction within three months, while longtime users were given up to six months by going to free treatment and detoxification clinics. After six months, any persons still using opium were imprisoned. This heavy-handed approach was evidently very successful; by the end of 1952 there were few opium users left in China (Rubenstein 1973).

Needle sharing was practiced by drug users as early as 1902 in China. Indeed, outbreaks of malaria in China between 1929 and 1937 were attributed to needle sharing and intravenous injection of opiates (Zule, Vogtsberger, and Desmond 1997). Heroin can be injected, inhaled, or smoked. Heroin smoking first originated in Shanghai, China, during the 1920s and involved the use of porcelain bowls, bamboo tubes, and heroin pills. The pills were often mixed with a base powder known as "daai fan," which contained barbiturates. Such usage rapidly spread to other parts of China, Hong Kong, and elsewhere in Eastern Asia and the United States. By the late 1930s, 4 million heroin pills were seized yearly by authorities in Hong Kong alone (Strang, Griffiths, and Gossop 1997).

The form of inhaling heroin, called "chasing the dragon," started in Hong Kong in the 1950s at a time when intravenous injection of heroin was still very rare, Chasing the dragon involves ingesting heroin by inhaling the vapors produced when the drug is heated on creased tin foil above a flame to the point it turns into a vapor. This practice grew in popularity throughout parts of East Asia and into Europe. Some have speculated the popularity of "chasing the dragon" was a response to the fear of injection from HIV-infected needles. However, the practice developed and grew long before HIV infection became known (Strang, Griffiths, and Gossop 1997).

Heroin injection emerged again in China during the late 1980s along the frontier of Yunnan Province in southwestern China near the borders of Myanmar (Burma), Laos, and Vietnam. The northern regions of these nations are collectively referred to as the "Golden Triangle," an area of major heroin production and international export. By the late 1980s, heroin addiction through shared needles became quite common, especially among the various ethnic populations of this region who often traveled outside China into neighboring countries. During the 1990s, heroin injection became very common throughout Yunnan Province and began to spread further into adjacent areas of mainland China. With the heroin came infected needles, syringes, and related drug paraphernalia (McCoy et al. in press). Currently, injection drug use is the major vector of HIV transmission in China (Ball 2000; Kumar, Shakuntala, and Daniels 2000; Wu 2000).

ISSUES RELATING TO HIV AND AIDS

The reopening of China to a global market economy in 1978 lowered the invisible shield protecting the Chinese from outside influences, including drug use, especially injection drug use, which continues to spread deeply into China. In the early 1980s, the drug problems seemed to be isolated in Yunnan Province, a southwestern province bordering Myanmar. However, drug use has spread rapidly throughout the country so that by 1995 major cities, autonomous regions, and all 31 Chinese provinces reported problems with drug abuse (Wu 2000).

In 1990, there were 70,000 registered drug users in China. By 1998, there were nearly 600,000 cases of registered drug users in China, an extremely conservative estimate, due in no small part to the fear of repercussion on the part of community leaders, should they report actual numbers of cases to supervisors (National Narcotic Control Committee 1999 as cited in Wu 2000). Far more realistic figures produced by experts and accepted by the National Narcotics Control Committee (NNCC) in China estimates an actual 6 million Chinese were drug users by the end of 1998 (Wu 2000).

The first AIDS case in China was reported in 1985. Since then, the reported AIDS cases have remained relatively low and epidemiologically unreliable. UNAIDS of the World Health Organization estimates the number of persons in China living with HIV/AIDS at the end of 1998 at 400,000, and at the end of 1999, 500,000 (UNAIDS/WHO 2000). More recent mid-2000 estimates for China are 600,000 (Rosenthal 2000). Most (77.8%) of the HIV-infected adults in China are males, with only 1 in 8 infected persons being female. Because of the low proportion of HIV-infected females, the number of infected children is also relatively low—estimated to be 4,800.

Since the AIDS epidemic is relatively new to China, the annual death toll has so far remained fairly low, with an estimated 17,000 AIDS deaths in 1999. Nevertheless, some 3,900 children have been orphaned by the disease (UNAIDS/WHO 2000). These figures are expected to grow rapidly as the epidemic matures.

The association of drug injection and HIV was first reported in 1989 (Wu 2000). During the late 1980s and early 1990s heroin injection began to spread rapidly through those counties within Yunnan Province closest to the southern border adjacent to Myanmar, Laos, and Vietnam. With the shared use of needles, syringes, and related paraphernalia, HIV infection rates began to climb rapidly (Ball 2000).

In China's HIV sentinel sites in April–June 1996, 43.8% of drug users injected drugs. By October–December 1999, 53.3% of drug users were injecting their drugs (Ministry of Health, National Center for AIDS Prevention and Control, 1997–2000, as cited in Wu 2000). In Longchuan County of southern Yunnan Province, of 433 male drug users (out of 1,548 persons interviewed in 82 rural villages), the annual incidence of injection drug use increased from 10% in 1991 to 30% in 1994. Risk factors for injection drug use among males included having had premarital or extramarital sex (condoms were used only 25% of the time during extramarital sex), having a family member who used drugs in 1991, being encouraged by friends or others to try drugs, smoking cigarettes, being a member of the Jingpo ethnic group, and being divorced, widowed, or separated (Z. Wu, Zhang et al. 1996). Jinpo men were six times more likely to share injecting equipment than others (Z. Wu, Detels et al. 1996). By 1994, of 192 injecting drug users (IDUs), 73% were sharing syringes with others (Z. Wu, Zhang, and Dong 1998).

In a broader study of three Yunnan Province rural counties, of 860 drug users, 33% reported injecting drugs, with 82% beginning injection drug use after 1988. Nearly two-thirds (64%) injected drugs at least once a day. All IDUs shared needles, but none cleaned the injection equipment with alcohol or bleach. Half (49%) tested positive for HIV. The epidemic also began to spread to the non-drug-using wives of the male IDUs. Among the 62 wives of HIV-positive IDUs, condoms were never used during sex, and 10% tested positive for HIV (Zheng et al. 1994). By 1997, 12.3% of the wives were HIV-positive (Zheng, Zhang, and Qu 1997).

Three recent outbreaks of HIV-1 among injection drug users in China appear linked to trafficking routes. In the first route, HIV-1 subtype B, and later subtype C, spread from Myanmar into China's Yunnan Province. In

CHINA 73

the second route, subtypes B, C, and a B/C recombinant subtype spread from Myanmar into Yunnan Province and then to Xinjiang Province. In the third route, subtype E spread from Myanmar and Laos through northern Vietnam to China's Guangxi Province (Beyer et al. 2000). By the end of the 1990s in Guangxi Province, subtypes E and C were circulating among injection drug users and their heterosexual partners, while subtypes B and D were circulating among commercial blood donors (Chen, Liu, and Nancy 1999). HIV-1 infection, subtypes B and C, have also spread to Sichuan Province from Yunnan Province, Thailand, Myanmar, and India (Qin, Shao, and Liu 1998).

HIV-1 subtype B has also recently spread from Yunnan Province into Hubei Province (Y. Li, Shao, Luo 1997). Subtype C appears to have taken hold of injection drug users in Yunnan Province. The HIV-1 infection rate among IDUs in Ruili county of Yunnan Province was 5.1% in 1992, 12.9% in 1993, and 31.9% in 1994 (D. Li, Zheng, and Zhang 1996). IDUs range between 44% and 85% HIV-positive in selected communities of drug users in Yunnan and Xinjiang Provinces (UNAIDS/WHO 2000). Subtype E in Yunnan Province, possibly entering the region from Thailand and northern Vietnam, appears to be more closely associated with female sex workers who are rarely IDUs (X. Yu et al. 1998).

In a recent study of 630 male and female heroin IDUs in Yunnan Province, injectors in the city of Kunming were compared with injectors in the rural communities of Dali and Dehong (McCoy et al. in press). Women in urban Kunming were much more likely to engage in injection drug use than women in Dali and Dahong. Over half (53%) of the 165 female subjects in Kunming were IDUs, but only one-quarter (27%) of the 30 female subjects in Dali and Dehong were injectors. Males are considerably more likely to be IDUs in rural Yunnan Province, but as injection heroin use continues to spread into urban areas throughout China, it appears likely we will see a more equivalent male/female ratio among IDUs.

Factors that appear to inhibit HIV transmission in the rural villages include greater education, Han (Chinese) ethnicity, not smoking cigarettes, traveling less to Myanmar (Zheng, Zhang, and Chen 1995), and boiling reusable needles and syringes. In a study of 182 drug users in Longdao village, Yunnan Province, 43% were HIV-positive. Among the 64 IDUs, reported sterilization of reusable injection equipment by boiling before intravenous drug use was associated with six times greater protection (Xia, Kreiss, and Holmes 1994). These figures are expected to grow rapidly as the epidemic matures.

Heroin users in China are at risk not only for HIV-1 but for several other viruses as well. Hepatitis B virus (HBV) infection is endemic at extraordinarily high rates throughout China, but even more common among IDUs. In a study conducted in Ruili County of Yunnan Province, 52% of non-IDU adults were positive for HBV, while an even greater proportion (68%)

of the IDU population was positive for HIV. Nearly all (92%) of the IDUs who were HIV-positive in the study were also anti-hepatitis C virus (HCV) antibody positive (Cheng 1993). In another Yunnan Province study conducted among 507 IDUs, 66.5% were HIV-positive, while 94.9% were HCV positive, with a very strong correlation between those who are co-infected (D. Li, Zheng, and Zhang 1996).

The newly described TT virus (TTV) has been found in 20% of 158 IDUs in Yunnan Province (Cao et al. 1999), and the GB virus C/hepatitis G virus (GBV–C/HGV) has been found in 64 of 85 HIV-IDUs in Nanning, southern China (R. Wu et al. 1997). While HBV and HCV have been demonstrated to cause increased morbidity and mortality over a prolonged period of time, the pathogenicity of these newly described viruses has yet to be ascertained.

Other Non–IDU Routes of HIV Transmission

Approximately 68% of all HIV-positive Chinese are IDUs who shared injection equipment, clearly the primary mode of HIV transmission in China today. Rosenthal (2000) recently builds a strong case for the view that the second largest source of HIV transmission can be attributed to donating and receiving blood for blood transfusions. The sale of blood was banned in China in 1998, but blood shortages are common, and illegal blood sales continue. An estimated 5 million Chinese regularly provide blood for pay each year. In rural China, blood gangs buy blood from farmers and then sell it to individual patients in need or to rural doctors. Since blood is drawn from unsterilized needles, blood donors can be exposed to the blood of between 6 and 12 other donors every time they sell their blood. While the risk for HIV is low in Chinese hospitals where blood is routinely screened, this may not be the case in some major rural areas of China.

Since 1978, the Chinese government has emphasized modernizing the nation. With this reform has come the reemergence of female and male commercial sex work throughout urban China. With the increase of Western influence, including satellite television, there has been an ideological shift by many away from traditional Chinese values of "jen" in which the personality is placed squarely within the context of the community (rather than the individual) and toward a more individualized model of personal values and freedom. Sex work can be seen in part as a by-product of this change, and the rate of arrests for female sex workers who are streetwalkers has rapidly increased.

Gil et al. (1996) distinguish between the "Pheasant (Yeh-Chi) prostitute," who is a streetwalker, and the "Plum Blossom (Mei Hua) prostitute," who is a call girl. Undoubtedly, more hotels will receive some marketplace pressure to provide sex services along with other "modern" services. The Yeh-Chi prostitute is more likely to be arrested and sent for six months to two years to the reeducation camps designed to reform female sex workers in the nation.

Most Chinese female sex workers are not IDUs and are not at very high risk for HIV at this time. However, the sexually transmitted disease (STD) rates are extraordinarily high, with gonorrheal infections among Yeh-Chi women at some 41.9% and trichomonas at 38.5%. Although 65% of female sex workers report they use condoms (UNAIDS/WHO 2000), a very high figure for China, it is likely HIV infection will become more common among both sex workers and their clients as the epidemic spreads.

Male homosexuality was very common during nineteenth-century Imperial China but became extremely hidden with the rise of Mao and Chinese communism in the middle of the twentieth century. With Western and modernizing influences, Chinese gay culture has cautiously begun to redevelop in key cities such as Shanghai, Beijing, and Wuhan (K. Zhang et al. 1999). Today, there are perhaps several million gay men, bisexuals, and lesbians in China. The very earliest cases of reported AIDS were among gay Chinese males who had contacts with HIV-positive European or North American men. Before 1987, reported cases were among homosexuals or persons with hemophilia (Chuang, Chang, and Lin 1993). Today, although little, if any, research is being conducted in this area, it is likely HIV infection is spreading in China among men who have sex with men. Based upon actual reported AIDS cases, E. Yu et al. (1996) classify male homosexuals as the third greatest risk group in China.

Sexual norms are changing in China, and it is likely these changes will increase the transmission of HIV and other sexually transmitted diseases throughout the heterosexual population during the coming decade (Gil 1991). In a recent study conducted in rural China among 886 sexually active persons, 22.8% had premarital sex, 7.8% had more than one sexual partner at the time of the survey, 2.4% had anal intercourse, 4.1% had oral sex, and 2.3% had both anal and oral sex (Liu et al. 1998). In a study conducted during 1995–1996 at four Guangzhou hospitals among pregnant women, the most common STD was cervical chlamydial trachomatis, occurring in 19.1% of the sample of 1,656 women (Fu, Huang, and Zhang 1997).

HIV Knowledge and Behavior in China

In spite of the rapidly expanding HIV epidemic in China, most Chinese—including those at very high risk—have only a very limited knowledge and awareness about HIV/AIDS. In a study conducted among 177 Dai villagers in southern Yunnan Province during 1994 (Liao et al. 1997), only 18% had heard of the disease, only 25% had heard of STDs, and only 28% had heard of condoms. Half (50%) of the Dai villagers had traveled to Laos in the previous six months and had access to heroin. While most watched television every day, the programming was conducted in Mandarin, and most of the villagers (66%) had difficulty in understanding spoken Mandarin. The villagers had numerous misconceptions about HIV transmission. Most incorrectly believed HIV could be transmitted by sharing eating utensils (84%), getting mosquito bites (84%) and by shaking hands (64%). A sizable minority of villagers incorrectly believed that HIV transmission could not be caused by sharing syringes (42%), through sexual contact (39%), and from mother to infant (45%).

In a study of 433 male drug users under the age of 30 in Yunnan Province (Z. Wu, Zhang et al. 1997), over half the individuals scored 0 on HIV knowledge, but knowledge was greater among nonsharing drug injectors. Most IDUs did not correctly know several crucial facts about AIDS. For example, most did not know that condoms can prevent AIDS or that shaking hands does not cause AIDS. Needle-sharing IDUs were less likely to correctly respond to questions about boiling equipment, water and soap cleaning, sharing needles, the purity of drugs, and sex with female sex workers than non-needle-sharing IDUs.

Different segments of the general Chinese population have been surveyed about their knowledge, attitudes, beliefs, and behaviors about HIV/AIDS. In a study conducted in Beijing among 448 taxi drivers and 556 hotel attendants (X. Zhang, Luo, and Zhang 1994), 37% of taxi drivers and 24% of hotel attendants did not know that contact with infected blood could transmit HIV. Many (42% of taxi drivers and 35% of hotel attendants) did not believe that IDUs were at high risk for HIV. About half of the sexually active respondents (56% of taxi drivers and 48% of hotel attendants) thought condom use interfered with sexual pleasure.

Chinese medical school students (N = 302) were also assessed about their HIV-related knowledge and attitudes (V. Li et al. 1993). While average scores on the knowledge scale were 80% correct, two-thirds of the medical students indicated they thought people with AIDS got what they deserve. Over 40% of the sample blamed female sex workers for AIDS in China, whereas 22% blamed IDUs and 6% blamed men who have sex with men. About one-third of the students supported quarantine measures and keeping infected students out of classrooms. About one-quarter (27%) thought the Chinese government was concealing information about AIDS.

In a similar study among 1,058 Chinese males in the military (Hang, Xu, and Gong 1996), most knew the risk of AIDS and its route of transmission, but only 8.5% of those surveyed answered all the questions in the survey correctly. Most thought they had little or no chance of contracting the illness. Several focus groups were also conducted in a study among Chinese college students at Xiamien University (Walsh-Childers et al. 1997). Most thought their personal risk from AIDS was very low because they felt distanced—either geographically or morally—from those at risk. Many believed that fate, not individual behavior, determines whether or not a person contracts HIV.

In a more general survey conducted in four major Chinese cities—Beijing, Shanghai, Guagzhou, and Wuhan—only 5% said they knew a lot about AIDS, whereas 69% said they had some understanding of the disease, 24% said they had heard about AIDS but knew little about it, and 2% had not even heard about it. Only one-third of the respondents were aware of the seriousness of AIDS in China (Diao 1997).

A study of 1,400 health care professionals (Z. Wu et al. 1999) indicated public health workers had more knowledge than clinicians, having attended training workshops was not associated with an adequate level of knowledge, and the level of knowledge about HIV/AIDS differed by professional level and by the geographical region in which they worked. Weaknesses in their knowledge included HIV transmission routes, the "window period," and the length of the incubation period. Clearly, on both the societal level and among various occupational and cultural groupings, HIV/AIDS awareness, knowledge, and compassion for people with AIDS are lacking, and educational/behavioral interventions are needed to give particularly those at high risk for HIV/AIDS—and those who help those at high risk—the skills and basic information to protect themselves from this epidemic.

RESPONSES TO HIV/AIDS

The Chinese Approach

In 1990, there were approximately 70,000 registered drug users in China; by 1995, this number had grown to some 520,000 (National Narcotic Control Committee 1999 as cited in Wu 2000). By 1999, the number of registered drug users grew to approximately 600,000 (National Narcotic Control Committee 1999 as cited in Wu 2000). Unofficial estimates place the current number of all drug users, registered and unregistered alike, as low as 3 million and as high as 12 million (Leicester 2000). During the 1990s the Chinese government confiscated almost 40 tons of heroin, 17 tons of opium, 15 tons of marijuana, and 23 tons of methamphetamine (Leicester 2000). The Chinese Ministry of Health in 1994 estimated that only 6.5% of the heroin smuggled into China from the Golden Triangle is interdicted. After the early 1950s, China had virtually eradicated cultivation of plants used in the production of drugs within its borders and now assists Myanmar and Laos with crop substitution and tourism promotion programs to discourage poppy growing (Leicester 2000).

China is facing an enormous emerging challenge as injecting heroin use spreads from areas such as the Yunnan Province countryside into the vast rural and highly populated urban regions of mainland China. The high purity of the drug (up to 80% pure compared to 6% to 25% in the United States) leads to rapid addiction and greater difficulties in treating withdrawal symptoms.

The government of China has recently taken dramatic steps to control the burgeoning growth of heroin and other drug addiction. Executions of major drug dealers have become more common. For example, in one week in June 2000, 38 drug traffickers were executed. Beginning in the late 1980s, the government began to develop a system of both compulsory rehabilitation centers as well as treatment and labor camps for "hard-core" users. Today, there are 746 compulsory rehabilitation centers and 168 treatment and labor camps throughout China. Private treatment centers are also being established. One model community outreach program for recovering drug users in Inner Mongolia Province has brought the relapse rate down to 30% (Leicester 2000).

McCoy et al. (1997) describe the Kunming Drug Rehabilitation Center, first opened in Kunming in 1989. In 1994, it accommodated 620 drug users, of which 500 were arrestees under a compulsory detoxification and rehabilitation process, with the remaining 120 voluntarily enrolled. Treatment begins with 12 to 15 days of detoxification. Methadone was first used at the rehabilitation center, but now herbal medications, referred to as the "626 series," are used to detoxify the drug users. The medications are believed by the treatment directors as safe, effective, easy to use, cost-effective, and free of side effects. Detoxification is followed by intensive psychological counseling as well as physical labor. Counseling includes education about drug laws and the dangers of drug use, moral education, and individualized counseling. Physical labor may include construction work or raising chickens or pigs. Family involvement is a very important element of the treatment program. The final phase of treatment includes preparing the former drug user to reenter society and to resist temptation to use drugs again. Sports, exercise, and self-evaluation are also important components of the treatment plan.

Despite a comprehensive approach, the Kunming Rehabilitation Center had a relapse rate of 80% within two years (McCoy et al. 1997). Most of the drug users return to the same social networks that promoted their addiction in the first place, jobs are difficult to find after they leave the center, drugs are still readily available, and they are often stigmatized by members of their community. By 1999, the Kunming center had grown to 2,000 drug users. The reputation as a relatively humane center had spread, and half of the inmates now come from other provinces. The Kunming center is perhaps atypical from other centers in that it practices a more humanitarian approach to drug addiction. This has been recognized, and the program has been singled out by the United Nations antidrug program (*The Economist* 1999).

Zhao and associates (2000) introduced a therapeutic community-based rehabilitation program to 198 heroin addicts in a correction camp in Hunan Province. The 96 members of the rehabilitation group underwent an intensive and comprehensive rehabilitation program incorporating the successful experiences of other programs in conjunction with therapeutic community-based principles. The control group, 102 camp members, underwent regular corrective training with work correction being emphasized. In order to assess the effectiveness of the rehabilitation program, 86 participants, 38 members of the rehabilitation group, and 47 members of the control group were followed three months after discharge from the camp. There was no significant difference between the two groups based upon baseline Addiction Severity Index (ASI) scores. Several differences, most notably drug use habits, family and social functions, criminal activity, and emotional states, indicated improvement at the time of the three-month follow-up. However, there was no significant difference in abstinence rates. This may be due to the small number of sample participants, four in the rehabilitation group and nine in the control group.

Wang (1999) evaluated drug treatment at two rehabilitation centers in Xian and in Shenzhen. Through interviews with 243 drug users at the sites, most resented their forced incarceration, which lasts between six months and a year. Counseling involves writing a "thought-change report" on a weekly basis, where they repeat the importance of living a drug-free life. There is also resentment that wealthier Chinese escape incarceration in the centers and that poorer Chinese are more likely to be arrested for their drug use. Those who are rearrested after receiving treatment are incarcerated for almost three years in the camps.

Zhou and Li (1999) conducted a study of 833 drug users at six drug rehabilitation centers in Yunnan and Guangxi Provinces. The majority were male, young, single, mostly heroin users, and with little education. About half were unemployed when they entered the programs. Two-thirds reported at least daily use, either through injecting, sniffing, or snorting heroin.

There appears to be a fundamental shift in Chinese culture away from a sense that people are fully imbedded within one's community and culture (the concept of "jen") and individuality should be suppressed to promote social order and harmony. As was expressed through the Tianamen Square events of 1989, many Chinese today are embracing the worldview that individual freedom and personal expression are paramount. As modern China is drawn ever closer to the West, it is likely this world view will grow even stronger among its citizens.

AIDS Prevention in China

In 1995, China's State Council established the Coordinating Conference System for the Prevention and Treatment of AIDS and Venereal Disease, which gave priority to the prevention and treatment of AIDS (*Beijing Review* 1997). In November 1998, China's Ministry of Health outlined a national program for HIV/AIDS control for the first decade of the twenty-first century, aimed at keeping the number of HIV-infected below 1.5 million by 2010. The project is based upon an understanding that the epidemic is preventable, and the focus is directed at curbing infections through reducing drug abuse and blood transfusions (*Beijing Review* 1998b).

Several critical steps in establishing a national HIV/AIDS program have already been taken. Many HIV hotlines have opened up throughout urban China during the 1990s to dispel many of the myths about the disease and to provide accurate information about HIV/AIDS (*Beijing Review* 1998a). At the Shanghai AIDS Monitoring Center, doctors tell patients how to avoid infecting others, stress the importance of follow-up visits, and provide consultations (Yang 1997). In 1999, Beijing opened its first AIDS patients club, called the Home of the Red Ribbon. The club is designed to encourage understanding and offers a tolerant atmosphere for persons with HIV/AIDS (*Beijing Review* 1999).

Chinese herbal medications are being developed to assist in the treatment of HIV/AIDS. In a study of 158 HIV-infected patients performed by the China-Tanzania Coordinating Group, it has been reported that 6 of the patients seroconverted to HIV-negative status and remained so for up to 15 months (Lu 1995). In another study with 104 Chinese AIDS patients conducted at the Shanghai Hospital for Infectious Diseases by the Heilongjiang Gongming Pharmaceuticals Company, an herbal medicine named "Gongming Anti-HIV" was reported to be effective in the treatment of AIDS. It was reported to have restored the immune system and eliminated herpes lesions among formerly immunocompromised AIDS patients (Kou 1999). However, Forney and Lawrence (1998) caution that "producers are taking advantage of China's largely ineffectual regulation of health products to offer dubious 'anti-AIDS' potions that could threaten lives." Certainly, double-blind placebo-controlled studies of herbal medicines are urgently needed to establish potential harm or efficacy of the medications.

CONCLUSION

During this first decade of the twenty-first century, China will need to squarely face the enormity of the threat of problems such as drugs, HIV/AIDS, and other consequences. Mass media campaigns are needed to reach every social strata, age, ethnic group, injecting drug users, urbanites, and rural dwellers throughout the entirety of China. The messages will need to be targeted toward specific groups in clear, comprehensive, language appropriate for each group. Alternative approaches to combating drug addiction will need to be developed. Condoms need to be made universally available to coordinate with innovative social marketing strategies to all sectors of the population. Behavioral interventions need to be developed that reach the new, younger populations who may be more sexually active and have more

Westernized values stressing individual freedom and personal choice (Ball 2000; Kumar, Shakuntala, and Daniels 2000).

Drug abuse programs need to be expanded to increase efficacy among those who are not being helped through the existing treatment rehabilitation centers. Programs need to be developed that emphasize the importance of using clean drug injecting equipment. One such strategy, "needle social marketing," is to be implemented by the Chinese government in association with the Department for International Development in the United Kingdom. Fifteen million pounds will be spent in an effort to support HIV/AIDS control in the provinces of Yunnan and Sichuan. It will be some time, however, for the effectiveness of such a strategy to be seen (Wu 2000). The growing gay community needs to be given direct government funding and assistance in promoting HIV prevention among men who have sex with men. Alternatives to paid blood donations need to be further developed. Sex workers need to be assisted through government-sponsored safer sex programs.

China has succeeded in the past in controlling drug use within its borders and in promoting health practices. It is reasonable to expect that China will again succeed in meeting the tremendous challenge that it currently faces in combating both the rapid acceleration in drug abuse and its consequences such as the spread of HIV/AIDS throughout the nation.

BIBLIOGRAPHY

Ball, A. 2000. "Epidemiology and Prevention of HIV in Drug-Using Populations: Global Perspective." Global Research Network in HIV Prevention in Drug-Using Populations Second Annual Meeting, National Institute on Drug Abuse, Washington, DC, pp. 45–47.
Beeching, J. 1975. *The Chinese Opium Wars.* New York: Harcourt Brace Jovanovich.
Beijing Review. 1997. "What China Has Done with AIDS." 10 February, p. 25.
Beijing Review. 1998a. "Ignorance Is Accomplice to AIDS." 1 June, p. 22.
Beijing Review. 1998b. "Program Launched to Curb AIDS." 30 November, p. 5.
Beijing Review. 1999. "Beijing Establishes First AIDS Club." 15 March, p. 31.
Beyer C., M.H. Razak, K. Lisam, J. Chen, W. Lui, and Yu X.F. 2000. "Overland Heroin Trafficking Routes and HIV-1 Spread in South and South-east Asia." *AIDS* 14 (1): 75–83.
Cao, K., M. Mizokami, E. Orito, X. Ding, X.M. Ge, G.Y. Huang, and R. Ueda. 1999. "TT Virus Infection among IVDUs in South Western China." *Scandinavian Journal of Infectious Diseases* 31(1): 21–25.
Chen, J., W. Liu, and L.Y. Nancy. 1999. "Molecular-Epidemiological Analysis of HIV-1 Initial Prevalence in Guangxi, China" (in Chinese). *Chung Hua Liu Hsing Ping Hsueh Tsa Chih* 20 (2): 74–77.
Cheng, H. 1993. "Epidemiologic Studies on HCV and HBV Infections among Intravenous Drug Users in the Area with High HIV Infection" (in Chinese). *Chung Hua Liu Hsing Ping Hsueh Tsa Chih* 14 (5): 275–278.

Chuang, C.Y., P.Y. Chang, and K.C. Lin. 1993. "AIDS in the Republic of China, 1992." *Clinical Infectious Diseases* 17 (Supp.) 2: S337–S340.

Diao, C. 1997. "Survey Reveals Public's View on AIDS." *Beijing Review*, 10 February, pp. 24–25.

The Economist. 1999. "The Kindness Treatment." 353 (8148): 42.

Forney, M., and S.V. Lawrence. 1998. "Impotent Potions: 'Anti-aids' Elixirs Confound Regulators and Threaten Lives in China." *Far Eastern Economic Review* 161 (32): 64–65.

Fu, Y.L., Y. Huang, and W.S. Zhang. 1997. "Risk Factor Scoring Model of STD for Pregnant Women in Antenatal Clinic" (in Chinese). *Chung Hua I Hsueh Tsa Chih* 77 (2): 87–90.

Gil, V.E. 1991. "An Ethnography of HIV/AIDS and Sexuality in the People's Republic of China." *Journal of Sex Research* 28 (4): 521–537.

Gil, V.E., M.S. Wang, A.F. Anderson, G.M. Lin, and Z.O. Wu. 1996. "Prostitutes, Prostitution and STD/HIV Transmission in Mainland China." *Social Science and Medicine* 42 (1): 141–152.

Guo, X. 1977. "Drug Related Crimes in China." In *From Hu Men Burning Opium to Drug Detoxification in Contemporary China*, Q. Ling and Q. Shao, eds., pp. 112–119. Sichan, China: Sichan People's Publisher.

Hang, G., J. Xu, and Z. Gong. 1996. "A Study on AIDS-Related Knowledge, Attitude and Behavior in Servicemen in China" (in Chinese). *Chung Hua Yu Fang I Hsueh Tsa Chih* 30 (2): 94–97.

Kou, Z. 1999. "Sheng Zhenming Challenges AIDS." *Beijing Review*, 25 January, pp. 22–23.

Kroll, C.J., E. Oppenheimer, and A. Reynolds. 2000. "Policies Related to Drug Use and HIV/AIDS in Asia." Global Research Network on HIV Prevention in Drug-Using Populations Second Annual Meeting, National Institute on Drug Abuse, Washington, D.C., pp. 45–47.

Kumar, M.S., M. Shakuntala, and D. Daniels. 2000. "Injection Drug Use and HIV Infection in South Asia: Opportunities and Challenges for Prevention Efforts." Global Research Network on HIV Prevention in Drug-Using Populations Second Annual Meeting, National Institute on Drug Abuse, Washington, DC, pp. 48–51.

Leicester, J. 2000. "China Executes Dealers on Drug Day." *The Associated Press*, 26 June.

Li, D.Q., X.W. Zheng, and G.Y. Zhang. 1996. "Study on the Distribution of HIV-1 C Subtype in Ruili and Other Counties, Yunnan, China" (in Chinese). *Chung Hua Liu Hsing Ping Hsueh Tsa Chih* 17 (6): 337–339.

Li, V.C., B.L. Cole, S.Z. Zhang, and C.Z. Chen. 1993. "HIV-Related Knowledge and Attitudes among Medical Students in China." *AIDS Care* 5 (3): 305–312.

Li, Y.W., Y.M. Shao, and X.G. Luo. 1997. "Subtype and Sequence Analysis of the C2-V3 Region of gp120 Genes among HIV-1 Strains in Hubei Province" (in Chinese). *Chung Hua Liu Hsing Ping Hsueh Tsa Chih* 18 (4): 217–219.

Liao, S., K.H. Choi, K. Zhang, T.L. Hall, B. Qi, Y. Deng, J. Fang, Y. Yang, J. Kay, Z. Qin, W. Liu and J.S. Mandel. 1997. "Extremely Low Awareness of AIDS, Sexually Transmitted Diseases and Condoms among Dai Ethnic Villagers in Yunnan Province, China." *AIDS* 11 (Supp. 1): S27–S34.

Liu, H., J. Xie, W. Yu, W. Song, Z. Gao, Z. Ma, and R. Detels. 1998. "A Study of Sexual Behavior among Rural Residents of China." *Journal of Acquired Immune Deficiency Syndrome and Human Retrovirology* 19 (1): 80–88.

Lu, W. 1995. "Prospect for Study on Treatment of AIDS with Traditional Chinese Medicine." *Journal of Traditional Chinese Medicine* 15 (1): 3–9.

McCoy, C.B., S. Lai, L.R. Metsch, X.-r. Wang, C. Li, M. Yang, and L. Yulong 1997. "No Pain No Gain, Establishing the Kunming, China, Drug Rehabilitation Center." *Journal of Drug Issues* 27 (1): 73–85.

McCoy, C.B., H.V. McCoy, S. Lai, Z. Yu, X. Wang, and J. Meng. In press. "Reawakening the Dragon: Changing Patterns of Opiate Abuse in Asia, with Particular Emphasis on China's Yunnan Province." *Substance Use and Misuse.*

Ministry of Health of the People's Republic of China. 1994. *National Strategic Plan for the Prevention of AIDS and STD in the People's Republic of China 1995–1999.* Beijing: Author.

Newman, R.K. 1995. "Opium Smoking in Late Imperial China: A Reconsideration." *Modern Asian Studies* 29 (4): 765–794.

Qin, G., Y. Shao, and G. Liu. 1998. "Subtype and Sequence Analysis of the C2-V3 Region of gp120 Genes among HIV-1 Strains in Sichuan Province" (in Chinese). *Chung Hua Liu Hsing Ping Hsueh Tsa Chih* 19 (1): 39–42.

Rosenthal, E. 2000. "Scientists Warn of Inaction as AIDS Spreads in China." *New York Times* 2 August, pp. A1, A8.

Rubenstein, A. 1973. "How China Got Rid of Opium." *Monthly Review* 25 (5): 58–63.

Strang, J., P. Griffiths, and M. Gossop. 1997. "Heroin Smoking by 'Chasing the Dragon': Origins and History." *Addiction* 92 (6): 673–683.

Suwanwela, C., and V. Poshyachinda. 1986. "Drug Abuse in Asia." *Bulletin on Narcotics* 38 (1–2): 41–53.

Tang, B., L. Tong, and Q. Tan. 1995. "A Survey on HIV and HIV Infection of Heroin Addicts in Linchang and Kunming" (in Chinese). *Chung Hua Yu Fang I Hsueh Tsa Chih* 29 (4): 228–230.

UNAIDS/WHO. 2000. *Epidemiological Fact Sheet on HIV/AIDS and Sexually Transmitted Infections: China.* 2000 Update. http://www.unaids.org/hivaidsinfo/statistics/june00/fact_sheets/pdfs/china.pdf

Walsh-Childers, K., D. Treise, K.A. Swain, and S. Dai. 1997. "Finding Health and AIDS Information in the Mass Media: An Exploratory Study among Chinese College Students." *AIDS Education Prevention* 9 (6): 564–584.

Wang, W. 1999. "Illegal Drug Abuse and the Community Camp Strategy in China." *Journal of Drug Education* 29 (2): 97–114.

Wu, R.R., M. Mizokami, K. Cao, T. Nakano, X.M. Ge, S.S. Wang, E. Orito, K. Ohba, M. Mukaide, K. Hikiji, J.Y. Lau, and S. Iino. 1997. "GB Virus C/Hepatitis G Virus Infection in Southern China." *Journal of Infectious Diseases* 175 (1): 168–171.

Wu, Z. 2000. "Preventing HIV Infection among Injection Drug Users in China." Global Research Network on HIV Prevention in Drug-Using Populations Second Annual Meeting, National Institute on Drug Abuse, Washington, DC, pp. 52–60.

Wu, Z., R. Detels, J. Zhang, S. Duan, H. Cheng, Z. Li, L. Dong, S. Huang, M. Jia, and X. Bi. 1996. "Risk Factors for Intravenous Drug Use and Sharing

Equipment among Young Male Drug Users in Longchuan County, Southwest China." *AIDS* 10 (9): 1017–1024.

Wu, Z., G. Qi, Y. Zeng, and R. Detels. 1999. "Knowledge of HIV/AIDS among Health Care Workers in China." *AIDS Education and Prevention* 11 (4): 353–363.

Wu, Z., J. Zhang, R. Detels, S. Duan, H. Cheng, Z. Li, L. Dong, S. Huang, M. Jia, and X. Bi. 1996. "Risk Factors for Initiation of Drug Use among Young Males in Southwest China." *Addiction* 91 (11): 1675–1685.

Wu, Z., J. Zhang, R. Detels, V.C. Li, H. Cheng, S. Duan, Z. Li, L. Dong, S. Huang, M. Jia, and X. Bi. 1997. "Characteristics of Risk-Taking Behaviors, HIV and AIDS Knowledge, and Risk Perception among Young Males in Southwest China." *AIDS Education and Prevention* 9 (2): 147–160.

Wu, Z., J. Zhang, and L. Dong. 1998. "Relationship between Risk-Taking Behavior and Knowledge for HIV Infection among Young Men in Longchuan, Yunnan of China" (in Chinese). *Chung Hua Yu Fang I Hsueh Tsa Chih* 32 (3): 171–173.

Xia, M., J.K. Kreiss, and K.K. Holmes. 1994. "Risk Factors for HIV Infection among Drug Users in Yunnan Province, China: Association with Intravenous Drug Use and Protective Effect of Boiling Reusable Needles and Syringes." *AIDS* 8: 1701–1706.

Yang, J. 1997. "Doctors and Patients Keep a Common Secrecy." *Beijing Review*, 10 February, p. 24.

Yu, E.S., Q. Xie, K. Zhang, P. Lu, and L.L. Chan. 1996. "HIV Infection and AIDS in China, 1985 through 1994." *American Journal of Public Health* 86 (8 pt. 1): 1116–1122.

Yu, X.F., J. Chen, Y. Shao, C. Beyer, and S. Lai. 1998. "Two Subtypes of HIV-1 among Injection-Drug Users in Southern China." *Lancet* 351 (9111): 1250.

Zhang, K., D. Li, H. Li, and E.J. Beck. 1999. "Changing Sexual Attitudes and Behaviour in China: Implications for the Spread of HIV and Other Sexually Transmitted Diseases." *AIDS Care* 11 (5): 581–589.

Zhang, X., B. Luo, and K. Zhang. 1994. "A KABP (Knowledge, Attitude, Belief and Behavior) Study about AIDS among Taxi Drivers and Hotel Attendants in Beijing" (in Chinese). *Chung Hua Liu Hsing Ping Hsueh Tsa Chih* 15 (6): 323–327.

Zhao, M., S.Y. Xiao, W. Haow, D.S. Yang, W.W. Chen, K. Deng, and X.X. Deng. 2000. "The Therapeutic Community-Based Rehabilitation Program in the Treatment of Individuals Addicted to Heroin in a Correction Camp: An Experience from Hunan." Global Research Network on HIV Prevention in Drug-Using Populations Second Annual Meeting, National Institute on Drug Abuse, Washington, DC, pp. 61–67.

Zheng, X., C. Tian, K.-H. Choi, J. Zhang, H. Cheng, X. Yang, D. Li, J. Lin, S. Qu, X. Sun, T. Hall, J. Mandel, and N. Hearst. 1994. "Injecting Drug Use and HIV Infection in Southwest China." *AIDS* 8: 1141–1147.

Zheng, X.W., J.P. Zhang, and Y.L. Chen. 1995. "A Cohort Study and KAP Investigation of HIV Infected Persons in Ruili, and Other Counties in Yunnan, 1994" (in Chinese). *Chung Hua Liu Hsing Ping Hsueh Tsa Chih* 16 (2): 67–70.

Zheng, X., J.P. Zhang, and S.Q. Qu. 1997. "A Cohort Study of HIV Infection among Intravenous Drug Users in Ruili and Other Two Counties in Yunnan Province, China, 1992–1995" (in Chinese). *Chung Hua Liu Hsing Ping Hsueh Tsa Chih* 18 (5): 259–262.

Zhou, Y., and X. Li. 1999. "Demographic Characteristics and Illegal Drug Use Patterns among Attendees of Drug Cessation Programs in China." *Substance Use and Misuse* 34 (6): 907–920.

Zule, P.H., K.N. Vogtsberger, and D.P. Desmond. 1997. "The Intravenous Injection of Illicit Drugs and Needle Sharing: An Historical Perspective." *Journal of Psychoactive Drugs* 29 (2): 199–204.

5

HAITI

Mary Comerford

INTRODUCTION

HIV and AIDS remain a challenge for the twenty-first century. HIV infection by the year 2020 is predicted to be the tenth leading cause of disease burden in the world (Murray and Lopez 1996). The priority is to find a cure and to continue to decrease transmission of the infection through health promotion and education. Nowhere is this challenge more difficult than in developing nations. Characterized by high infant mortality rates and low gross national product (GNP), these nations are faced with the difficult task of HIV prevention with minimal resources as their populations continue to grow at exponential proportions. In addition to the rising rates of HIV and AIDS, these nations must also continue to deal with three persistent health problems: high rates of infectious diseases, malnutrition, and an uncontrollable population growth. These forces make it difficult for advancement in the global economic world. Haiti, located in the Caribbean, is one of these nations facing the daunting task of eliminating the increasing rate of HIV and AIDS. In Haiti, in addition to HIV and AIDS, adults continue to be affected by malaria, tuberculosis, and malnutrition, and children continue to be affected by diarrhea, malnutrition, and respiratory infections.

Haiti occupies the western half of the island of Hispaniola, which it shares with the Dominican Republic. Cuba lies only 80 kilometers to the west of the island. Being surrounded by the Atlantic Ocean to the north, and the Caribbean Sea to the south, along with its mountainous terrain, helps reduce the tropical heat in the mountainous areas. Haiti is geographically separated into nine administrative sections or departments, and its capital, Port-au-Prince, is situated in the west department. In order to understand the HIV/AIDS epidemic in Haiti, it is necessary to examine its history and current economic and political conditions. Unlike industrialized countries in which mechanisms to control the disease have been instituted, Haiti has no resources to invest. The HIV/AIDS epidemic has added an additional layer of misery to the lives of the Haitian people with little hope of recovery.

Colonized by the French in 1659, Haiti was one of the first colonies to seek independence through the uprising of African-descendant slaves, a free nation as of 1804 (*European World Year Book* 1999). Although once referred to as the "Pearl of the West Indies," more recently Haiti has been plagued by political instability resulting in lack of economic growth and is now characterized as the "poorest nation in the Western Hemisphere." Jean-Jacques Dessaline became the first African-descendant leader of a free, previously colonized nation. Regrettably, unrest between blacks and mulattoes led to U.S. military intervention lasting from 1915 to 1934. In 1946, President Dumarsais Estimé removed political power from the mulatto descendants. Other presidents were in administration until 1957 when François Duvalier became "president for life" and established a repressive dictatorship. His successor and son Jean-Claude Duvalier fled from Haiti in 1985 due to public unrest and protests. Governed by dictatorships since its independence, the nation is attempting to achieve democracy. In 1991 populist leader Jean-Bertrand Aristide was elected, an event that led to civil unrest, which resulted in a coup d' état by Duvalier supporters and the establishment of a military junta. Aristide was forced to flee the country. After numerous acts of terrorism and human rights abuses by the coup leaders, an international embargo was placed on the nation from 1991 through 1994, which ended with the return of Aristide to the presidency. The second democratically elected president René Preval was inaugurated on 17 December 1995.

International economic sanctions from 1991 through 1994 further crippled the impoverished nation, and conditions on the island deteriorated. The embargo affected the poor and disadvantaged by impacting food, medical, and vaccine supplies. Child mortality increased during the embargo (Gibbons and Garfield 1999). The effect of the sanctions on the rate of HIV and AIDS is unknown. Yet unquestionably with the banned foreign aid to Haiti, the freezing of Haitian government assets in the United States, and decreasing commercial air transport and oil shipments (Gibbons and Garfield 1999), the probable impact on HIV and AIDS was significant. Foreign aid was restored after the return of Aristide and remains the key source of health care funding in the area of HIV and AIDS prevention. However, most foreign aid and loans were again withheld during Preval's regime because of political instability in the nation. Irregularities in the 2000 election have further eroded international confidence in the future of Haiti, and international support is once again being withheld.

There are a variety of factors that come to play in HIV and AIDS prevention in Haiti, including poverty, the limited number of health care facilities, low levels of education, high levels of illiteracy, and cultural beliefs. HIV and AIDS in Haiti are changing demographically similar to other nations, increasingly affecting women and children. But the resources to stem this tide are unavailable at the present time.

ISSUES RELATED TO HIV AND AIDS

Health Status

Haiti has a population estimated to be over 8 million persons. With an annual growth of 2.1%, the population is expected to double by the year 2025 (Maynard-Tucker 1996). A total of 40% of inhabitants are aged 14 and younger, 56% are between the ages of 15 and 64, and only 4% are 65 years and older. More than 70% of the population lives below the poverty line (Institut Haitien de l'Enfance 1995). Of the total population in 1994, one-third lived in urban areas and two-thirds of the population in rural areas. The level of urbanization is one of the lowest in the developing nations (Pan American Health Organization [PAHO] 1998). The capital, Port-au-Prince, has a total of 2 million inhabitants, and the population density in Haiti is one of the highest in Latin America and the Caribbean. In 1994 the gross domestic product decreased (one of the primary ways of determining the level of development of a nation) to levels prior to 1980 (PAHO 1998) and has continued decreasing each year since (UNAIDS/WHO 2000). In 1999 the gross national product per capita was estimated to be U.S. $380. Only 30% of Haitians are employed, resulting in an unemployment rate of 70%. In 1999 the life expectancy at birth was 54, the infant mortality rate was 66 deaths per 1,000 live births, and the under-5 mortality rate was 134 deaths per 1,000. The fertility rate was 4.3, the crude birthrate was 32 per 1,000, and the crude death rate was 12 per 1,000. The maternal mortality rate is high, 1,000 deaths per 100,000 live births (UNAIDS/WHO 2000).

In Haiti, land is difficult to cultivate because of mountainous conditions and soil erosion caused by deforestation. These factors cause an estimated 20,000 tons of arable land to be lost annually. The level of deforestation is aggravated by the use of charcoal burning as a main source of fuel. The electricity supply remains scarce on the island, reaching only the urban areas and only sporadically. Other necessities such as the availability of a potable water supply and sanitary disposable sites remain poor. Only 30% of the population has access to potable water situated at least 15 minutes from their homes, and only 25% of the population has access to proper sanitary disposable facilities (Institut Haitien de l'Enfance 1995).

Barriers to Health

Education

An estimated 45% of the population is illiterate, and the rate of illiteracy is highest in rural areas. The official languages of Haiti are French and Creole. Many schools teach in French, yet the majority of Haitians speak Creole. The state and religious organizations, particularly the Roman Catholic Church, provide education. Although most inhabitants do not have the funds, many of the schools charge for tuition, books, and uniforms (*Europa World Year Book* 1999). Education is divided into primary, secondary, and tertiary levels. Only 26% of the children in 1990 attended and completed primary school, which is mandatory from ages 6 to 12, and only 22% of children attended secondary school. Tertiary schools provide vocational and professional training. There are a total of 18 vocational schools, 42 schools called domestic science schools, and one university for the 8 million inhabitants on the island. A study conducted by Behets et al. (1995) found that of the women receiving antenatal services in two clinics in Cité Soleil, a poverty-stricken slum area outside of Port-au-Prince, only 33% were functionally literate (defined in the study as being able to write a letter).

Health Care System and Resources

The health care system in Haiti is composed of public, private, and public/private organizations. Only a small segment of the population is reached through the public health care system. At least 1.5 million inhabitants are served by private and nongovernmental organizations (NGOs). These organizations have traditionally functioned independently (UNAIDS/WHO 2000), with little or no planning coordination between the agencies. Those who have access to health care services are located mainly in the Port-au-Prince area, leaving a large portion of the people of Haiti without access to health care services. In 1998, an estimated 40% of the population of Haiti had no access to primary care (UNAIDS/WHO 2000). Other indicators also provide a picture of the difficulty in treating HIV and AIDS. These indicators include number of physicians and other health professionals, actual number of hospitals, and the expenditure on health. In 1994, reports indicated that there were an estimated 49 hospitals in Haiti, slightly lower than the number of hospitals reported in 1980; 52 NGOs operate 32% of these health facilities (PAHO 1998). In 1990 there were 16 physicians and 13 nurses for every 100,000 inhabitants. Expenditure on health is only U.S.$2 per capita annually. It is estimated that the Haitian government provides 16% of total expenditures on health, and external donors provide the remaining health expenditures. Reports indicate that in 1994, in addition to hospitals, there were 61 inpatient facilities. In all, including inpatient and hospitals, these facilities provided 90 beds per

100,000 population; however, these health delivery system indicators are expected to improve over the coming years. In 1996, the Ministry of Health introduced a health policy that recognized the right of all to have access to care. This reform would decentralize the health care system in the hope of ensuring equal access to all Haitians. The reform priorities focused on strengthening the Ministry of Health itself, establishing and developing a primary health care system, strengthening health promotion activities, and improving environmental health. Hopefully these reforms will provide the infrastructure needed in the health care system. However, unless the economic and political conditions in Haiti improve dramatically, they will be impossible to implement.

Many Haitians receive care through an informal health care system, utilizing both home remedies and traditional healers. It is important to note that although Catholicism is the most practiced religion in Haiti, the practice of voodoo along with Catholicism remains high. The number of different healers may never fully be known; healers include traditional birth attendants (Barnes-Josiah, Myntt, and Augustin 1998), leaf doctors (who use leaves in traditional medicine), and voodoo priests and priestesses (DeSantis 1989). This level of care provides access for those who are unable to receive health care services. Traditional medicine provides "the need for psychosomatic explanations for illness" (Barnes-Josiah, Myntt, and Augustin 1998) and accessible inexpensive health services. No research has examined the use or role of these traditions in treating HIV and AIDS (Barnes-Josiah, Myntt, and Augustin 1998).

The previous information has provided the social and political context in which HIV and AIDS are situated in Haiti. Haiti suffers from many barriers to the prevention and control of HIV infection including low literacy rate, low levels of education, and limited access to health care for its inhabitants. These factors are similar to other developing nations.

History of HIV and AIDS

Initial reports from *developed* nations found that men having sex with men were at risk for HIV and AIDS. It soon became apparent that in the developed nations other groups such as injection drug users and persons receiving blood transfussions or blood products were also at high risk for AIDS.

The *developing* nations followed a different track. In the developing world, specifically in Africa, the equal rate of female and male infection indicated a more heterosexual mode of transmission, and AIDS spread with the rapidity of other sexually transmitted diseases (STDs). HIV transmission in Haiti is mainly heterosexual, and evidence shows that it has moved from a predominantly male disease to one affecting women and infants at an alarming rate.

Early in the epidemic, Haiti received blame for the HIV and AIDS crisis in the United States and Canada (Farmer 1994). When a number of Haitian immigrants were determined to be positive in the United States in 1982 (Centers for Disease Control [CDC] 1982), Haitians were considered to be an independent risk group for AIDS. Individuals of Haitian descent and those who had traveled to Haiti were not permitted to donate blood in the United States during the 1980s for fear of transmitting the virus through blood products. The erroneous belief that Haitians were at higher risk than other ethnic groups for HIV further stigmatized both Haitians living in Haiti and Haitian immigrant communities living in the United States.

Information on the extent of HIV/AIDS in Haiti is sparse. No surveillance system is in place and operating in the country. There are nine sentinel sites across the country, but reporting is intermittent and inconsistent. Haiti has reported no figures on AIDS to the Pan American Health Organization (PAHO 1998) since 1995. It has been estimated that the prevalence of HIV infection among the adult Haitian population rose from 2% in 1989 to 5% by 1994. Current estimates range from 5% to 10%. It is further estimated by the Joint United Nations Programme on HIV/AIDS/World Health Organization (UNAIDS/WHO 2000) that there were 210,000 people living with HIV/AIDS in Haiti at the end of 1999, 5,200 of whom were children under the age of 15. The estimated number of deaths due to AIDS for the year 1999 was 23,000. In addition, an estimated 74,000 Haitian children under the age of 15 have lost their mother or both parents to AIDS during the epidemic.

Risk Groups

Few studies have examined the likely source of HIV transmission among Haitians. The available evidence, however, suggests that heterosexual transmission is the primary route of infection. For example, Deschamps et al. (1996) found that 90% of AIDS patients in Haiti were infected through heterosexual contact.

Sex workers in Haiti have been found to have a high prevalence of HIV. For example, a 1986 study found that 49% of Haitian prostitutes in Port-au-Prince were infected with HIV (Pape, Stanback, and Pamphile 1990). Prostitution is widespread in Haiti, and because of the general state of health and health care, reciprocal health risks between clients and prostitutes are of great concern.

The HIV infection rate among women is rising dramatically. In 1986 for the urban area of Cité Soleil and Port-au-Prince, the HIV prevalence among antenatal women ranged between 8% and 9%. Women in rural areas who underwent testing in 1986 and 1990 had a prevalence rate of 3% to 4%. The primary age group among women with HIV is 20 to 24 (R. Boulos et al. 1990). The WHO estimates an infection rate of 53% among female partners of males infected with HIV. A total of 4,967 AIDS cases (46% women) were reported in Haiti between 1982 and 1992. Rural prevalence rates ranged from 3 to 5%, and prevalence rates in urban areas ranged from 7 to 10%.

STDs are a major problem in Haiti, and attempts at prevention have not been extremely successful. In Haiti, STDs are difficult to monitor because of the lack of reporting mechanisms and accessibility to health care. The level of STDs is unknown because many affected by STDs receive treatment and care from non-Western services (Behets et al. 1995). In a study conducted by Behets et al. (1995), the prevalence detected in an antenatal clinic for syphilis was as high as 6 to 8%.

One of the difficulties in controlling STDs including HIV/AIDS are cultural beliefs related to sex and condom use. Many interventions have been established to promote condom use. Among Haitian males in Cité Soleil the knowledge concerning condom use was extremely high, yet the use of condoms was low (M. Boulos, Boulos, and Nichols 1991). The rate of condom use among males was estimated to be between 5% and 6%. The minimal use of condoms reported did not relate to issues of efficacy. The report indicates that the men were well aware of the protective nature of condoms for STDs and pregnancy. Of those reported ever using condoms, contraception was the primary reason for 85% of those surveyed; those reporting use for STD prevention accounted for only 2%.

Much work has been done in Haiti to increase condom use, and it appears as if there is some success in this area. While the traditional view that condoms decrease pleasure is still prevalent, information on the benefits of condom use not only as a form of birth control but as a method to prevent HIV infection has been disseminated. Many organizations supply condoms at no charge, and condoms remain relatively cheap in Haiti compared to the cost in some developing countries (International Planned Parenthood Federation 2000).

RESPONSES TO HIV/AIDS

Governmental Efforts

The government of Haiti has made periodic attempts to control AIDS through education. Education campaigns have taken place in the past, and an official governmental agency was established for HIV/AIDS education. However, due to lack of funding, the agency is no longer operative. Previous educational campaigns have been more successful within major cities than in rural areas.

Nongovernmental Organizations

Four international agencies have supported HIV and AIDS prevention in Haiti: the PAHO, the U.S. Agency for International Development

(USAID), WHO, and the United Nations Fund for Population Activities (UNFPA). Through the support of these international organizations, 20 NGOs are surveying HIV infection (PAHO 1998). These NGOs, in addition to surveillance, provide educational campaigns and materials for distribution, training for health care workers and leaders in the community, and psychological and clinical care for clients afflicted with the disease. The NGOs are also responsible for distribution of condoms and the prevention of STDs. In 1996, UNAIDS officially began to operate in Haiti. In 1996 the World Health Organization and UNAIDS initiated a working group. The main purpose is to improve data collection, in order to make informed decisions, and to strengthen networks and infrastructure to improve surveillance of STDs and HIV. The objective is to improve decision making by establishing quality data collection mechanisms (UNAIDS/WHO 2000).

CONCLUSION

At the present time, the HIV/AIDS epidemic has not devastated Haiti to the same extent as it has many other developing nations such as those in Africa. But the full extent of the epidemic is still unknown. Many Haitians acquire HIV, become symptomatic, and die without ever encountering the health care system. Many others who are most probably HIV-positive die from other diseases or causes prior to becoming symptomatic. Considering the multitude of problems in Haiti, HIV/AIDS does not receive high priority. The HIV/AIDS epidemic has added to the untold suffering and misery of the Haitian people. It is an additional burden on a country and health care system that cannot perform even basic health care and health maintenance for its people.

BIBLIOGRAPHY

Barnes-Josiah, Debora, Cynthia Myntt, and Antoine Augustin. 1998. "The Three Delays as a Framework for Examining Maternal Mortality in Haiti." *Social Science Medicine* 46: 981–993.

Behets, Frieda M.-T., Julio Desormeaux, Dania Joseph, Mario Adrien, Gessie Coicou, Gina Dallabetta, Holli Hamilton, Stoffel Moeng, Homer Davis, Myron S. Cohen, and Reginald Boulos. 1995. "Control of Sexually Transmitted Diseases in Haiti: Results and Implications of a Baseline Study among Pregnant Women Living in Cité Soleil Shantytowns." *Journal of Infectious Diseases* 172: 764–771.

Boulos, Michaelle L., Reginald Boulos, and Douglas J. Nichols. 1991. "Perceptions and Practices Relating to Condom Use among Urban Men in Haiti." *Studies in Family Planning* 22: 318–325.

Boulos, Reginald, Neal A. Hasley, Elizabeth Holt, Andrea Ruff, Jean-Robert Brutus, Thomas C. Quinn, Mario Adrien, Carlos Boulos, and the Cité Soleil/JHU

AIDS Project Team. 1990. "HIV-1 in Haitian Women 1982–1988." *Journal of Acquired Immune Deficiency Syndromes* 3: 721–728.

Centers for Disease Control (CDC). 1982. "Opportunistic Infections and Kaposi's Sarcoma among Haitians in the United States." *Morbidity and Mortality Weekly Report* 31: 353–354, 360–361.

Coreil, Jeannine, Phyllis Losikoff, Rachel Pincu, Gladys Mayard, Andrea J. Ruff, Harry P. Hausler, Julio Desormeau, Homer Davis, Reginald Boulos, and Neal A. Halsey. 1998. "Cultural Feasibility Studies in Preparation for Clinical Trials to Reduce Maternal-Infant HIV Transmission in Haiti." *AIDS Education and Prevention* 10: 46–62.

DeSantis, Lydia. 1989. "Health Care Orientations of Cuban and Haitian Immigrant Mothers: Implications for Health Care Professionals." *Medical Anthropology* 12: 69–89.

Deschamps, Marie-Marcelle, Jean William Pape, Alice Hafner, and Warren D. Johnson, Jr. 1996. "Heterosexual Transmission of HIV in Haiti." *Annals of Internal Medicine* 125: 324–330.

Europa World Year Book. 1999. Pittsburgh, PA: Europa Publications.

Farmer, Paul. 1994. *The Uses of Haiti.* Monroe, ME: Common Courage Press.

Gibbons, E., and Richard Garfield. 1999. "The Impact of Economic Sanctions on Health and Human Rights in Haiti, 1991–1994." *American Journal of Public Health* 89: 1499–1504.

Institut Haitien de l'Enfance. 1995. *Demographic and Health Surveys.* Enquête Mortalité, Morbidité et Utilisation des Services EMMUS II 1994/1995. Calverton, MD: Macro International.

International Planned Parenthood Federation. 2000. "Country Profiles: Haiti." Available on the World Wide Web at: http://www.ippf.org

Manyard-Tucker, Gisèle. 1996. "Haiti: Unions, Fertility and the Quest or Survival." *Social Science Medicine* 43: 1379–1387.

Murray, Christopher J.L., and Alan D. Lopez, eds. 1996. *The Global Burden of Disease: A Comprehensive Assessment of Mortality and Disability from Diseases, Injuries, and Risk Factors in 1990 and Projected to 2020.* Cambridge, MA: Harvard University Press.

Pan American Health Organization (PAHO). 1998. *Country Health Profiles for Haiti.* http://www.paho.org/English/SHA/prfhai.htm

Pape, Jean W., Bernard Liautaud, Frank Thomas, Jean-Robert Mathurin, Marie-Myrtha A. St. Amand, Madeline Boncy, Vergniaud Pean, Moliere Pamphile, A. Claude Laroche, and Warren D. Johnson, Jr. 1983. "Characteristics of the Acquired Immunodeficiency Syndrome (AIDS) in Haiti." *New England Journal of Medicine* 309: 945–950.

Pape, J.W., M.E. Stanback, and M. Pamphile. 1990. "Prevalence of HIV Infection and High-Risk Activities in Haiti." *Journal of Acquired Immunodeficiency Syndromes* 3: 995–1001.

UNAIDS/WHO. 2000. *Epidemiological Fact Sheet on HIV/AIDS and Sexually Transmitted Infections:* Haiti. 2000 Update. http://www.unaids.org/hivaidsinfo/statistics/june00/fact;sfsheets/pdfs/haiti.pdf

6

IRELAND

Karen McElrath

INTRODUCTION

The island of Ireland consists of 32 counties. The border separating the
north and south regions of Ireland has been in place since 1922. The six
counties located in the northeastern region of the island are referred to
officially as Northern Ireland[1] and are currently ruled by the British government. The remaining 26 counties, referred to officially as the Republic of
Ireland,[2] are located largely in the southern region and are represented by
the Irish government. This chapter addresses issues pertaining to HIV and
AIDS as they relate to the 26 countries in the south of Ireland. Major
differences exist between Northern Ireland and the Republic of Ireland in
terms of the prevalence and incidence of HIV and AIDS. Although relationships between the primary health agencies in the north and south of
Ireland have been described as "excellent" (Department of Health and Children 2000b: 15), vast differences exist in terms of service provision, as well
as related health policies with respect to HIV and AIDS. Additionally, linkages in service provision have not been firmly established, and little collaborative (north-south) research into HIV and AIDS has been conducted.
Thus, the border reflects real differences in terms of issues relating to HIV
and AIDS. Some of these differences are discussed in this chapter. Elsewhere
in this volume, Higgins and Haw address issues pertaining to HIV and AIDS
in Northern Ireland in the context of the United Kingdom.

ISSUES RELATING TO HIV AND AIDS

Reported AIDS Cases

The 26 counties of the Republic of Ireland are divided into 10 health boards that have the responsibility for overseeing and providing a range of health services within their areas. The Eastern Regional Health Authority encompasses three health boards and includes Dublin city, the largest metropolitan area on the island. The reporting of AIDS cases can be characterized as a two-stage process whereby medical diagnoses are reported first to the Regional AIDS coordinators from each of the health boards. In turn, the Regional coordinators report the information to the National AIDS Coordinator, Department of Health and Children. In many instances, reporting occurs well after the year of diagnosis. For example, O'Sullivan and Barry (1999) found that nearly 40% of all AIDS cases were reported 1 year or more after the initial diagnosis. Approximately 10% of all cases were reported between 6 and 11 years after the diagnosis. These discrepancies pose problems for monitoring AIDS cases in Ireland (O'Sullivan and Barry 1999). The European Centre for the Epidemiological Monitoring of AIDS includes AIDS incidence data reported by the year of diagnosis. In their most recent report, the (Ireland) National AIDS Strategy Committee recommended that the country comply with the reporting criteria issued by the European Centre and report cases by year of diagnosis as opposed to year of report (Department of Health and Children 2000a). The proposed change would allow for more accurate use of epidemiological trend data and would be more useful for drawing international comparisons.

AIDS cases in the Republic of Ireland were reported first in 1983, having been diagnosed in 1982 (Department of Health and Children 2000a). The number of new cases increased slowly, and the cumulative total had reached 37 cases by December 1987 (Department of Health and Children 2000a: 23). Data on likely mode of transmission for these early cases suggested that the syndrome disproportionately affected three groups: injecting drug users (IDUs), gay men, and hemophiliacs (O'Briain et al. 1990).

Despite the limitation with respect to reporting delays, the available data indicate a total of 691 AIDS cases in the 26 counties of Ireland from 1983 to December 1999 (UNAIDS/WHO 2000a). An estimated 350 people had died of AIDS-related illnesses by year-end 1999.

Exposure Categories

Table 6.1 describes the cumulative AIDS cases through 1999. The data indicate that injecting drug use is the leading category of exposure, representing 42% of all reported AIDS cases (UNAIDS/WHO 2000b). Sexual contact between men represented 34.3% of all cases through 1999. An ad-

IRELAND   99

ditional 13.3% of all reported AIDS cases were transmitted through heterosexual contact, 5.2% via receipt of blood or blood products, and 3.3%
through perinatal transmission.

Injecting drug use emerged as a growing problem in Ireland in the early
1980s but was confined largely to the Dublin area (Butler 1991). In 1996,
capture-recapture methods[3] identified an estimated 13,460 opiate users in
Dublin in 1996, for an estimated prevalence rate of 21 opiate users per
1,000 population (Comiskey forthcoming). As shown in Table 6.1, IDUs
represent a large proportion of the cumulative AIDS cases. This proportion
is higher than that found in several other European countries. O'Gorman
(1998) suggested that the high rate of IDUs among AIDS cases is the result
of two factors. First, although various harm reduction measures have been
implemented in Ireland, these interventions were introduced well after the
development of an injecting drug use culture. Second, O'Gorman suggested
that several gay males from Ireland had emigrated to other regions—areas
that might be characterized as being more tolerant of gay lifestyles. Indeed,
acts of anal intercourse were illegal in the Republic of Ireland until 1993
(Smyth 1998). Assuming that this emigration pattern had occurred, we
would expect that the proportion of gay males among the cumulative AIDS
cases would be lower had the emigration not occurred. In turn, the proportion of IDUs would be inflated in the cumulative case total.

In the 1990s, the lowest proportion of IDUs transmission occurred in
1997 and 1998 (28%, 27%, respectively); however, the proportion increased
substantially in 1999 when IDUs accounted for 37% of all AIDS cases. The
tabular data show that the proportion of IDUs by year peaked in 1993
(63%). However, in that year the number of new AIDS cases among gay
males declined substantially (N = 13), and that decline represented the
lowest number of new AIDS cases within this group since 1987. Thus,
changes in one group can affect the representative proportion of another
group.

In 1990, transmission through heterosexual contact was not viewed as a
major problem in Ireland (O'Briain et al. 1990). By December of that year,
a cumulative total of 12 cases were thought to be exposed through heterosexual contact. The data in Table 6.1 show that between 1990 and 1999
the number of AIDS cases ranged from 5 to 11 for this exposure category.
Thus, although the proportion of cases from heterosexual contact in 1999
reached its highest level ever (27%), the actual numbers do not reflect a
major increase since 1990.

Transmission through blood and blood products (e.g., transfusion) accounted for 5.2% of the cumulative total as of December 1999. AIDS cases
in this category peaked in 1989 and 1994 (N = 6 for each year), and four
cases were recorded in 1998. Perinatal exposure has been low relative to
other categories of transmission. The highest number of cases was observed
in years 1994 (N = 6) and 1998 (N = 4).

Table 6.1
Reported AIDS Cases by Exposure Category and Year (actual numbers in parentheses)

Probable Mode of Transmission

	Injecting Drug Use[a]	Sex between Men	Heterosexual	Blood/Blood Products	Perinatal	Unknown	TOTAL[b,d]
1982	0 (0)	100% (2)	0 (0)	0 (0)	0 (0)	0 (0)	100% (2)
1983	100% (1)	0 (0)	0 (0)	0 (0)	0 (0)	0 (0)	100% (1)
1984	33% (1)	33% (1)	0 (0)	33% (1)	0 (0)	0 (0)	100% (3)
1985	40% (2)	20% (1)	0 (0)	0 (0)	20% (1)	20% (1)	100% (5)
1986	17% (1)	17% (1)	0 (0)	50% (3)	17% (1)	0 (0)	100% (6)
1987	50% (10)	30% (6)	5% (1)	15% (3)	0 (0)	0 (0)	100% (20)
1988	29% (11)	55% (21)	3% (1)	8% (3)	5% (2)	0 (0)	100% (38)
1989	45% (23)	33% (17)	4% (2)	12% (6)	2% (1)	4% (2)	100% (51)
1990	44% (27)	36% (22)	13% (8)	2% (1)	3% (2)	2% (1)	100% (61)
1991	44% (31)	32% (23)	16% (11)	4% (3)	3% (2)	1% (1)	100% (71)
1992	54% (27)	30% (15)	14% (7)	2% (1)	0 (0)	0 (0)	100% (50)
1993	63% (43)	19% (13)	16% (11)	2% (1)	0 (0)	0 (0)	100% (68)
1994	31% (21)	40% (27)	11% (7)	9% (6)	9% (6)	0 (0)	100% (67)

	Injecting Drug Use[a]	Sex between Men	Heterosexual	Blood/Blood Products	Perinatal	Unknown	TOTAL[b,d]
1995	42% (23)	29% (16)	18% (10)	5% (3)	4% (2)	2% (1)	100% (55)
1996	43% (34)	43% (34)	14% (11)	0 (0)	0 (0)	0 (0)	100% (79)
1997	28% (9)	38% (12)	22% (7)	3% (1)	3% (1)	3% (1)	100% (32)
1998	27% (11)	32% (13)	12% (5)	10% (4)	10% (4)	10% (4)	100% (41)
1999	37% (15)	32% (13)	27% (11)	0 (0)	2% (1)	2% (1)	100% (41)
Cumulative	42.0% (290)	34.3% (237)	13.3% (92)	5.2% (36)	3.3% (23)	1.9% (13)[c]	(691)

[a]Includes male injectors who have had sex with men.
[b]Some row percentages do not total 100% due to rounding.
[c]One AIDS case of unknown mode of transmission is missing from the annual data.
[d]Cumulative percentages are taken directly from data reported in UNAIDS/WHO (2000a), and those original figures were rounded to one decimal point.

Sources: Department of Health and Children 2000a; UNAIDS/WHO 2000a.

101

HIV

An estimated 200,000 tests for HIV antibodies have been conducted each year in Ireland since the mid-1990s, and positive results within the health boards are sent to a single agency for confirmation (Department of Health and Children 2000a). A total of 2,195 positive tests have been recorded from 1985 to year-end 1999 (Department of Health and Children 2000a). An estimated 2,200 persons were living with HIV/AIDS at year-end 1999, including 170 children aged 15 or younger (UNAIDS/WHO 2000a). The absolute number of HIV cases has increased each year since 1994 (Department of Health and Children 2000a), in comparison to the number of AIDS cases, which peaked in 1996. Thus, the data suggest that while the number of AIDS cases in the Republic of Ireland have somewhat stabilized, the number of HIV infections has increased in recent years. Similar patterns have been documented in other European countries, and these patterns have been explained by the availability of antiretroviral therapies designed to slow the progress of HIV infection and in turn delay the onset of AIDS-related illnesses (Mocroft et al. 2000). Indeed, antiretroviral therapies have increased survival rates for persons in Ireland (Dunne, Rushkin, and Mulcahy 1997). Because these treatments do not prevent the spread of HIV infection, one might expect that AIDS incidence might be lowered but with little effect on the number of HIV infections.

The available data on HIV infections are collected and reported differently than reported AIDS cases in the Republic of Ireland. The latter identify the probable mode of transmission based on medical or clinical diagnoses. Alternatively, HIV antibody test results are identified by laboratories, whereby technicians will often report the site from the blood samples derived.

Table 6.2 describes HIV-positive tests by various categories of exposure. Comparing the annual data over time suggests a number of concerns. First, the cumulative test data suggest that injecting drug users represent the group for which the highest number of positive tests have been recorded (N = 913; 41.6%). Males who have sex with other males represent 498 (22.7%) of the cumulative cases, and heterosexuals account for 412 (18.8%) of all cases. The cumulative data indicate that children account for 172 (7.8%) of the positive antibody tests; however, these data are not adjusted for cases in which children subsequently test negative (Department of Health and Children 2000a). The cumulative data also indicate that HIV-positive antibody tests have been recorded for hemophiliacs and their contacts (N = 118; 5.4%), prisoners (N = 39; 1.8%), and blood donors (N = 29; 1.3%). Positive test results for each of the other categories (i.e., recipients of blood transfusion, organ donors, visa requests, occupational hazards among persons working in medical settings) represent less than 1% of the cumulative total.

Excluding the cumulative pre-1986 data, the number of positive tests for

HIV antibodies peaked in years 1986 (N = 112) and 1992 (N = 82) among IDUs. Compared to 1998 figures (N = 26), a substantial increase within this group was recorded in 1999 (N = 69), following five years during which the number of positive tests had stabilized. Among gay males, the number of positive tests for HIV antibodies peaked in 1992 (N = 58).

Prior to 1986, there were no reported cases of HIV infection transmitted through heterosexual contact, and the cumulative total for this category through December 1991 suggests that 10.4% of HIV infections (N = 116) were the result of heterosexual contact. This figure increased to 18.8% in the cumulative totals as of 1999. The number of new HIV infections in 1999 transmitted through heterosexual contact reached 59—the highest number since data collection commenced. Additionally, the percentage of females found in new cases of HIV increased from 24% in 1992 to 31% in 1998 (Virus Reference Laboratory 1999). However, these numbers and percentages should be interpreted with caution in that changes could reflect an increase in the number of heterosexuals and women being tested for HIV antibodies.

In the Republic of Ireland, more than 100 hemophiliacs who have used contaminated blood products have become infected with HIV, and approximately 260 have become infected with hepatitis C. Most of the blood products were imported from other countries. A class-action civil suit was filed in 1992 on behalf of these individuals. A Hemophilia Tribunal is currently under way in the Republic of Ireland in order to investigate how such a large number of hemophiliacs became infected with HIV and hepatitis C from contaminated blood products. At this writing, a final settlement has not been reached. In addition to costs awarded to the plaintiffs, the Irish government is considering its own compensation scheme for these persons.

Stigma Surrounding HIV and AIDS

Service workers in the area of HIV and AIDS have described the public perception that people living with HIV or AIDS generally are viewed in terms of either "guilty" or "innocent" victims (Smyth 1998). Stigma surrounding HIV and AIDS remains, particularly against injectors. In Dublin, an IDU with HIV infection was beaten to death by a group of six males in 1996. Further, government proposals that have called for an expansion of methadone clinics in the Dublin area have been met by resistance from residents in these localities (ffrench-O'Carroll 1997; *Irish Medical Times* 2000). Discrimination against persons living with HIV and AIDS was designated a priority area of importance by the National AIDS Strategy Committee in its latest report (Department of Health and Children 2000a). However, the Discrimination Sub-Committee has proposed that it be dissolved, with the assumption that the Equality Authority would address discrimination against persons living with HIV and AIDS.

Table 6.2
Number of Positive Tests for HIV Antibodies

			Group Category or Site from which Specimen Was Obtained						
	IDUs	Gay Males	Heterosexuals	Hemophiliac & Contacts	Children	Prisoners	Blood Donors	Other[a]	TOTAL
Pre-1986	221	39	0	92	8	0	3	0	363
1986	112	11	21	13	11	0	1	0	169
1987	72	21	26	7	16	0	3	0	145
1988	58	17	20	0	18	0	2	0	115
1989	57	33	0	0	10	12	4	0	116
1990	50	25	24	0	11	0	1	0	111
1991	34	27	25	0	4	1	1	0	92
1992	82	58	50	1	7	0	2	1	201
1993	52	48	21	1	12	1	1	1	137
1994	20	31	22	0	10	0	2	0	85
1995	19	33	30	1	4	2	0	2	91
1996	20	41	27	1	8	2	5	2	106

	IDUs	Gay Males	Heterosexuals	Hemophiliac & Contacts	Children	Prisoners	Blood Donors	Other[a]	TOTAL
1997	21	37	40	1	10	5	1	4	119
1998	26	37	47	0	20	3	2	1	136
1999	69	40	59	1	23	13	1	3	209
Cumulative	913	498	412	118[b]	172	39	29	14	2195

[a]Includes recipients of blood transfusion, organ donors, visa requests, insurance, and hospital/occupational hazard/needlestick.
[b]The majority (N = 114) are hemophiliacs.

Source: Department of Health and Children 2000a: 26; original data reported by the Virus Reference Laboratory.

Selected Research Findings

Studies have examined aspects of HIV among various groups and sub-cultures within the Republic of Ireland. Some of this research has concentrated on women. For example, a study conducted between 1987 and 1990 based on data collected from 109 HIV-antibody positive women attending a Dublin sexually transmitted disease (STD) clinic found that 93% of the women were injecting drug users (Mulcahy, Kelly, and Tynan 1994). A lower figure was reported in a study of attendees from a Dublin STD clinic between 1992 and 1995. In that study, 70% of women were injecting drug users (Study Group for the MRC Collaborative Study of HIV Infection in Women 1999). Nevertheless, these studies suggest that most women who test positive for HIV antibodies and who attend STD clinics in Dublin have a history of injecting drug use.

Other research has shown that women in the Republic of Ireland who have tested positive for HIV antibodies typically are of childbearing age. One study found an average age of 25.6 years (range 19–41 years) among women in this category who had attended an STD clinic in Dublin (Mulcahy, Kelly, and Tynan 1994). A second study, based on data collected in 1991, reported similar findings whereby the average age of women who had tested positive for HIV antibodies and who had presented for treatment was 25 years (Murphy et al. 1993). Although few studies have examined safe-sex practices among this group of women, one study found that only 22% of women who had tested positive for HIV antibodies reported regular use of condoms (Murphy et al. 1993).

Some studies have focused on women sex workers in the Republic of Ireland. McDonnell et al. (1998) examined case records of female sex workers who attended the Dublin Women's Health Project between 1991 and mid-1997. Eight percent reported current injection drug use. Among those women who were tested for various infections, 2.5% were positive for HIV, and 8.1% were positive for hepatitis C. Moreover, while the vast majority of these women reported using condoms during sexual contacts with clients, only 19.5% reported condom use with their significant other.

In October 1992, voluntary perinatal HIV testing (anonymously and un-linked) was implemented in various clinics throughout the south of Ireland. Between 1992 and 1998, 354,223 perinatal tests had been conducted, of which 90 were positive (Department of Health and Children 2000a). Compared to previous years, increases in the number of positive perinatal were observed in 1997 (.042%) and 1998 (.039%).

A Dublin study of 109 women who tested positive for HIV antibodies found that 40% of the women had given birth to children since they first learned of their HIV status (Mulcahy, Kelly, and Tynan 1994). A surveillance system designed to monitor children born to HIV-infected mothers was introduced in the Republic of Ireland in 1985. Although not all children have become infected with HIV, Nourse et al. (1998) examined data pertaining to 29 children in the Republic of Ireland who were infected with HIV. Although 48% were born to mothers who injected drugs, 65% were born to fathers who injected drugs. Those authors also found that in two-thirds of all cases involving school-age children (i.e., 12 of 18 children) parents had *not* disclosed the child's illness to school authorities. The low percentage of disclosure to school authorities suggests that some parents might perceive that children could face additional stigma if disclosure occurs.

Prisoners in the Republic of Ireland, and in particular those inmates incarcerated in Dublin's Mountjoy Prison, represent a group disproportionately affected by HIV infection. A study of Mountjoy prisoners was conducted in 1996 (O'Mahony 1997). Data were collected through interviews with prisoners, who were selected by a systematic random sample (N = 108). Sixty-six percent of the sample had used heroin, and most of the respondents had injected the substance. Thirty-four percent of the overall sample had injected heroin during their incarceration, and several had borrowed or loaned a needle/syringe while in prison. Although a number of prisoners had never undergone testing for HIV, 9% of the full sample reported that they had at some point tested positive for HIV antibodies.

A study of inmates incarcerated in several Irish prisons supports the earlier findings. Allwright et al. (2000) collected self-report data and oral fluid specimens in their study of prisoners in Ireland conducted in 1998. A total of 43.2% of the prisoners had injected drugs during the lifetime, and females (59.7%) were significantly more likely than males (42.4%) to have had injected drugs. Two percent of the overall sample tested positive for HIV antibodies, and among self-identified injectors, the prevalence rate for HIV infection was 3.5%.

RESPONSES TO HIV/AIDS

Similar to other developed countries, nongovernment organizations (NGOs) in the south of Ireland responded quickly and proactively to the emerging AIDS problem. This history as well as selected agencies are described here. Gay activists were instrumental in these efforts, and in the mid-1980s, several individuals formed the Gay Health Action, designed to increase awareness and provide information about AIDS. However, the organization was initially refused funding by the government; at that time Irish legislation prohibited homosexuality as well as acts of anal intercourse (Smyth 1998). Although the Gay Health Action no longer exists, it has been credited with assisting the development of several other NGOs designed to assist people with HIV infection and AIDS (Smyth 1998). Several other community agencies currently cater to gay individuals in the Republic of Ireland; however, as of 1996 the Dublin-based Gay Men's Health Project was the only organization for which primary activities focused on HIV and

AIDS (Gay and Lesbian Equality Network and the Nexus Research Co-operative 1996). Similar to the earlier funding difficulties, other community agencies, while catering to the gay community, have lacked the funding to implement services for HIV and AIDS (Gay and Lesbian Equality Network and the Nexus Research Co-operative 1996).

Cáirde (the Irish word for "friends") was established in Dublin in 1985 to provide assistance to adults and children with HIV and AIDS and their families (http://www.cairde.org). A nongovernment agency, its services include the provision of information, counseling, referral material, home care, and various other forms of support. The agency utilizes trained volunteers who provide extensive support to individuals and families (e.g., during hospitalization and in bereavement). The program's Child and Family Project was established in 1997 and represented the first service of its kind in Ireland, offering various outings for children.

Dublin AIDS Alliance, a nongovernment organization, was established in 1987 (formerly known as AIDS Action Alliance) and provides referrals, information, education, support, and related services to persons living with HIV and AIDS and their families. The agency has been proactive in its lobbying efforts, and one of its primary objectives is to monitor and reduce discrimination against persons who live with HIV and AIDS. The Dublin AIDS Alliance also provides funding for informal initiatives, such as the publication of *Brass Munkie*, a "user friendly" news periodical containing articles and various information pertaining to injection drug use, treatment, HIV and AIDS, and related issues. Similar to the Dublin AIDS Alliance, other agencies operate in Cork (i.e., AIDS and Sexual Health Resource Centre, formerly Cork AIDS Alliance), Galway (AIDS Help West) and Limerick (Limerick AIDS Alliance).

The responses by government occurred much later than those efforts initiated by NGOs. Government strategies to assist drug injectors commenced in the late 1980s. Butler (1991) noted that one Dublin hospital offered methadone on a limited basis to some clients in 1987. That site closed shortly thereafter, and methadone services were moved to the National Drug Treatment Centre. By 1991, the Centre was the only site in Dublin that provided for methadone maintenance (ffrench-O'Carroll 1997), and allegations surfaced that the Centre failed to incorporate a harm reduction ideology (Butler 1991). In 1992, methadone maintenance was implemented on a larger scale, and subsequently, mobile methadone units were placed in circulation in the Dublin area. Additionally, in the 1990s the health board representing the Dublin area actively encouraged physicians to prescribe methadone for patients in need. However, physicians are not required to prescribe the drug, nor are pharmacists required to dispense methadone when physicians provide prescriptions (ffrench-O'Carroll 1997). The central methadone treatment list included approximately 4,300 persons at year-end 1999 (Department of Health and Children 2000a). However, the demand

for methadone maintenance in Dublin exceeds the number of available treatment slots (ffrench-O'Carroll 1997).

Needle exchange schemes have been in operation in Dublin since 1989.
Most schemes operate within government health centers; however, one nongovernment agency—the Merchant's Quay Project—also provides for needle exchange (Smyth 1998). The Project was established in Dublin in 1990
by the Franciscan Friars in their effort to assist drug users. It offers drug
treatment services (including alternative or complimentary treatments, e.g.,
acupuncture), family support, and a women's project and distributes various
harm reduction materials. Day care is available for clients with children.

Other programs also offer a range of services. For example, the Baggot
Street Clinic—a government service located in Dublin—offers HIV testing,
HIV counseling, needle exchange, and programs specifically geared to particular groups. One of its more progressive programs is the Women's Health
Project. Established in 1991, the program serves women sex workers and
now offers various services, example, referral information, education, testing
for HIV, and family planning. Condoms as well as a needle exchange are
available from the Project. One study found that although women generally
were satisfied with the service provision of the Women's Health Project,
several suggested that operating hours be extended (Commission of the
European Community 1994).

Testing for HIV antibodies is conducted in various health clinics and in
Genitourinary Medicine (GUM) clinics, located in hospitals throughout Ireland. Many of these clinics provide for HIV testing without a prior appointment. Some sites, however, have very limited hours of operation, and at
other clinics, entry and exit into and from the clinic can hardly be described
as private. The HIV Outpatient Clinic located in the Department of Genitourinary Medicine at St. James' Hospital in Dublin provides several services
to persons living with HIV and AIDS and also offers in-patient treatment.
Specialist treatment interventions, such as antiretroviral therapy, are available, and the government assumes the treatment costs when a physician recommends this treatment (Department of Health and Children 2000a).
Antiretroviral therapy has also been available to pregnant women in the
Republic of Ireland who have tested positive for HIV antibodies. As of
1998, no cases of perinatal transmission in Ireland were recorded among
women who opted for this intervention (Bichard 1998).

In the late 1980s and early 1990s, the Irish government was considerably
more responsive to implementing harm reduction services for injecting drug
use as a means of reducing the spread of HIV infection than it was with
respect to promoting safe sex practices. Although methadone maintenance
and needle exchange were implemented well after the emergence of injecting subcultures, efforts by the Irish government contrast greatly with service
provision in Northern Ireland, where methadone maintenance and needle

exchange are not available and the availability of diverse drug treatment modalities is extremely limited.

In the Republic of Ireland prior to 1993, condoms could be sold only to married persons, by selected pharmacies or family planning agencies, and could not be sold to youth under the age of 17. These restrictions resulted from the tremendous influence of the Catholic Church on Irish legislation and policy (Smyth 1998). In 1992 the National AIDS Strategy Committee recommended changes to existing legislation that would permit condoms to be sold from vending machines. More recently, fewer legislative restrictions are in place regarding the sale and distribution of condoms. However, the costs of condoms are reportedly higher in Ireland than in other European countries (Department of Health and Children 2000a).

Confidential telephone helplines are in operation, and government efforts have included strategies to increase public knowledge about HIV and AIDS. For example, three media campaigns have been implemented since 1992. Early government-endorsed media campaigns, however, were alarmist in nature, linking HIV and AIDS with death (Smyth 1998). AIDS information pamphlets are in circulation, and although currently available government pamphlets that focus on HIV and AIDS are far more progressive than information presented in the earlier campaigns, attention still focuses on issues of morality (Smyth 1998). For example, a 1997 pamphlet produced by the government's Health Promotion Unit states that the "most effective way" to avoid HIV transmission through sexual contact is to "stay with one partner" and to "remain faithful to that one partner" (Health Promotion Unit 1997). The government's pamphlet on hepatitis C provides similar moralistic advice (Department of Health and Children n.d.). Government-sponsored educational literature intended for school-age children still reflects traditional Catholic morals, although some progress has been made (Smyth 1998).

Representatives from both government and nongovernment agencies came together in 1991 to form the (Irish) National AIDS Strategy Committee. The Committee's first report was issued in 1992 and included several recommendations for improving and expanding services for HIV and AIDS. However, five years after the report was published, some of the recommendations had not been fully implemented (Smyth 1998). A second report was published in June 2000 (Department of Health and Children 2000a) and is composed of information compiled by four subcommittees (1) Surveillance, (2) Education and Prevention, (3) Care and Management, and (4) Discrimination. Each subcommittee has offered recommendations pertaining to HIV and AIDS. Although these recommendations are not binding, the goal of the Committee is to implement as many recommendations as possible.

CONCLUSION

Ireland has thus far maintained a low prevalence of HIV and AIDS in comparison to other European countries (UNAIDS/WHO 2000b). However, data are collected and reported differently, and these factors make it difficult to compare across countries. In the Republic of Ireland, injecting drug users represent the largest proportion of cumulative cases for both HIV and AIDS, and despite several harm reduction measures already in place, the latest figures on new HIV infections are particularly worrisome. Additional research is needed to investigate the extent to which IDUs utilize available programs and why some IDUs apparently continue to engage in behaviors that pose risk for HIV infection. Waiting lists for treatment space must be eliminated so that injectors, in particular, can receive drug treatment on demand.

HIV incidence through heterosexual contact also has increased, but it is not known whether the change reflects an increase in testing among non-injecting heterosexuals. Prevention programs must place more emphasis on promoting safe sex practices but without the moralistic advice inherent in traditional Catholic ideology. Another challenge concerns the stigma surrounding HIV and AIDS. Innovative strategies that seek to reduce this stigma might need to be localized, taking into account the (possibly diverse) beliefs and attitudes of communities. The degree to which the Irish government addresses these emerging problems will have considerable effect on the future epidemiological trends.

NOTES

1. The term *Northern Ireland* is rejected by most Irish Nationalists, who perceive it as a British label imposed on them without their consent.

2. The official title *Republic of Ireland* also is rejected by many Irish Nationalists who prefer the term *26 counties* or, more simply, *the south of Ireland*.

3. A methodological approach used to estimate prevalence by using two or more samples. The technique adjusts for cases that appear in more than one sample (Comiskey forthcoming).

BIBLIOGRAPHY

Allwright, Shane, Fiona Bradley, Jean Long, Joseph Barry, Lelia Thornton, and John V. Parry. 2000. "Prevalence of Antibodies to Hepatitis B, Hepatitis C, and HIV and Risk Factors in Irish Prisoners: Results of a National Cross Sectional Survey." *British Medical Journal* 321: 78–82.

Bichard, Karen. 1998. "Ireland's Success with HIV Pregnancies." *Lancet* 352: 796.

Butler, Shane. 1991. "Drug Problems and Drug Policies in Ireland: A Quarter of a Century Reviewed." *Administration* 39: 210–233.

Comiskey, Catherine M. Forthcoming. "Methods for Estimating Prevalence of Opiate Use as an Aid to Policy and Planning." *Substance Use and Misuse.*

Commission of the European Community. 1994. *AIDS Prevention for Prostitutes. Final Report Europap 1994: Country Report of Ireland.*

Department of Health and Children. 2000a. *AIDS Strategy 2000: Report of the National AIDS Strategy Committee.* Dublin: Stationery Office.

———. 2000b. *National Health Promotion Strategy, 2000–2005.* Dublin: Author.

———. n.d. *Living with Hepatitis C: Information about Hepatitis C for People with the Virus, Their Family and Friends.* Dublin: Author.

Dunne, M.T., H.J. Rushkin, and F.M. Mulcahy. 1997. "Survival with AIDS in Ireland." *AIDS* 11: 1281–1290.

ffrench-O'Carroll, Michael. 1997. *The Irish Drugs Epidemic.* Cork: Collins' Press.

Gay and Lesbian Equality Network and Nexus Research Co-operative. 1996. *HIV Prevention Strategies and the Gay Community. Phase One Report: A Baseline Study.* Dublin: Authors.

Health Promotion Unit. 1997. *AIDS: The Facts* (October). Dublin: Author.

Irish Medical Times. 2000. "HIV Figures Are a Major Concern." 30 June.

McDonnell, R.J., P.M. McDonnell, M. O'Neill, and F. Mulcahy. 1998. "Health and Risk Profile of Prostitutes in Dublin." *International Journal of STD and AIDS* 9: 485–488.

Mocroft, A., C. Katlama, A.M. Johnson, C. Pradier, F. Antunes, F. Mulcahy, A. Chiesi, A.N. Phillips, O. Kirk, and J.D. Lundgren. 2000. "AIDS across Europe, 1994–98: The EuroSIDA Study." *Lancet* 356: 291–296.

Mulcahy, F., G. Kelly, and M. Tynan. 1994. "The Natural History of HIV Infection in Women Attending a Sexually Transmitted Disease Clinic in Dublin." *Genitourinary Medicine* 70: 81–83.

Murphy, D., M. Lynch, N. Desmond, and F.M. Mulcahy. 1993. "Contraceptive Practices in HIV Seropositive Females in Ireland." *International Journal of STD and AIDS* 4: 107–109.

Nourse, C., E. Hayes, R. Travers, S. McConkey, and K.M. Butler. 1998. "Paediatric HIV Infection in the Republic of Ireland and the Need for Antenatal Screening." *International Journal of STD and AIDS* 9: 587–590.

O'Briain, D.S., F. Jackson, M.G. Courtney, F. O'Malley, G.S. McDonald, E.M. Mulvihill, J.J. Dinn, I.J. Temperley, and F. Mulcahy. 1990. "The Emerging AIDS Epidemic in Ireland—Clinicopathological Findings in 23 Early Cases." *Irish Medical Journal* 83: 50–53.

O'Gorman, Aileen. 1998. "Illicit Drug Use in Ireland: An Overview of the Problem and Policy Responses." *Journal of Drug Issues* 28: 155–166.

O'Mahony, Paul. 1997. *Mountjoy Prisoners: A Sociological and Criminological Profile.* Dublin: Stationery Office.

O'Sullivan, P., and J. Barry. 1999. "Reporting Delay in the AIDS Surveillance System of the Eastern Board." Research Correspondence. *Irish Medical Journal* 92: 405.

Smyth, Fiona. 1998. "Cultural Constraints on the Delivery of HIV/AIDS Prevention in Ireland." *Social Science and Medicine* 46: 661–672.

Study Group for the MRC Collaborative Study of HIV Infection in Women. 1999. "Survival and Progression of HIV Disease in Women Attending GUM/HIV Clinics in Britain and Ireland." *Sexually Transmitted Infections* 75: 247–252.

Virus Reference Laboratory. 1999. *Analysis of HIV Data Held by the Virus Reference Laboratory over the Period 1–7-92 to 31–12–98.* June. Dublin: Author.

UNAIDS/WHO. 2000a. *Epidemiological Fact Sheet on HIV/AIDS and Sexually Transmitted Infections: Ireland.* 2000 Update. Geneva: Joint United Nations Programme on HIV/AIDS.

———. 2000b. *Report on the Global HIV/AIDS Epidemic—June 2000.* Geneva: Joint United Nations Programme on HIV/AIDS.

7

KENYA AND UGANDA

Elizabeth Pisani

INTRODUCTION

Kenya and Uganda, neighbors in East Africa, have much in common historically and culturally. As HIV began its spread through the populations of the region, its epidemiology in these two countries was remarkably similar. Driven by early age at first sex for both men and women, high rates of partner exchange, low condom use even in commercial and extramarital sex, and high background levels of other sexually transmitted infections (STIs), HIV spread rapidly throughout the general heterosexual population of both countries.

Kenya and Uganda have, however, diverged widely in their approach to the HIV epidemic. Uganda felt the effects of AIDS earlier than Kenya and tackled HIV head-on at a relatively early stage. Strong political leadership fertilized an active response at the community level, and everyone from religious leaders to the private sector became involved in national HIV prevention and care efforts. Kenya, by contrast, reacted to the epidemic with denial, both at the political and at the community levels. By the late 1990s, it was clear that these differences in approach had significantly affected the course of the epidemic in each country. Figure 7.1 illustrates these differences. While in Kenya HIV prevalence has continued its steady upward trend, in Uganda it has apparently been curbed. HIV prevalence began to fall among pregnant women in their teens and early twenties in urban areas as early as the mid-1990s. By the end of the decade, large population-based

Figure 7.1
HIV Prevalence in Kenya and Uganda: Mean Values for Urban Sentinel Sites*

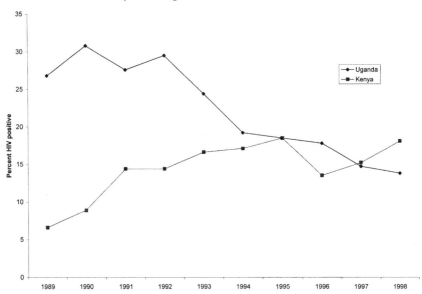

*The data for Kenya are for the two largest cities in the country (Nairobi and Mombasa) only. These are the cities used to give estimates for urban prevalence in official statistics, including those published by UNAIDS. Table 7.1 shows that several other areas that could be considered urban (including the nation's third and fourth largest cities, Kisumu and Nakuru) have far higher prevalence levels than this figure suggests.

Source: Data drawn from spreadsheets provided to the author by the National AIDS programs.

studies in rural areas of Uganda confirmed that drops in HIV infection rates among young women were not confined to the urban elite.

ISSUES RELATING TO HIV AND AIDS

Sources of Information

Uganda reported its first AIDS case in 1982, and Kenya two years later. Both countries maintain AIDS case reporting systems. By June 1999, some 87,000 AIDS cases had been reported to the Ministry of Health in Kenya. Since health information systems are poor, diagnostic facilities limited, case definitions unclear, and HIV-related stigma pronounced enough to discourage AIDS diagnosis in many situations, it is recognized that these AIDS case reports provide limited information. Kenya, for example, estimates only 1 in 8 AIDS cases is reported (National AIDS Control Programme, Kenya [NASCOP] 1999). Uganda reported just 53,306 AIDS cases by the end of

1997 (Uganda AIDS Commission 1999). The Joint United Nations Programme on HIV/AIDS (UNAIDS) estimated that in fact over 30 times that many Ugandans had already died of AIDS by the end of 1997 (UNAIDS/WHO 1998).

In order to improve information about the spread of HIV, Uganda established a sentinel surveillance system for HIV in 1989 and has since conducted annual rounds of unlinked anonymous HIV surveillance on blood taken from pregnant women for syphilis screening (Asiimwe-Okiror et al. 1997). Kenya began its sentinel surveillance in urban centers a year later, expanding the system to include peri-urban and rural sites in 1994 (NASCOP 1999).

Both countries have among the most reliable sentinel surveillance data (and among the longest time series data) anywhere. However, data from sentinel surveillance among pregnant women are subject to a number of limitations (Gray et al. 1998; Zaba and Gregson 1998). Pregnant women have by definition had unprotected sex in the recent past. In terms of exposure to HIV, they are not representative of all women in the general population and are clearly not representative of men. Differences in antenatal service use, interactions between HIV, other STIs, and infertility, and associations between contraceptive use and risky sexual behavior are among the factors that contribute to limit the generalizability of sentinel surveillance data for HIV. Uganda, in particular, has minimized these limitations by supplementing HIV sentinel surveillance systems with two long-term population-based cohorts, established in rural areas in 1989 (Mulder et al. 1994; Musagara et al. 1989) These studies, which follow individuals over time, have provided invaluable information about HIV incidence and prevalence among men and women in the general population in rural areas. In Kenya, a single, cross-sectional HIV-prevalence study conducted in the western city of Kisumu in 1997 provides the only population-based seroprevalence information in the country (NASCOP and the Population Council 1999). In both cases, population-based studies have confirmed that data generated by sentinel surveillance systems are generally rather robust (UNAIDS/WHO 2000).[1]

HIV Prevalence Levels and Risk Behavior

What, then, do these information systems tell us about HIV prevalence in the two countries? Table 7.1 shows HIV prevalence in Kenya's antenatal sentinel sites. Clearly, HIV prevalence varies widely throughout the country. It was first recorded at high levels in the western province of Nyanza. The rapid growth of the epidemic in this area may be related in part to its geographic proximity to Uganda, which experienced an explosive epidemic early on, and partly to cultural practices of the Luo ethnic group that dominate the area. The Luo are the only major ethnic group in Kenya among

Table 7.1
HIV Prevalence among Women Aged 15–49 in Selected Urban Sentinal Sites, Kenya

Sentinel Site	1990	1993	1996	1998
Busia	17	22	28	29*
Garissa	5	4	5	8*
Kakamega	5	9	10	16
Kisii	2	2	16	16*
Kisumu	19	20	27	29
Kitale	3	7	2	18
Kitui	1	7	4	10
Meru	3	2	15	23
Mombasa	10	16	12	17*
Nairobi**	6	16	16	16*
Nakuru	10	22	27	26
Nyeri	3	3	9	17
Thika	2	27	13	34

*1997 data
**Data for Nairobi from University of Nairobi study clinics. These are clinics in areas where enhanced HIV prevention programs have been in place for eight years.

Source: Baltazar et al. 1999.

whom male circumcision is not the norm. Evidence from a growing number of studies—including one important study comparing circumcised and uncircumcised Luo men—(Kahindo, Nyang, and Chege 1998) confirm that prepubertal circumcision is independently associated with lower HIV incidence as well as lower prevalence (Kelly et al. 1999; Quinn et al. 2000; Weiss, Quigley, and Hayes 2000). The lack of circumcision among a large majority of Luo men may have contributed to the rapid spread of HIV in western Kenya. In recent years, however, many other parts of the country have reached similarly high rates of HIV prevalence, even in areas where male circumcision is the norm.

Clearly, HIV prevalence is high and rising in a majority of sites across Kenya. Overall, Kenya's national AIDS program estimated that around 2 million citizens were living with HIV by the end of 1998, 90,000 of them children. A year later, UNAIDS estimated 2.1 million adults and children were living with HIV in Kenya, where adult prevalence was estimated at 14%. The UN body further estimates that close to 500 HIV-infected Kenyans died every day of 1999. These deaths, 29% higher than deaths estimated for 1997, bring to 960,000 the number of AIDS-related deaths in the country since the start of the epidemic. These deaths, most of them in adults, imply that 440,000 Kenyan children have lost their mothers before their fifteenth birthday because of AIDS (UNAIDS/WHO 2000).[2]

The only area of Kenya for which population-based data on HIV prevalence are available is Kisumu, and these data, collected from around 890 women and 620 men in randomly selected households, confirm the extremely high HIV prevalence levels recorded in pregnant women (NASCOP and the Population Council 1999). Some 30.1% of women and 19.8% of men in this study tested positive for HIV. As Figure 7.2 shows, there was a striking difference in HIV prevalence among men and women in the youngest age groups. Twenty-three percent of girls aged 15 to 19 were infected with HIV, compared with just 4% of boys of the same age. By the early twenties, the ratio of female to male infection had diminished, but the absolute difference had grown.

A combination of physical and behavioral factors contribute to these large age differences in infection. Women become infected more easily in any act of sex with an infected partner than men do (Downs and de Vincenzi 1996). But, crucially, young women often have sex with much older men, either within marriage or outside it (Glynn 2000). HIV prevalence among these older men is far higher than prevalence among younger men. The population-based study in Kisumu found that no teenage women married to men 3 years or less their senior were infected with HIV. By contrast, among teenage women married to men 10 years or more older than them, HIV prevalence was 50% (Glynn 2000). The study also found that older men who have sex with younger women may also have other high-risk partners.

Figure 7.2
**HIV Prevalence among Men and Women in a Household Study in Kisumu,
Kenya, by Age, 1997**

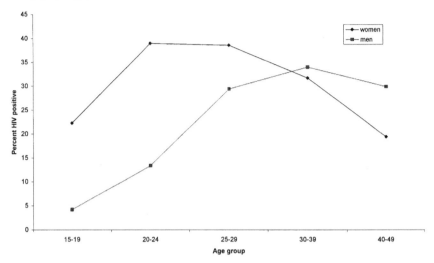

Source: NASCOP and the Population Council 1999.

Because of these very high levels of HIV infection in young women, more
women are living with HIV in Kenya than men. This difference is partly
because the age group in which they become infected accounts for a larger
proportion of the population than the age group in which men typically
become infected. And it is partly because individuals who are infected at a
younger age tend to survive longer (Phillips et al. 1991). On average, it is
estimated that there are around 122 women living with HIV in Kenya for
every 100 men (UNAIDS/WHO 1999).

Behavioral data suggest that most young people in Kenya are sexually
active long before marriage (Erulkar et al. 1998; Kenya 1999; NASCOP
and the Population Council 1999). According to one study, women are
active for an average of three years before marriage, while men have sex for
close to nine years on average before getting married (Egesah et al. 1999).
It is clear that many young women are becoming infected with HIV during
these premarital sexual encounters. Among married teenage women in the
Kisumu population-based study, nearly two-fifths of those who had had
premarital partners were HIV-positive, whereas none of the women who
had been virgins at marriage were infected with the virus (Glynn 2000).
This finding suggests that these women were infected before marriage. If
they had married a man who was not himself infected with HIV, they would
certainly have put him at risk of infection. And indeed there is some evidence
from this same study that women may be passing HIV on to their new

Table 7.2
HIV Prevalence among Women Aged 15–49 in Selected Peri-Urban and
Rural Sentinel Sites, Kenya

Sentinel Site	District	1994	1995	1997
Chulaimbo [r]	Kisumu	49	22	27*
Kaplong [r]	Bomet	N/a	4*	6
Karurumo [r]Embu	Embu	2	10	27
Maragua [p/u]	Muranga	7	13	11
Mbale [p/u]	Vihiga	12	11	16
Mosoriot [r]	Uasin Gishu	2	12	9
Motomo [r]	Kitui	0	5	6
Njambini	Nyeri--	--	--	4
Tiwi [p/u]	Kwale	12	24	--

p/u = Peri-urban.
r = Rural
*1996 data.

Source: Baltazar et al. 1999.

husbands. In Kisumu, over a quarter of married men aged 20 to 24 tested
HIV-positive, compared with fewer than 10% of single men (Glynn 2000).
This finding suggests that marriage may well be a major risk factor for young
men. (Tables 7.1 and 7.2 show HIV prevalence rates among women aged
15–49 in various Kenyan sentinel sites.)

The HIV epidemic appears to have established itself earlier in Uganda
than in Kenya. By the time sentinel surveillance among pregnant women
began in 1989, three out of four sites were already registering HIV prevalence levels of over 20% in women aged 15 to 49 (Asiimwe-Okiror et al.
1997). Because of this earlier start, more Ugandans than Kenyans have died

Table 7.3
HIV Prevalence among Pregnant Women in Various Sentinel Sites, Uganda, 1989–1996

	1989	1990	1991	1992	1993	1994	1995	1996
Site								
Nsambya	24.5	25.0	27.8	29.5	26.6	21.8	16.8	15.4
Rubaga	---	---	27.4	29.4	24.4	16.5	20.2	15.1
Mbarara	21.8	23.8	24.3	30.2	18.1	17.3	16.6	15.0
Jimja	24.9	15.8	22.0	19.8	16.7	16.3	13.2	14.8
Tororo	---	4.1	12.8	13.2	11.3	10.2	12.5	8.2
Mbale	3.8	11.0	12.1	14.8	8.7	10.2	7.8	8.4

Source: Asiimwe-Okiror et al. 1997.

of HIV since the epidemic began: some 1.2 million by the end of 1999, according to UNAIDS estimates (UNAIDS/WHO 2000). However, unlike Kenya, Uganda appears to have passed the peak of mortality. UNAIDS estimated that 110,000 HIV-infected Ugandans died in 1999, down from 160,000 in 1997.

HIV prevalence in Uganda is believed to have peaked at around 15% in 1990. At the start of 2000, adult prevalence stood at 8.17%, according to UNAIDS estimates (UNAIDS/WHO 2000). Table 7.3 describes HIV prevalence among pregnant women in various sites within Uganda.

Falling prevalence among pregnant women of all reproductive ages says little about changing patterns of HIV infection. Lower prevalence may be the result of fewer new infections, but it may also be the result of a rise in mortality among HIV-infected women, rising infertility associated with HIV infection, or lower sexual activity among those with symptomatic infection (Kilian et al. 1999). These biases are less likely to affect women in the younger age groups, among whom most infections are relatively recent and among whom mortality and HIV-related infertility are likely to be low. A look at the age disaggregated data for one site, Nsambya, suggests that HIV prevalence also fell most significantly over time in the youngest age groups. Figure 7.3 illustrates falling prevalence rates among women in their teens and early twenties. Nationally representative behavioral studies record a rapid rise in condom use among young people during this period. Sixty-one percent of boys and 44% of girls aged 15 to 19 reported in 1995 that they had ever used condoms, compared with just 20% of boys and 10% of women six years earlier (Asiimwe-Okiror et al. 1997). However, it should be noted

Figure 7.3
HIV Prevalence among Young Women at Nsambya Sentinel Surveillance Site, Uganda, 1991–1996

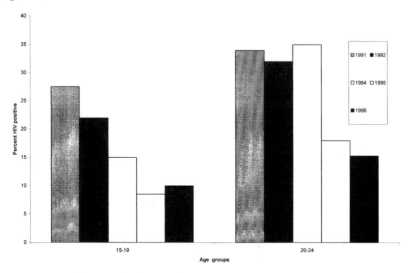

Source: Asiimwe-Okiror et al. 1997: 1760.

that the falls in prevalence occurred in women who were pregnant and who must therefore have had unprotected sex.

Recent data show that the fall in HIV prevalence among young pregnant women in urban Uganda is mirrored among young women in the general population in rural areas. In the rural district of Rakai, HIV prevalence among teenage women in 1989–1990 was 4.4%, compared with just 0.2% among teenage men. Seven years later, prevalence in teenage women had fallen steadily to 1.4% (X^2 for trend 8.97, p 0.003), whereas among men little significant difference was recorded over time (Kamali et al. 2000). Figure 7.4 illustrates the trends in prevalence over time in these groups. In this case, too, a large increase in condom use probably contributed to these lower rates of infection (and to the significant fall in teenage pregnancy that accompanied it). The percentage of teenage women who had ever used a condom tripled between 1994 and 1997. And the proportion of teenage women who had ever used a condom was higher than the proportion who had ever used a condom in any other age group, indicating that the acceptability of condom use is growing more rapidly among young people than among older people. Among the men who have sex with these women, lifetime condom use rose, too, more than doubling in all age groups between 1994 and 1997.

Figure 7.4
**HIV Prevalence among Men and Women Aged 13–19, Rural Uganda,
1989–1997**

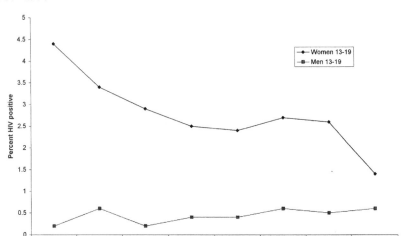

Source: Kamali et al. 2000: 429.

HIV-Related Stigma: Efforts to Break the Silence Pay Off

As some of the data cited above suggest, sexual mixing in East Africa is widespread enough to constitute a norm. This behavioral norm remains at odds, however, with the socially accepted (and largely rhetorical) ideal of virginity at marriage and mutual faithfulness within marriage, promoted by religious leaders. Associated with "unacceptable" behaviors, HIV is heavily stigmatized in most communities. People infected with HIV and their families are subject to discrimination in a number of fields, including employment and education. HIV-related stigma and discrimination are usually hidden, and they can easily be disguised with rational explanations. It is therefore almost impossible to quantify HIV-related stigma (Goldin 1994; Malcolm et al. 1998). The willingness to find out one's HIV status, to share results with partners, and to openly acknowledge infection in oneself, one's family, and one's community are therefore often taken as proxy markers for the level of HIV-related stigma in a community. Official attitudes to HIV are most easily gauged from the existence and enforcement of laws preventing discrimination and protecting the rights of infected individuals.

Kenya has no such laws. While the Sessional Paper on AIDS of 1997 includes a policy banning compulsory HIV testing, the paper (and therefore the policy) has no legal standing. Anecdotal evidence suggests that preemployment testing for HIV is common practice in many Kenyan firms. A negative HIV test is also a prerequisite for most life and health insurance policies issued in the country. The country continues to debate the limits of confidentiality and is considering instituting a policy of mandatory notification of primary sexual partners for anyone who tests positive for HIV. A study conducted between 1989 and 1993 in Nairobi suggests that such a policy might prejudice the well-being of people, and especially women, who test HIV-positive. In the study, just 66 out of 243 HIV-positive women counseled chose to share their results with their partners. Nearly one-third of those who did later said they had been abandoned or beaten as a result (Temmerman et al. 1995).

The possibility of mandatory partner notification may well further dent the uptake of counseling and voluntary testing, which is already low. An inventory of HIV counseling and testing services in Nairobi published in 1999 found that city's only full-service VCT (voluntary counseling and testing) center for HIV was serving just 20 clients a week (Population Council and Family Health International 1999). Among pregnant women in Nairobi offered counseling and HIV testing in a study on the transmission of HIV from mother to child in 1997, 99% accepted a test. However 30% never returned for their test result. Interestingly, the return rate was much lower among women who were HIV infected—just 54% (Cartoux et al. 1998). This finding suggests that women who knew or believed themselves to be at high risk for HIV were especially reluctant to be confronted with their HIV status, even in the context of a free intervention that might save their baby from infection. Clearly, with an extremely low proportion of Kenyans aware of their HIV status, the demand for HIV-related care is limited.

Perhaps one of the most graphic illustrations of the denial common even in areas where HIV is extremely prevalent comes from a study in Rusinga, an island in Lake Victoria that is part of the western Kenyan province of Nyanza. Among 1,137 pupils in the last three years of primary school, 34.5% had lost at least one parent, so orphanhood is not a rare event (Ferguson and Johnston 1999). While not all of these deaths have been HIV related, AIDS is overwhelmingly the most common cause of adult death in the area. A supplementary study of 72 children confirmed as AIDS orphans showed that knowledge about AIDS was more or less universal among these children (Johnston and Ferguson 1999). As Figure 7.5 shows, high proportions were also prepared to recognize that AIDS was a problem in the community. The closer the questioning came to home, however, the lower the willingness to acknowledge the impact of the disease. Not one of the 72 AIDS orphans in the study said their parents had died of AIDS. This is a powerful indication of people's willingness to accept the epidemic as long at it is "not in my back yard."

Efforts to break the silence surrounding AIDS in Kenya were given a boost in February 2000, when the government pledged U.S.$80,000 a month's worth of free air time on the country's only nationally broadcast television station for campaigns related to HIV. The country is also sup-

Figure 7.5
Beliefs of AIDS Orphans Concerning AIDS in Their Communities and
Families, Rusinga, Kenya, 1999

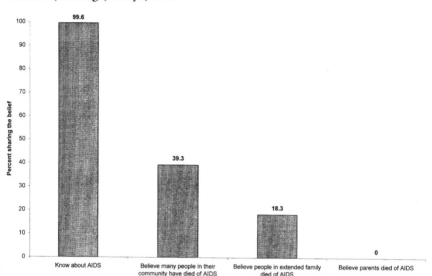

Source: Johnston and Ferguson 1999.

porting research into the integration of voluntary counseling and HIV testing services into primary health services. To date, demand has been low, but
there is evidence that people are more willing to seek testing at health service
sites than in more stigmatized HIV-related service sites (Gilly Arthur, personal communication, March 2000).

In Uganda, active promotion of counseling and voluntary HIV testing
has been successful in increasing the proportion of people in society who
know their HIV status and who can thus act to protect themselves and their
partners while planning for their family's future. These efforts were led by
a nongovernmental organization (NGO), the AIDS Information Center,
and are discussed later in the chapter.

RESPONSE TO HIV/AIDS

National Responses

Falling HIV prevalence rates among young people can only be seen as a
vindication of Uganda's frontal assault on HIV (Nsubuga et al. 1998).
Uganda was the first African country publicly to recognize the gravity of
the threat posed by the AIDS epidemic. In 1986, Ugandan President Yoweri
Museveni stood against the tide of denial engulfing other African nations,

speaking openly about sexual behavior and cultural norms and endorsing condom promotion. Museveni initially faced opposition from religious leaders and other conservative voices in society. But the country, recovering from decades of political turmoil, appeared ready for messages that overturned the old order. Other cabinet ministers fell in behind the president; by 1987 AIDS featured in the speeches of all cabinet ministers, and HIV and AIDS became a regular feature of public discourse. Donors were keen to support Uganda's bold stance against HIV, and funding for HIV programs was readily available (Uganda AIDS Commission 1999). It is difficult to determine how much is spent on HIV and AIDS programs, especially when AIDS-related interventions are integrated into the work of other sectors such as education and industry. One study has tried to estimate spending by looking at the records of both national governments and international development agencies (UNAIDS and Harvard School of Public Health 1999). This study shows that by 1996 Uganda was spending U.S.$37.6 million a year on HIV prevention and care, 93% of it from foreign loans or grants. This figure equates to around U.S.$40 per HIV-infected person: three times as much as Kenya spent. The Ugandan government estimates that it spent U.S.$117 million on HIV/AIDS activities between 1994 and 1996 and predicted spending of U.S.$131 million between 1998 and 2001 (Uganda AIDS Commission 1999).

Active political support for HIV-related activities and the availability of resources encouraged other sectors of society to become involved in efforts to reduce the spread and impact of HIV in Uganda. In 1992, the Uganda AIDS Commission—a statutory body established by act of Parliament and answering directly to the President's Office—was formed to broaden the response to HIV beyond the biomedical. AIDS programs were established within 10 ministries, ranging from defense to justice to gender and community development. NGOs including organizations of people living with HIV were included in the AIDS Commission (Uganda AIDS Commission 1999). Although resistance to sex education and condom promotion from some quarters was initially fierce, religious leaders of all denominations have eventually become active in confronting AIDS. The head of the country's Islamic community, for example, declared a Holy War on HIV as early as 1989. Islamic leaders at all levels were trained to incorporate accurate and nonstigmatizing information about HIV in their religious teachings, and by 1993 they were encouraging condom use as a third-line defense against AIDS after abstinence and faithfulness within marriage (UNAIDS and Islamic Medical Association of Uganda 1998).

Political commitment to confronting AIDS has been slower to develop in Kenya, where HIV was from the start branded a disease of homosexual men and foreigners. By the late 1980s, studies of stored sera taken from female sex workers in Nairobi showed that HIV prevalence had risen from 4% in 1981 to over 80% just two years later (Piot et al. 1987). By 1990, a sentinel surveillance site in western Kenya had recorded HIV prevalence of 19% among pregnant women (NASCOP 1999). The country's leaders were not, however, prepared openly to acknowledge the extent of the threat. Kenya earned U.S.$454 million from tourism in 1995—its single biggest source of foreign exchange (Britannica 2000), and senior politicians were loathe to jeopardize that by putting AIDS high on the national agenda. For the best part of a decade, HIV was a virtually untouchable subject for politicians (Rau and Forsythe 1994). A World Bank appraisal conducted in 1991 noted that Kenya's Ministry of Health was not adequately planning for HIV/AIDS (World Bank 1991).

Many attempts have been made to increase the response to HIV in Kenya. Notably, efforts were made to introduce "Family Life Education," including information on reproductive health and HIV/AIDS into the school curriculum. These efforts met with fierce opposition from parents and from the powerful religious lobby—over two-thirds of Kenyans are practicing Christians—and after three attempts, the efforts were abandoned (Rau 1997). This is perhaps surprising in the light of an evaluation of a family life education program, published while the debate about the virtues of reproductive health education was at its height (Marie Stopes International 1996). The educational program was provided together with reproductive health services to young people aged 16 to 26 engaged in Kenya's Youth Training Service (YTS). Compared with students of the same age in similar vocational colleges who had received no family life education, more young people in YTS colleges reported safe sexual behavior, including prolonged abstinence. This self-reported reduction in risk was reflected in STI rates. College medical records show that where 20% of students in Youth Training Service colleges suffered from STIs in 1990, the proportion dropped by more than half by 1995, after family life education was instituted. In colleges with no special programs, a nearly constant 16% of students were infected with STIs over the five-year period.

In 1997, after two years of debate, the Kenyan Parliament passed a sessional paper on AIDS in Kenya (Kenya 1997). This paper lays out a national policy on HIV, but it does not have the force of law. It recommends establishing a multisectoral national AIDS council, something that was finally budgeted for in 1999–2000. The council was constituted in early 2000. Three years after the sessional paper was passed, however, none of its other provisions had been implemented. These included policies prohibiting pre-employment HIV testing, providing free schooling to AIDS orphans, adopting a national policy to prevent mother-to-child transmission of HIV, and designing a "culturally, morally and scientifically acceptable AIDS education programme for youth in and out of school" (Kenya 1997: 28). Little activity was seen, even though after the sessional paper was passed AIDS became a regular topic for comment in the speeches of Kenyan President Daniel arap Moi. Perhaps in an attempt to encourage implementation, Moi declared

AIDS a national disaster at the end of 1999 (Achieng 1999). This generated a burst of debate about the subject, and for several weeks the media were dominated by discussion of how best to respond to AIDS. There were many calls for greater openness about AIDS, but religious leaders continued to express vocal opposition to any AIDS prevention campaign that promoted condom use (*East African Standard* 2000a). President Moi, himself a devout and conservative Christian, at first concurred that condom promotion would be culturally inappropriate in Kenya. NGOs and international organizations weighed in along with many domestic commentators to plead for a less moralistic and more pragmatic response. Within days, the president reversed his position, declaring that condoms would be actively promoted in the country.

Since its inception, Kenya's National AIDS Control Programme has been placed low in the political hierarchy. It is currently a division of the Ministry of Health, headed by midlevel civil servants. Technical capacity within the program has been limited, and most AIDS prevention activities are driven by donors and executed through local or international NGOs. At the start of 2000, considerable effort was being put into improving the structure of the AIDS program and increasing its technical as well as its administrative capacities. Part of this effort is centered around the creation of the multisectoral National AIDS Council. It remains to be seen whether these efforts will raise the capacity of government institutions to respond to HIV in Kenya. Interestingly, the strategic framework developed by Uganda to guide the national response to HIV between 1998 and 2002 has restructured the Ugandan AIDS Commission, limiting its "multisectoral role." While the commission is still charged with coordinating the national response in different sectors and receives funding directly from the treasury, it now answers on policy matters to the Health Ministry, which has assumed responsibility for HIV/AIDS issues at cabinet level (Uganda AIDS Commission 1999).

There has been little systematic attempt to evaluate the impact of Kenya's response to HIV, although individual donors have attempted to track the success of the projects they fund. One initiative with measurable success is the social marketing of condoms, supported by the U.S. government through Population Services International (PSI). PSI has been marketing Trust brand condoms since 1995, targeting young people in urban areas. By the first quarter of 2000, sales had risen to 1.1 million a month—an 18% rise on the previous year (PSI, John Berman, personal communication). In the 1998 Kenya Demographic and Health Survey (KDHS) (Kenya 1999), 81.9% of Kenyan men and 55.6% of women in urban areas reported that they had heard of Trust condoms, which are widely advertised on television and other media. Time series data for self-reported condom use are not available in Kenya, but cross-sectional data suggest that a high proportion of the rising number of condoms sold are used with casual sex partners. Only 3% of women and 7% of men in the nationally representative KDHS said they had used a condom the last time they had sex with their spouse, while with nonregular partners use was much higher—15% among women and 43% among men. These figures are considerably lower than in Uganda, where 66% of men and 49% of women said they used a condom with their most recent casual partner in 1995—but they almost certainly represent a rise from pre-AIDS days. Despite any advances, however, the figures indicate that an extremely high proportion of sex with casual partners remains unprotected in Kenya.

Neither these figures nor President Moi's commitment to support condom promotion appear to have dented opposition from church leaders. Following the declaration of AIDS as a national emergency, a German company announced plans in early 2000 for a US$2.5 million investment in a condom factory in Kenya (Reuters 2000). These plans were aggressively opposed by the Kenyan Council of Churches and other religious organizations on the basis that opening a condom factory in the country would promote promiscuity (*East African Standard* 2000b).

Nongovernmental Organizations

Even in Uganda where political will created the will and the space to respond to AIDS, much of the work itself has been done by nongovernmental organizations. In 1990, for example, an NGO known as the AIDS Information Center established the continent's first anonymous counseling and testing service. The organization has provided anonymous counseling and HIV testing to 350,000 clients over the last decade. The proportion of those getting tested because they are considering marriage has risen steadily over time, from 6% in 1992 to 33% in 1997 (Turyagyenda 1999). Two-thirds of these men and women came with their prospective partners, and the vast majority tested negative. Indeed, people taking these "precautionary" tests were far less likely to be infected with HIV than people tested for other reasons. In 1997, just 6% of premarital tests were positive, compared to a quarter of clients who chose to be tested for other reasons.

It is difficult to quantify the effects of such services on behavior and harder still to measure an impact on HIV-related stigma. But Uganda visibly differs from other countries where the vast majority of tests are ordered by physicians for diagnostic purposes, usually when a person is already suffering from symptomatic disease. Although data are scarce, it appears that the median survival time from symptomatic AIDS to death in East Africa lies between 9 and 18 months (Boerma et al. 1998). It is not surprising, then, that where diagnostic testing is the norm, a positive HIV test result is equated in the public mind with near-instant death. High demand for voluntary counseling and HIV testing in Uganda results in far earlier diagnosis and far greater potential for positive living among the HIV-infected. Antiretroviral treatment remained virtually nonexistent throughout the late 1990s, and a World

Health Organization (WHO) survey found that management of common opportunistic infections was altogether inadequate. However, large nongovernment organizations such as The AIDS Support Organization (TASO) provide active support for healthy diets and safer sexual behavior and have begun stepping up pressure for better access to care for opportunistic infections.

The lobbying power of TASO and other nongovernmental groups has also contributed significantly to efforts to protect the rights of HIV-infected people in Uganda. The Uganda Network on Law, Ethics and HIV/AIDS has been active in lobbying for stronger property rights for widows and orphans. Members of the network have also invoked the law to protect those who suffer discrimination in the workplace as a result of their HIV status; cases of sexual abuse and violence are also actively prosecuted. The high profile given to prosecution of those abusing the rights of people with AIDS has encouraged others to come forward in defense of their own rights (Mayambala et al. 1998; Nsubuga and Bossa 1996).

It would be wrong to give the impression that Uganda has overcome the stigma associated with AIDS (Uganda AIDS Commission 1999). Most support services are aimed at people of lower socioeconomic status, with the result that AIDS remains particularly stigmatized among the social elite (Okou 1998). While uptake of voluntary HIV testing has risen dramatically in urban areas over the last decade, it remains very low in rural areas. In one study area where free HIV counseling and testing are made universally available, researchers estimate that well under 10% of the population avail themselves of the service (James Whitworth, personal communication). However the vocal engagement of high-profile political, religious, and cultural leaders in combating AIDS and AIDS-related stigma in Uganda has certainly taken the country much further than any of its neighbors in protecting the rights and improving the lives and prospects of people living with the virus and their families.

In Kenya, very few indigenous NGOs have arisen to meet the needs of HIV-affected communities. Those that do exist are often church based, which limits their role in HIV prevention activities, for reasons given above. Church-based organizations are more likely to provide care to people who are already dying and to the families of those who are dead. Many bilateral donors, finding government structures corrupt and inefficient, are seeking to channel funds for HIV prevention and care through NGOs. Because local capacity is limited, this means working principally through large international organizations such as Family Health International and Population Services International. While some of these organizations work to increase local capacity to manage HIV prevention and care services, they tend to be locked into funding cycles that are independent of a community's will or capacity to confront HIV.

One umbrella organization, the Kenya AIDS NGO Consortium, has been working actively to increase the capacity of local organizations to respond to the epidemic. But the conspiracy of silence and denial surrounding AIDS in Kenya continues to undermine the likelihood that community organizations will mobilize effectively to confront the epidemic.

CONCLUSION

Kenya and Uganda have among the most severe AIDS epidemics in the world, surpassed only by the countries of southern Africa. The two heterosexually driven epidemics share common roots, but they have taken different paths. In Uganda, HIV prevalence is still unacceptably high, and high rates of teen pregnancy and STIs indicate that risky sexual behavior remains common. However, under the umbrella of strong political leadership, an extremely active response to the epidemic from different social sectors has succeeded in reducing the stigma associated with the disease. At the end of the twentieth century, Uganda was the only African nation that had clear evidence that HIV prevalence was falling among young people in the general population.

Kenya was slower to respond to the epidemic. There are signs that political commitment to confronting the AIDS epidemic is on the rise, but by mid-2000 these signs were largely confined to rhetoric. HIV prevalence continues to rise in most sites, and at least in some areas of the country, it has reached levels among young people that surpass anything ever recorded in Uganda. As background HIV prevalence rises, the likelihood of one's sexual partner being HIV-infected rises also, so even quite low levels of risk behavior are able to perpetuate the epidemic. To be successful, prevention programs therefore have to achieve ever greater levels of success. And yet important HIV prevention strategies, including condom promotion in rural areas and sexual health education in schools, remain crippled in Kenya by active opposition from politically important constituencies. Unless Kenyan society confronts the HIV epidemic in the same way that Uganda has done, there seems little prospect that it will see a similar downturn in prevalence of the virus in the foreseeable future.

NOTES

1. Comparison between sentinel surveillance and general population data in a number of mature, high-prevalence HIV epidemics in Africa suggests that sentinel surveillance systems underestimate HIV prevalence among women ages 20 to 49, while overestimating it in the smaller group of teenagers. HIV prevalence among men tends to overtake prevalence among women at ages over 35, but for the entire 15–49 age range, HIV prevalence is lower among men than among women. These two effects—underestimation of female prevalence and overestimation of male prevalence—tend to balance out, and estimates of HIV prevalence provided by sentinel

surveillance systems in African epidemics are remarkably similar to prevalence measured in the male and female population as a whole.

2. In this chapter, all prevalence figures refer to adults aged 15 to 49 unless otherwise stated.

BIBLIOGRAPHY

Achieng, Judith. 1999. "President Moi Joins the Campaign against AIDS." *InterPress Services*, 3 December.

Asiimwe-Okiror, Godwil, Alex A. Opio, Joshua Musinguzi, Elizabeth Madraa, George Tembo, and Michael Caraël. 1997. "Change in Sexual Behaviour and Decline in HIV Infection among Young Pregnant Women in Urban Uganda." *AIDS* 11:1757–1763.

Baltazar, G.M., J. Stover, T.M. Okeyo, B.O.N. Hagembe, and K. Mutemi (eds.), 1999. *AIDS in Kenya: Background, Projections, Impact and Interventions*. Nairobi: Kenya National AIDS/STDs Control Programme, Available on the World Wide Web at: http://www.arce.or.ke/nascop/1999pub.html.

Boerma, JTies, Andrew Nunn, and James Whitworth. 1998. "Mortality Impact of the AIDS Epidemic: Evidence from Community Studies in Less Developed Countries." *AIDS* 12 (Supp. 1): S3–S14.

Britannica. 2000. *2000 Britannica Book of the Year*. Chicago: Author.

Cartoux, Michel, Nicolas Meda, Philippe Van de Perre, Maria Louise Newell, Isabelle de Vincenzi, and François Dubís. 1998. "Acceptability of Voluntary HIV Testing by Pregnant Women in Developing Countries: An International Survey." *AIDS* 12: 2489–2493.

Downs, Angela, and Isabelle de Vincenzi. 1996. "Probability of Heterosexual Transmission of HIV: Relationship to the Number of Unprotected Sexual Contacts." *Journal of Acquired Immune Deficiency Syndrome and Human Retrovirology* 11: 388–395.

East African Standard. 2000a. "Catholic Bishop Says AIDS Scourge Created to Boost Condom Sales." 28 January.

———. 2000b. "Church Official Opposes Building of Condom Factory." 14 February.

Egesah, O., M. Ondiege, H. Voeten, et al. 1999. "Sexual Behaviour of Young Adults, Commercial Sex Workers and Their Clients in Nyanza." Presentation of preliminary results, sponsored by Erasmus University, Kisumu.

Erulkar, Annabel, J.P.M. Karueru, George Kaggwa, Nzloki King ola, and Frederick Nyagah. 1998. *Adolescent Experiences and Lifestyles in Central Province, Kenya*. New York: Population Council.

Ferguson, Alan, and Tony Johnston. 1999. *AIDS, Gender and School Drop-out: A Rusinga Island Study*. Nairobi: Population Communication Africa.

Glynn, Judith. 2000. "Sexual Behaviour and HIV Risk in Young Adults in Kisumu, Kenya and Ndola, Zambia." Paper presented at the Conference on Partnership Networks and Spread of HIV and Other Infections, Chiang Mai.

Goldin, Carol. 1994. "Sigmatization and AIDS: Critical Issues in Public Health." *Social Science and Medicine* 39 (9): 1359–1366.

Gray, Ronald H., Maria J. Wawer, David Serwadda, Nelson Sewan Kambo, Chuajun

Li, Frederick Wabwire-Mangen, Lynn Paxton, Noah Kiwanuka, Godfrey Ki-
    gozi, Joseph Korde-Lule, Thomas C. Quinn, Charlotte A. Gaydos, and Denise
    McNairn. 1998. "Population-Based Study of Fertility in Women with HIV-1
    Infection in Uganda." *Lancet* 351(9096): 98–103.
Johnston, Tony, and Alan Ferguson. 1999. *Adolescent AIDS Orphans: A Profile.*
    Nairobi: Population Communication Africa.
Kahindo, Maina, Johnson Nyang, and Jane Chege. 1998. "Multicentre Study on
    Factors Determining the Differential Spread of HIV in Africa—Preliminary
    Results of the Kisumu Site Study (Biomedical Data)." Paper presented at Sec-
    ond National HIV/AIDS/STDs Conference, Nairobi.
Kamali, Anatoli, Lucy Mary Carpenter, James Alexander Grover Whitworth, Robert
    Pool, Anthony Ruberantwan, and Amato Ojwiya. 2000. "Seven-Year Trends
    in HIV-1 Infection Rates, and Changes in Sexual Behaviour, among Adults
    in Rural Uganda." *AIDS* 14 (4): 427–434.
Kelly, Robert, Noah Kiwanuka, Maria J. Wawer, David Serwadala, Nelson K., So-
    wankambo, Fred Webwire-Mangen, Chuanjun Li, Joseph K. Konde-Lule,
    Tom Lutalo, Fred Makumbi, and Ronald H. Gray. 1999. "Age of Male Cir-
    cumcision and Risk of Prevalent HIV Infection in Rural Uganda." *AIDS* 13
    (3): 399–405.
Kenya. 1997. "Sessional Paper No. 4 of 1997 on AIDS in Kenya." Ministry of
    Health. Nairobi: Government Printer.
———. 1999. *Kenya Demographic and Health Survey 1998.* National Council for
    Population and Development. Calverton, MD: Macro International.
Kilian, H.D. Albert, Simon Gregson, Bannet Ndyanabangi, Kenneth Walusaga, Wal-
    ter Kipp, Gudrun Sahlmuller Geoffrey P. Garnett, Godwil Asiimwe-Okiror,
    Geoffrey Kabagambe, Peter Weiss, and Frank von Sonnenburg. 1999. "Re-
    ductions in Risk Behaviour Provide the Most Consistent Explanation for De-
    clining HIV-1 Prevalence in Uganda." *AIDS* 13 (3): 391–398.
Malcolm, Anne, Peter Aggleton, Mario Bronfman, Jane Galvão, Purnima Mane, and
    Jane Verrall. 1998. "HIV-Related Stigmatization and Discrimination: Its
    Forms and Contexts." *Critical Public Health* 8 (4): 347–370.
Marie Stopes International. 1996. "A Family Life Education Programme for Kenyan
    Youth: Assessment of Programme Impact." Nairobi: Author.
Mayambala, Esther, K.Y. Nsugba, R. Mutyaba, et al. 1998. "The Role of the Law
    in Fighting HIV/AIDS: The Case of Uganda." Paper presented at the 12th
    International Conference on HIV/AIDS, Geneva.
Mulder, Daan, Anthony Nunn, Hans-Ulrich Wagner, Anatoli Kamali, and Jane-
    Frances Kengeya-Kayondo. 1994. "HIV-1 Incidence and HIV-Associated
    Mortality in a Rural Ugandan Population Cohort." *AIDS* 8: 87–92.
Musagara, M., S. Musgrave, B. Biryahwaho, et al. 1989. "Seroprevalence of HIV-1
    in Rakai District, Uganda." Paper presented at the Fourth International Con-
    ference on AIDS and Associated Cancers in Africa, Marseille.
National AIDS Control Programme, Kenya (NASCOP). 1999. *AIDS in Kenya.* Nai-
    robi: Author.
National AIDS Control Programme, Kenya and the Population Council. 1999. "The
    Multi-Center Study on Factors Determining Differential Spread of HIV In-
    fection in African Towns. Kisumu: Population-Based and Commercial Sex

Workers Survey Findings." Paper presented at a public dissemination meeting, Nairobi.

Nsubuga, Yusuf, and S.B. Bossa. 1996. "The Cultural, Legal and Ethical Issues in the Wake of HIV/AIDS: Which Way for African Women?" Paper presented at the 11th International Conference on HIV/AIDS, Vancouver.

Nsubuga, Yusuf, John Rwomushana, Elizabeth Madra, et al. 1998. "The Role of Appropriate Policies in the Fight against HIV/AIDS: Uganda's Experiences and the Way Forward." Paper presented at the 12th International Conference on HIV/AIDS, Geneva.

Okou, Richard. 1998. "Coping with HIV/AIDS as an Elite in the Workplace without any Intervention—10 Years Experience of an HIV Positive Bank Employee." Paper presented at the 12th International Conference on HIV/AIDS, Geneva.

Phillips, A.N., C.A. Lee, J. Elford, et al. 1991. "More Rapid Progression to AIDS in Older HIV-Infected people: The Role of CD4+ T-cell Counts." *Journal of Acquired Immune Deficiency Syndrome* 4 (10): 970–975.

Piot, Peter, Francis Plummer, M. Rey, et al. 1987. "Retrospective Seroepidemiology of AIDS Virus Infection in Nairobi Populations." *Journal of Infectious Disease* 155: 1108–1112.

Population Council and Family Health International. 1999. *HIV/AIDS Couselling, Testing, Care and Support Services in Nairobi.* Nairobi: Population Council.

Quinn, C. Thomas, Maria J. Wawer, Nelson Sewankambo, David Serwadda, Chuanjun Li, Fred Wabwire-Mangen, Mary O. Meehan, Thomas Lutalo, Ronald H. Gray, for the Raka Project Study Group 2000. "Viral Load and the Risk of Heterosexual Transmission of HIV-1 among Sex Partners." *New England Journal of Medicine* 342: 921.

Rau, Bill. 1997. *HIV/AIDS Policy in Kenya: A Review of Changes, 1994–1997.* Arlington, VA: AIDSCAP.

Rau, Bill, and Steven Forsythe. 1994. *A Review of Policy Dimensions in Kenya.* Arlington, VA: AIDSCAP.

Reuters. 2000. "German Condom Maker to Build Kenya Factory." 11 February.

Temmerman, Marleen, Jackoniah Ndinya-Achola, Joan Ambani, and Peter Piot. 1995. "The Right Not to Know HIV Test Results." *Lancet* 345: 969–970.

Turyagyenda, James. 1999. "Planning for Marriage and HIV Counselling and Testing in Uganda." Paper presented at the XIth International Conference on AIDS and STDs in Africa, Lusaka.

Uganda AIDS Commission. 1999. *Facts about AIDS.* Kampala: National AIDS Documentation and Information Centre.

UNAIDS and Harvard School of Public Health. 1999. *Level and Flow of National and International Resources for the Response to HIV/AIDS, 1996–1997.* Geneva: UNAIDS.

UNAIDS and Islamic Medical Association of Uganda. 1998. *AIDS Education through Imams: A Spiritually Motivated Community Effort in Uganda.* Geneva: UNAIDS.

UNAIDS/WHO. 1998. *Epidemiological Fact Sheet: Uganda.* Geneva: UNAIDS.

———. 1999. *AIDS Epidemic Update: December 1999.* Geneva: UNAIDS.

———. 2000. *Report on the Global HIV/AIDS Epidemic, June 2000.* Geneva: UNAIDS.

Weiss, Helen, A. Maria Quigley, and Richard J. Hayes. 2000. "Male Circumcision and Risk of HIV Infection in Sub-Saharan Africa: A Systematic Review and Meta-analysis." *AIDS* 14: 2361–2370.

World Bank. 1991. *Kenya: Health Rehabilitation Project.* Washington, DC: Author.

Zaba, Basia, and Simon Gregson 1998. "Measuring the Impact of HIV on Fertility in Africa." *AIDS* 12 (Supp. 1): S41–S50.

8

MEXICO

Roberto Castro and René Leyva

INTRODUCTION

AIDS is one of the most important public health problems in Mexico due
to the growing number of people affected by the epidemic as well as the
heavy social and economic toll that the disease is taking on medical institutions and society as a whole. In this chapter we will discuss the development of the disease since its appearance in Mexico in 1983. First we will
present statistics on AIDS in Mexico. These data will in turn allow us to
form a complete picture regarding how the epidemic has evolved in this
country and what to expect in the immediate future.

Next we concentrate on a description of the social and cultural context
in which the epidemic developed in Mexico. We emphasize various social
processes that are closely linked to AIDS: the dominant cultural dynamics
that work to the detriment of women and minority groups; the processes
of discrimination and paradoxically of support and solidarity toward people
who have AIDS; the massive migration of temporary Mexican workers to
the United States; the situation of women in relationship to AIDS; and the
ways in which health services in Mexico have faced the disease.

Then we describe the principal actions taken on by the state in its efforts
to fight the disease. The emphasis is placed on the educational policies that
have been implemented for the population at large. There is also a discussion
of some of the recent problems faced by the state in implementing its official
policy regarding AIDS.

Another section discusses the role that nongovernmental organizations

(NGOs) have played in Mexico with regard to this disease, identifies the main NGOs that work in the AIDS arena in Mexico, and analyzes some of the principal limitations and difficulties that these organizations face today in their efforts to work more efficiently.

Finally, the chapter concludes with a discussion of the four critical aspects that need to be addressed as priority concerns in future research and public policy concerning AIDS in Mexico.

ISSUES RELATING TO HIV AND AIDS

History of HIV/AIDS

While it has been established that the AIDS epidemic began in Mexico in 1981, the first diagnosed case was not registered until 1983. From that moment on, cases were registered, but it was not until 1997 that there was a computerized database of cases. From 1983 until the end of 1999, 42,762 cases have been registered, at a rate of 43.5 cases for every 100,000 persons in the period mentioned. Nevertheless, this figure is only an estimate of the real magnitude of the epidemic due to the delay in notification and the underreporting of cases (Magis et al. 1998). In 1983, the estimate of underreported cases was 33%, with a backlog of five years on average; in 1999 it was estimated that the System for Epidemiological Surveillance had coverage of 82% of cases and the backlog had been reduced to eight months. This Surveillance System includes studies in hundreds of special populations, undertakes active searches for cases in hospital units, periodically reviews death certificates, and screens donors at blood banks, among other actions that support the accurate reporting of AIDS cases in Mexico (Kuri 1999). Despite these efforts, there is still a significant number of AIDS cases, 26%, that are registered through death certificates, and in some states, this percentage can be as high as 40% (Magis et al. 1998: 237).

The results of Sentinel Surveillance undertaken in 1991–1997 have contributed to the monitoring of HIV infection rates in different groups in the general population and serve as additional information when trying to estimate the magnitude of the problem in the general population in Mexico. The results of these surveys show the differences in HIV prevalence rates by sex. In the groups studied, men predominate, except among prison populations where the numbers are similar (Table 8.1). In 1998 the number of persons infected with HIV was estimated at between 116,000 and 174,000. These estimates take into account the results of HIV detection among donors, sentinel surveillance among pregnant women, and serostatus epidemiological surveys in specific populations (Magis et al. 1998).

The distribution of HIV/AIDS cases in Mexico, according to the cases registered until 1999, is concentrated in three states (the Federal District, State of Mexico, and Jalisco). Fifty percent of all cases have been reported

Table 8.1
HIV Prevalence in Men and Women, Sentinel Surveillance, 1991–1997

Group	Men			Group	Women		
	Prevalence HIV	n	HIV+		Prevalence HIV	n	HIV+
Homosexuals and Bisexuals	15	7,747	1,102	Pregnant	0.09	11,488	10
Sex worker	12.2	872	106	Sex worker	0.35	28,099	98
IV drugs	6	1,099	66	—	—		
Tuberculosis	2.1	1,500	32	Tuberculosis	0.6	1,154	7
Prisoners	1.6	1,538	25	Prisoners	1.4	290	4

Source: Magis et al. 1998: 226–244.

Map 8.1
Distribution of AIDS in Mexico, Cumulative Incidence Rates, 1983–1999

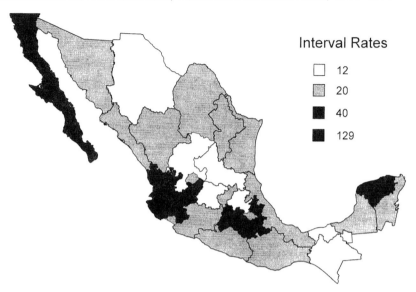

Rate per 100,000 inhabitants.

Source: CONASIDA 2000.

in these three states in the period between 1983 and 1999 (see Map 8.1) even though only 28% of the total population lives there; it is important to note that the main cities in Mexico are in these three states. With respect to the regional distribution, until 1994 only 3.7% of the cases were registered as residents of rural areas (areas with less than 2,500 inhabitants); the majority of cases were concentrated in the major cities in Mexico and in the northern border with the United States, with a higher percentage of cases among men. In the southern part of the country, which is largely rural, the epidemic has a higher proportion of cases among women (21%) than in urban areas (14%). In some states in Mexico, up to 25% of the cases in rural areas involve prior temporary immigration (Magis, del Río, and Valdespino 1995).

In Mexico, 80% of the AIDS cases registered in the beginning of the year 2000 are among persons between 15 and 44 years old; persons under 15 years old represent less than 2% of the total cases. Looking at risk factors, 80% of the cases result from sexual transmission, 18% list the method of transmission as unknown, and perinatal and blood transmissions account for 2.5% of the cases (CONASIDA 2000).

Gradually, AIDS has become one of the major health problems in Mexico. In 1997, Mexico was thirteenth in the world in total number of AIDS cases

Figure 8.1
Trends in AIDS Mortality Proportionally Women/Men, by Place of
Residence, 1988–1997

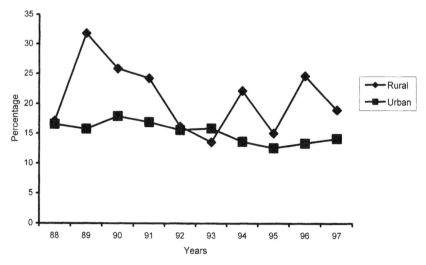

Source: Secretaria de Salud 1998.

and third in the continent; however, when using the cumulative incidence
rate Mexico occupies the sixty-ninth place in the world and twenty-ninth
place in Latin America and the Caribbean. Mexico is considered among the
countries with a very low incidence rate (Magis et al. 1998). It is estimated
that since 1996 the AIDS epidemic in Mexico has stabilized, with an average
of 4,000 new cases every year.

Mortality due to AIDS in Mexico

Until 1992, AIDS was not reported among the most frequent causes of
death in Mexico; however, it has increasingly occupied an important place
among certain age groups and by sex (Izazola et al. 1995). Figure 8.1 indicates the mortality rates for AIDS proportionally for men and women
according to their place of residence (rural and urban areas). This figure
shows that the proportion of women who die from AIDS is smaller in urban
areas than in rural areas. On average, in urban areas 14.5 women died from
AIDS for every 100 men, and in rural areas, 20 women died for every 100
men during the period analyzed. Nevertheless, the distribution of deaths
due to AIDS according to place of residence and sex has not changed for
the period under investigation (Table 8.2). In rural areas (localities with less
than 2,500 inhabitants), women who die from AIDS represent approximately 1%, whereas men in urban areas (localities with greater than 15,000

Table 8.2
AIDS Mortality in Mexico, by Sex and Place of Residence, 1988–1997

Year	Urban[1]		Rural[2]		TOTAL
	Men (%)	Women (%)	Men (%)	Women (%)	(n)
1988	71.9	11.9	6.2	1.1	562
1989	69.0	10.9	4.0	1.3	1,093
1990	68.3	12.3	5.7	1.5	1,500
1991	68.7	11.7	5.3	1.3	2,017
1992	86.5	13.5	5.5	0.9	2,118
1993	73.2	11.6	5.1	0.7	3,162
1994	71.8	9.8	5.4	1.2	3,514
1995	74.1	9.3	5.8	0.9	4,029
1996	71.0	9.5	6.0	1.5	4,369
1997	69.4	9.8	6.8	1.3	4,200

[1]Urban: Included areas with more than 15,000 inhabitants.
[2]Rural: Included areas with less than 2,500 inhabitants.

Source: Secretaria de Salud 1998.

inhabitants) represent 65% of the total deaths due to AIDS in the period studied.

Looking at age as a factor, deaths due to AIDS predominate in persons in the age groups 20–34 and 35–44, which together represent 80% of the deaths due to AIDS in Mexico (see Figure 8.2). During the period 1988–1997, when looking at sex and marital status as factors in deaths due to AIDS, the results show that most of the men who die from AIDS are single. Married women exhibit the highest mortality rates, though this tendency is declining; at the same time, among widowed women the percentage of deaths due to AIDS is increasing (see Figure 8.3).

The Social Context for AIDS in Mexico

Since its appearance in Mexico, various researchers have warned about the social nature of the epidemic. It was obvious from the very beginning that this disease was mobilizing processes of discrimination and stigmatization against diverse minority groups (Castro 1988; Monsiváis 1988) and that many of the social reactions that were developing surrounding the disease were similar to those seen in Mexico with other epidemics, like the plague (Pescador and Bronfman 1989). The mass media, particularly the press, played a pivotal role in the misinformation that ruled the early stages of the epidemic and participated in the spread of prejudice and myths surrounding the disease (Lozano 1994; Pamplona 1989).

Figure 8.2
Percentage Distribution of AIDS Mortality in Mexico, by Age Group,
1988–1997

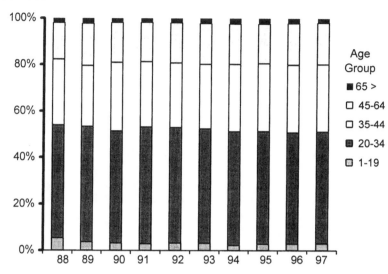

Source: Secretaria de Salud 1998.

Figure 8.3
Trends in AIDS Mortality Rates in Mexico, by Marital Status, 1988–1997

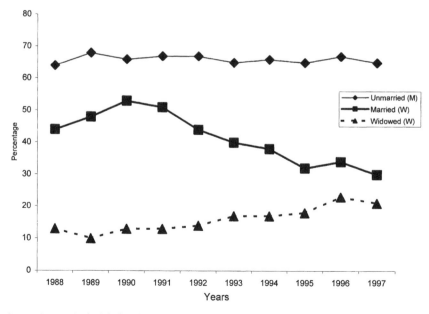

Source: Secretaria de Salud 1998.

Recent research has shown not only that discrimination occurs from hegemonic groups toward minority groups but also that it is reproduced within marginalized groups. That is to say, that within gay groups, and among women in Mexico—groups that are in some ways subordinate to the dominant heterosexuality and to men, respectively—there is discrimination and stigmatization of those who are living with AIDS. These persons are subject to a double marginalization (Castro, Orozco, and Eroza 1996). Fifteen years after the epidemic's appearance in Mexico, it was clear that the defense of human rights is a key piece in any effective public health strategy with regard to AIDS (Rico et al. 1995).

There are a number of myths and beliefs, among diverse sectors of the Mexican population, that function as cultural barriers, making it difficult for people to receive educational messages and adopt safer sex behaviors. For example, a research study among adolescents in a marginalized neighborhood in Mexico City discovered that their religious background favors women's reproductive function as well as a gender identity that is characterized by their orientation toward others. In this type of setting, for a woman to take care of herself, instead of adopting the typical attitude of placing others before herself, translates into a questioning of her own identity that can result in serious intra- and interpersonal conflicts (Rodríguez et al. 1995). Other research has confirmed the need to develop strategies for educational interventions that are sensitive to the cultural and socioeconomic characteristics of the targeted groups (Caballero, Villaseñor, and San Marín 1997).

It has been suggested that the very way in which Mexican men are socialized constitutes in and of itself a major risk factor for HIV/AIDS. Such socialization gives rise to a hegemonic masculinity that associates unsafe sexual practices with a form of "courage" appropriate and expected of "real men" (De Keijzer 1995).

Research has also been conducted concerning the social processes that give rise to both supportive behaviors toward and rejection of people who are living with AIDS. The results indicate that in traditional communities solidarity is borne basically from a culture of kinship, typical of countries with a community orientation such as Mexico. In gay communities, solidarity is based on the types of social networks (of friendship) that individuals may have (Castro, Orozco, Aggleton, et al. 1998). Supportive behaviors toward and rejection of people living with AIDS are social roles that are interchangeable and allow the same person to offer economic support to someone who is sick while at the same time morally rejecting him or her, or allows one person to alternate between being supportive and rejecting the person who is living with AIDS. This pattern varies according to the family history and the resources each family has at their disposal (Castro, Orozco, Eroza et al. 1998). The most important aspect of this research is that it identified critical points, in the course of dealing with the disease for both the patient and his or her family, where specific support interventions could be undertaken by the health services systems as well as the educational and social assistance sectors.

Immigration

Various authors have begun to document the ways in which the AIDS epidemic in Mexico is related to the immigration of undocumented Mexicans to the United States (Bronfman, Sejenovich, and Uribe 1998). This form of immigration is very frequent and is mostly practiced by poor, unemployed Mexicans who are looking to better their economic fate by getting hired as farmhands in jobs that most U.S. citizens scorn.

Immigration to the United States provides a propitious moment for many Mexicans to transform their sexual habits and to adopt behaviors that place them at greater risk for contracting HIV than those that they normally practice in their home country (Bronfman and Minello 1993). These changes are due to various factors: First there is the social context. Places like California, for example, are more sexually permissive than the immigrants' communities of origin. Second is their condition as foreigners who generally immigrate alone, without their families, linked to the undocumented nature of their stay in the United States. Many of them quickly enter into a situation where they are deprived of affection and seek sexual contact, many times occasional contact, as a form of refuge. Third, immigrants are exposed to new sexual practices that were previously unknown or unacceptable in their communities of origin. Finally, the economic exclusion in which many temporary immigrants live drives them to exchange sexual favors for money, food, or lodging, a practice that has been labeled "survival sex" (Bronfman and Rubin-Kurtzman 1999). Research has shown that workers who are temporary immigrants in the United States often use the services of commercial sex workers and that unmarried men are more likely to use a condom than married men, which points to the urgent need for educational strategies that stimulate consistent condom use with occasional sex partners (Organista et al. 1997).

Women and AIDS in Mexico

The situation of Mexican women with regard to AIDS is particularly critical. For a number of years now, the double discrimination that HIV-positive women in Mexico suffer (as women and as persons living with HIV) has been documented and there is an urgent need to defend their human rights (Márquez and Licea 1992; Uribe-Zúñiga, and Panebianco 1997).

As is the case in other countries, there are a host of gender expectations and conditioning that influence this group's vulnerability to the disease. There have been a number of studies with groups of women who are particularly at risk for HIV infection, such as commercial sex workers and partners of polygamous males. Among the first group, it was found that while on many occasions they negotiate condom use during sexual relations, they do so to prevent pregnancy and not to protect themselves from sexually transmitted diseases (STDs) (Allen et al. 1995; Uribe-Zúñiga 1994).

Public AIDS prevention and attention efforts directed at Mexican women have not centered on women as such but rather have seen women as "transmitters" so that the majority of the interventions in this category have made reference to perinatal transmission and to commercial sex workers. To make matter worse, the vast majority of the feminist groups in the country have not adopted AIDS as a central theme in their struggles (Campero and Herrera 2000) despite the fact that given the gender disparities in Mexico, women constitute a group that is particularly vulnerable to this disease. This vulnerability is due not only to biological reasons already outlined in the international literature (Berer and Sunanda 1993; Eng and Butler 1997) but also due to cultural norms and values that regulate in different ways sexual conduct among men and women. The dominant culture in Mexico promotes among men an active sexual conduct where the existence of various partners—simultaneously or throughout one's life—is tacitly approved. Women, on the other hand, must remain virgins until they marry and be faithful and submissive. In this context, it is extremely difficult for them to play an active role in securing their sexual health by, for example, demanding their partner use a condom or that fidelity be reciprocal within the relationship (Liguori 1999; Martina 1994; Salgado 1998). The risk for infection among women by their partners rises due to the high incidence of bisexuality among Mexican men (Carrier 1985; González-Block and Liguori 1992). This is a practice in which only the men who play a "receptive" role see themselves as bisexual or homosexual, while the men who penetrate other men find that this behavior confirms their masculinity and their dominant role in sex.

The Doctor-Patient Relationship and Health Services

Since the beginning of the epidemic in Mexico, patient care for people who are living with AIDS has been an important problem. Studies found that the cost of caring for a patient in 1992 was over U.S.$4,000 annually (Tapia-Conyer 1992), while in 1997 the cost was at least U.S.$1,200 (Saavedra et al. 1997). For patients who do not have access to the public health system, the cost of care becomes another factor in their social exclusion. Public health institutions must bear the burden of treatment costs, which demand that they search for alternative sources of funding for these services.

From the early stages of the epidemic, studies have been undertaken among health care providers to determine their level of knowledge concerning the disease and their attitudes toward people living with AIDS. In the beginning, the levels of misinformation regarding the disease within this population were significantly high (Izazola et al. 1988). Later studies have documented the importance of educational intervention for health care professionals designed to increase the quality of care and have described diverse strategies that are effective in changing the negative attitudes in this population (García et al. 1994).

Despite these efforts, there is still a high level of discrimination toward patients who are HIV-positive in health care institutions in Mexico. The staff in many of the hospitals have not been trained to deal adequately with the notification of an AIDS diagnosis or with patients who have AIDS (Liguori 1994). There are a number of documented cases where medical care was denied or patients were mistreated during their care. The abundance of cases has led to the development of various nongovernmental initiatives to counteract and compensate for the limitations inherent in public health institutions (Castro, Orozco, and Eroza 1997). While the levels of knowledge about AIDS have increased among health care providers, there is still a significantly high percentage of health care professionals who are not willing to provide care to a person who has AIDS (Fusilier et al. 1998). For example, among dentists in Mexico City, one study found that 26% refuse to treat persons living with AIDS (Irigoyen, Zepeda, and López-Cámara 1998).

RESPONSES TO HIV/AIDS

Governmental Efforts in Facing the Epidemic

In the early stages of the epidemic the Mexican government created first informally (1986) and later through a Presidential Decree (1988) the National Council for AIDS Prevention and Control (its acronym in Spanish is CONASIDA—Consejo Nacional para la Prevención y Control del SIDA), whose principal mission is to coordinate all prevention, epidemiological surveillance, and biomedical, clinical, and social research in the battle against AIDS.

CONASIDA has spearheaded various legal reforms that have been crucial in the fight against the epidemic, among these the compulsory monitoring of all blood and plasma units as stipulated in the General Health Law (1986) and the prohibition of the commercialization of blood (1987) and the publication of the Official Mexican Norm for the prevention and control of AIDS in Mexico (1993).

From its start, CONASIDA instigated a massive communication campaign about AIDS, which can be divided over the years into various stages. The first stage (1987–1988) began with polls to determine the general public's level of knowledge about AIDS. A massive educational campaign followed and among other things, looked to legitimize the use of the word *condom*, which at the time was considered "vulgar" by the more conservative circles in the country. These conservative groups found the educational campaign intolerable and argued that the government through its campaign to promote condoms was actually promoting promiscuity. The second stage (1989–1992) began with a consultation with various sectors of diverse groups in society concerned about the epidemic to develop an "intermediate" campaign that combined messages inviting the general population to seek more information about the disease with positive messages that informed about the need to prevent the disease and the importance of condom use (Rico, Bronfman, and del Río 1995). The third phase (1992–1994) developed messages targeting different sectors of society including parents and heads of households and tried to encourage the general population to be supportive of people living with AIDS. Finally, the fourth stage (1995–2000) concentrated on massive campaigns targeting adolescents and seeking to turn schoolteachers and parents into support groups (Pérez, Luna, and Hernández 2000).

At the same time, as the epidemic grew, a social movement developed to pressure the government and demand that it intervene in making access to treatment a reality for everyone living with HIV/AIDS. Approximately half of those living with HIV/AIDS have access to the social security system and thus access to treatment. The other half is completely unprotected. In February 1998, CONASIDA and the National Autonomous University of Mexico created a trusteeship called Fonsida to raise funds earmarked for the purchase of the costly retroviral medications. In June 1999, Fonsida announced that there were close to 1,000 persons in their program. However, in December of the same year, Fonsida made public their real financial situation: They had been unable to raise enough money and their future remains uncertain.

Finally, the government has promoted other types of support, particularly in the biomedical, clinical, epidemiological, and social research arenas with regard to AIDS. These efforts have contributed valuable information in the control of the epidemic, but they are insufficient in terms of the magnitude of the public health problem in the country. The principal objectives established by CONASIDA for the year 2000 included: reducing by 50% the number of cases of children infected with HIV during pregnancy, birth, or nursing; reducing blood transmission of the virus to 0.1%; reducing the incidence of HIV to 2%; increasing condom use by 30%; providing appropriate and timely care to 80% of the people living with HIV and other STDs; and eliminating from the health sector all human rights violations of persons with HIV (Uribe, Magis, and Bravo 1998).

Nongovernmental Organizations Confront AIDS

As soon as AIDS made its appearance in Mexico, various NGOs developed to construct spaces for civil society to organize against and fight the disease. Currently there are more than 300 NGOs throughout the country distributed among most of the 32 states of the republic, but with a high concentration in Mexico City (Colectivo Sol 1999).

As del Río (1998) points out, it is possible to identify four stages in the development of Mexican NGOs that work in the AIDS arena:

1. The first stage (1984–1988) begins with the appearance of the epidemic in Mexico and can be called a *social reaction phase*. The central feature of this stage is the initiative on the part of gay and lesbian groups and sex worker groups to add to their work programs information, prevention, and training in AIDS.
2. The second phase, which runs from 1988 to 1990, is characterized by the development of coordinating committees of NGOs and can be called the *grouping phase*. In this stage, the objectives of the NGOs are information, prevention, and defense of the human rights of people living with AIDS—the battle for civil society to have a greater presence in and influence over public policies and to strengthen their own institutions.
3. The third phase (1991–1993) can be called the *purging and breaking-up stage*. In this period many organizations disappear, but many new groups interested in the topic appear on the scene.
4. Finally, in the fourth stage (1993–2000), both conservative and liberal forces have been consolidated, and a growing number of NGOs dedicated to AIDS have been forming networks.

The origins of these NGOs are varied. In some cases the disease and deaths of certain notable activists in the gay movement led group members to become conscious of the problem and drove them to form NGOs; a similar thing happened in the women's movement. In other cases, the persistent difficulty in finding adequate medical attention drove various citizens to create NGOs that serve both to pressure the authorities to offer these much-needed services and, in some cases, to offer the minimum necessary themselves. Finally, other NGOs have emerged to promote a greater consciousness about the impact of the disease, to train the general population about preventive measures with regard to HIV/AIDS, and to strengthen the fight in favor of sexual, reproductive, labor, and human rights of people living with AIDS.

As time has passed, NGOs have also increased their participation in research activities related to AIDS. In 1994, 20% of the papers presented at national AIDS conventions were presented by NGOs, and they covered such topics as women, human rights, health care and pharmacy personnel, quality of life of persons living with AIDS, patient care, and others (Magis et al. 1995).

There are approximately 30 NGOs in the country dedicated to working on both AIDS issues and women's health. The majority of these organizations first developed with the purpose of defending women's rights, gender equality, and sexual freedom and only later incorporated AIDS into their agendas. Other organizations have centered their work in the defense of health and the rights of commercial sex workers (Hernández and Casanova 1999). A recent study reports that there is an almost absolute absence of organizations created specifically for and by women in relationship to HIV/AIDS. This study also documents that the programs developed by the majority of NGOs that work with women and AIDS continue to target specific populations such as adolescents or commercial sex workers while all but forgetting homemakers and housewives (Herrera and Campero 2000).

Currently, some of the more representative NGOs working on AIDS in Mexico are the following:

- *Ave de México (Mexico City)*. Works on issues of sexuality and prevention.
- *Fundación Mexicana para la Lucha contra el SIDA (Mexico City)*. Focuses its efforts on attention to persons living with AIDS, particularly psychosocial.
- *Colectivo Sol (Mexico City)*. Supports people living with AIDS and disseminates information about AIDS.
- *Frente Nacional de Personas Afectadas por el VIH (Mexico City)*. Works to ensure access to treatment for people living with AIDS.
- *Red Mexicana de Personas que Viven con el VIH (Mexico City)*. Is involved in health promotion and prevention.
- *Amigos contra el SIDA (Mexico City)*. Publishes a magazine for people living with AIDS.
- *Unidad de Atención Psicológica, Sexológica y Educativa para el Crecimiento Personal (Merida)*. Concentrates its efforts on such topics as women and AIDS and has a great deal of influence in the southeastern part of Mexico.
- *Abrazo (Monterrey)*. A radical organization that targets its activities in the struggle against conservative groups and the church in Mexico and has a great deal of influence in the northern part of the country.
- *Checos (Guadalajara)*. Focuses its efforts on attention and support of people living with AIDS and is influential in western Mexico.

The AIDS NGOs (more than 300) in the country have to face diverse problems and opportunities. A recent study concerning the situation of these agencies points out that many of them lack a clear mission and clear goals, which translates into difficulties in trying to consolidate their institutional development (Pérez, Luna, and Hernández 2000). The same study posits other realities: (1) Most NGOs concentrate their efforts on social welfare tasks, and very little is done to force a structural transformation in the public policies concerning AIDS; (2) there is little involvement of persons living with HIV/AIDS in the organization and direction of these NGOs; (3) many NGOs lack a clearly defined target audience, mechanisms for evaluating their work, and adequate salaries for their staff, all of which results in a lack of efficiency in their work; and (4) the "survival" conditions typical of these

NGOs create an atmosphere of intense competition among them, making it difficult for them to develop a solid network of NGOs that could lead to their enrichment.

Special mention must be made of the newspaper supplement *Letra S*, which is currently published by the *La Jornada* newspaper once a month. This supplement, which first appeared on the scene in 1994, has become an important journalistic space that reports diverse scientific, social, and cultural news related to AIDS and that at the same time constitutes a space for expressing the most cutting-edge positions regarding the epidemic and sexuality.

CONCLUSION

Given the panorama described, this final discussion will center on what, in our opinion, constitute the four most important aspects in explaining the path that the epidemic will follow in the near future.

The Problem Regarding AIDS Information

This problem has two parts: on the one hand, the issues of collecting and disseminating epidemiological information about the disease and, on the other hand, the problem of disseminating educational information about the disease. In terms of the first aspect, it is of fundamental importance that the Mexican state, through CONASIDA, improve its systems for the capture, registration, and follow-up of cases of people living with HIV/AIDS and those who have died from AIDS. Information regarding AIDS is being systematically collected in Mexico. However, it is worth asking: How useful is this information in making decisions or prioritizing regarding the epidemic or in developing prevention strategies? In the priorities defined by CONASIDA for the year 2000, all the indicators focus their activities on medical prevention strategies but do not target socially vulnerable groups. The information available does not seem to take priority groups into account when formulating programs or making decisions. The information that is disseminated through their Web page http://www.ssa.gob.mx.conasida can be considered a step forward. However, it is important to think about such spaces in terms of its users so that the Web page responds to their needs in both form and content. Aside from offering a "snapshot" of the AIDS epidemic, this space should include useful information for fund-raising, drawing epidemiological analyses, and making appropriate decisions in the development of local and regional strategies for controlling HIV.

As we pointed out earlier, the official AIDS informational and educational campaigns have gone through various stages that have combined, in varying degrees, aggressive and relatively open strategies with more conservative and ambiguous ones. The fundamental problems that all these campaigns face is the opposition of conservative groups, in particular, ProVida and the Catholic Church. ProVida, an antichoice, anticontraception, antigay organ- ization, and the Church believe that it is inappropriate for the state to take on these topics; they claim that AIDS is above all an issue of morality in society and therefore should be fought with similar measures. Prevention campaigns will be able to have serious impact only to the extent that they openly challenge these conservative positions.

Quality-of-Life Issues for People Living with HIV/AIDS

As is well known, every day the number of people living with HIV/AIDS as a chronic illness is growing. Various social and anthropological investi- gations have documented the economic, emotional, and social difficulties faced by the chronically ill in their daily lives in developed countries. There is growing documentation of the intense suffering in the lives of the "hidden victims" of the epidemic—the wives, daughters, mothers, and all other per- sons involved in accompanying and taking care of the chronically ill. The situation for the chronically ill and those who take care of them is, needless to say, imminently worse in countries like Mexico that do not have the support and counseling services that exist in the so-called developed coun- tries. In the coming years, as the number of chronically ill persons living with HIV/AIDS continues to grow, we will see an increase in social tension regarding this issue. The state and NGOs that work with AIDS will need to develop interventions that offer direct support to this population.

The Problem of Resources and the Relationship between CONASIDA and the NGOs

In the early stages of the epidemic and in response to a recommendation from the World Health Organization, the Mexican government created CONASIDA. In recent years, however, there has been a tendency to weaken this effort, which threatens to undo its accomplishments. One the one hand, there are plans to decentralize this institution in an effort to encourage local health services to assume their responsibilities. On the other hand, the de- cision has been made to lower the profile of this institution by subsuming it as one more division within the Head Office of Epidemiology in the Ministry of Health. Neither decision is in and of itself open to censure; however, they become highly risky, given the conditions under which they happen. Decentralization of CONASIDA could end up merely transferring the AIDS problem to the local level, where it must compete with other problems and other organized groups for the few available resources. This decentralization has not been accompanied by the necessary technical train- ing to assist health professionals at the local level in appropriately addressing the problem. This lack of training has led to the emergence of a series of false "dilemmas" and unnecessary competition for resources. The battle for resources takes place not only within the state. The competition among the diverse NGOs and the various social sectors concerned about the epidemic has frankly begun to take on dangerous nuances. For example, the gay men's movement argues that women are not a priority in the AIDS epidemic. Women, on the other hand, argue that gay groups have received far more support for AIDS programs. Another dilemma that is beginning to gather force has to do with the preference among AIDS funding sources for spending on preventive and educational measures as opposed to spending for retroviral medications to subsidize people living with HIV/AIDS. To the extent that these false alternatives are not uncovered—and one should investigate who stands to gain by them—it will be difficult to build the atmosphere of support and solidarity that is needed for people with HIV/ AIDS.

The Problem of the Link Between the Epidemiology of AIDS and the Public Policies Needed to Fight AIDS

Aside from giving us information about the epidemiological situation, the data obtained from the different HIV/AIDS monitoring systems could also shed light on the relationship between the epidemiological situation and the various initiatives undertaken by different government, nongovernment, national, and international agencies in Mexico. How have governmental and nongovernmental programs contributed to the stabilization of the AIDS epidemic in Mexico? What impact have these initiatives had on the understanding and behavior of the general population with regard to HIV and to people who live with AIDS? These questions and others related to the type, magnitude, and sustainability of a response to AIDS in Mexico are critical in the identification of the course to follow in future AIDS policy in Mexico. Understanding that the AIDS epidemic is *concentrated* in certain groups does not favor the development of strategies that limit information dissemination about the infection to the general public or to groups socially vulnerable to HIV. The quantification of the HIV problem is only useful to the extent that it contributes to qualifying the analysis of the situation. The task at hand is not to generate more information but rather to have better epidemiological information. This information can then be used to better understand the situation and to respond with better practices in a timely fashion and with the greatest benefit possible. The seriousness of the problem demands no less.

BIBLIOGRAPHY

Allen, Betania, María Arana, Roberto Castro, Mauricio Hernández-Avila, Victor Or-
    tíz, and Barbara de Zalduondo. 1995. "La autoimagen de las mujeres que

trabajan en el comercio sexual en la ciudad de México, como determinante de las conductas de riesgo de transmisión del VIH/SIDA" (Self-image in women who work in the sex industry in Mexico City as a determinant of their risk behaviors in HIV/AIDS transmission). Paper presented at the VI National Congress of Research on Public Health, México.

Berer, Marge, and Ray Sunanda. 1993. *Women and HIV/AIDS. An International Resource Book.* London: Pandora.

Bronfman, Mario, and Nelson Minello. 1993. "Hábitos sexuales de los migrantes temporales Mexicanos a los Estados Unidos de América: Prácticas de riesgo para la infección por VIH" (Sexual habits among Mexican temporary immigrants to the United States: Risk behaviors for HIV infection). In *El SIDA en México: Migración, adolescencia y género*, Mario Bronfman, Ana Amuchástegui, Rosa María Martina, Nelson Minello, Martha Rivas, and Gabriela Rodríguez, eds., pp. 19–89. México: Información Profesional Especializada, S.A. de C.V.

Bronfman, Mario, and Jane R. Rubin-Kurtzman. 1999. "Comportamiento sexual de los migrantes Mexicanos temporales a Los Angeles: Prácticas de riesgo para la infección por VIH" (Sexual behaviors among Mexican temporary immigrants to Los Angeles: Risk behaviors for HIV infection). In *México diverso y desigual: Enfoques sociodemográficos*, Beatriz Figueroa Campos, ed. pp. 39–56. México: El Colegio de México, Sociedad Mexicana de Demografía.

Bronfman, Mario, Gisela Sejenovich, and Patricia Uribe. 1998. *Migración y SIDA en México y América Central. Una revisión de la literatura* (AIDS and immigration in Mexico and Central America. A literature review). México: Consejo Nacional para la Prevención y Control del SIDA.

Caballero, Rubén, Martha Villaseñor, and Alfredo San Marín. 1997. "Sources of Information and Their Relationship to the Degree of Knowledge about AIDS in Mexican Adolescents." *Salud Pública de México* 31(4): 351–359.

Campero, Lourdes, and Cristina Herrera. 2000. "Improving Communication Based on the Needs of Latin-American Women in the Face of AIDS." Paper presented at the XIII World Conference on AIDS, Durban.

Carrier, John M. 1985. "Mexican Male Bisexuality." In *Two Lives to Lead: Bisexuality in Men and Women*, F. Klein and T. Wolf, eds., pp. 183–203. New York: Hawthorn Books.

Castro, Roberto. 1988. "Aspectos psicosociales del SIDA: Estigma y prejuicio" (Psychosocial aspects of AIDS: Stigma and prejudice). *Salud Pública de México* 30(4): 629–634.

———. 1989. "La educación como estrategia prioritaria contra el SIDA: Retos y dilemas" (Education as a priority strategy against AIDS: Challenges and dilemmas). In *SIDA, ciencia y sociedad en México*, Jaime Sepúlveda, Mario Bronfman, Guillermo Ruiz, and Estanislao Stanislawski, eds., pp. 413–433. México: Fondo de Cultura Económica.

Castro, Roberto, Emmanuel Orozco, Peter Aggleton, Enrique Eroza, and Juan Jacobo Hernández. 1998. "Family Responses to HIV/AIDS in Mexico." *Social Science and Medicine* 47 (10): 1473–1484.

Castro, Roberto, Emmanuel Orozco, and Enrique Eroza. 1996. "A Qualitative Study on the Household and Community Responses to HIV/AIDS in Mexico."

Paper presented at the III Qualitative Health Research Conference, Bourne-mouth, United Kingdom.

———. 1997. "Patrones de interacción entre enfermos de SIDA y prestadores de servicios de salud en México" (Patterns of interaction between patients with AIDS and health care providers in Mexico). Paper presented at the VII National Congress of Research on Public Health, Cuernavaca, Mexico.

Castro, Roberto, Emanuel Orozco, Enrique Eroza, María Cristina Manca, Juan Jacobo Hernández, and Peter Aggleton. 1998. "AIDS-Related Illness Trajectories in Mexico: Results from a Qualitative Study in Two Marginalized Communities." *AIDS Care: Psychological & Sociomedical Aspects of AIDS/ HIV* 10 (4): 583–598.

Colectivo Sol. 1999. *Directorio de Organizaciones Mexicanas con Trabajo con VIH/ SIDA* (Directory of Mexican Organisations Working in HIV/AIDS). México: Colectivo Sol, AC.

CONASIDA. 2000. Available on the World Wide Web at: http://www.ssa.gob.mx./ conasida/estadis/1999/trim-4/9912–03.htm.

De Keijzer, Benno. 1995. "Morir como hombres. Socialización y mortalidad masculina en México" (Dying like men. Socialization and male mortality in Mexico). Paper presented at the VI National Congress of Research on Public Health, Mexico.

Del Río, Carlos. 1998. *Directorio de Organizaciones no Gubernamentales con Trabajo en SIDA en México* (Directory of Organisations Working in AIDS in Mexico). Mexico: CONASIDA.

Eng, Thomas R., and William T. Butler, eds. 1997. *The Hidden Epidemic.* Washington, DC: National Academy Press.

Fusilier, Marcelline, Michael R. Manning, Armando J. Santini, and Daniel Torres. 1998. "AIDS Knowledge and Attitudes of Health-care Workers in Mexico." *Journal of Social Psychology* 138 (2): 203–210.

García, Lourdes, José Luis Valdespino, Manuel Palacios, José Antonio Izazola, and Jaime Sepúlveda. 1994. "Educación del personal de México sobre el SIDA" (Education for the Mexico staff about AIDS). *Boletin de la Oficina Sanitaria Panamericana* 117 (3): 213–219.

González-Block, Miguel Angel, and Ana Luisa Liguori. 1992. *El SIDA en los estratos socioeconómicos de México* (AIDS in the social-economic strata in Mexico). Mexico: Instituto Nacional de Salud Pública (Perspectivas en Salud Pública, 16).

Hernández, Ana María, and Esther Casanova. 1999. "Las ONG que trabajan con el SIDA y las mujeres" (The NGOs that work with AIDS and women). In *Las organizaciones no gubernamentales Mexicanas y la salud reproductiva*, Soledad González, ed., pp. 97–123. México: El Colegio de México.

Herrera, Cristina, and Lourdes Campero. 2000. "Needs of Latin-American Women in the Face of AIDS and the NGO Response." Paper presented at the XIII World Conference on AIDS, Durban.

Irigoyen, M., M. Zepeda, and V. López-Cámara. 1998. "Factors Associated with Mexico City's Dentists' Willingness to Treat AIDS/HIV-Positive Patients." *Oral Surgery, Oral Medicine, Oral Pathology, Oral Radiology, Endodontics* 86 (2): 169–174.

Izazola, José Antonio, José Luis Valdespino, Mario Mondragón, and Jaime Sepúl-

veda. 1988. "Conocimientos y actitudes sobre el SIDA en el personal médico
y paramédico de instituciones del sector salud en seis ciudades de la República
Mexicana" (Knowledge and attitudes about AIDS in medical and paramedical
staff in health institutions in six cities in the Mexican Republic). Paper presented at the I National Congress on AIDS, Ixtapa, México.

Izazola, José Antonio, Mary Cruz Valdez, Héctor Javier J. Sánchez, and Carlos del
Río. 1995. "La mortalidad por el SIDA en México de 1983–1992. Tendencias
y años perdidos de vida potencial" (Mortality due to AIDS in Mexico 1983–
1992. Tendencies and years of potential life lost). *Salud Pública de México* 37
(2): 140–148.

Kuri Morales, Pablo. 1999. "Fortalecimiento de la vigilancia epidemiológica del
VIH/SIDA" (Strengthening the epidemiological surveillance of HIV/AIDS).
Boletín Epidemiológico Semanal (Semana 02: del 10 al 16 de enero de 1999).
Available on the World Wide Web at: http://www.ssa.gob.mx/conasida/
eventos/prosalud/fortalec.htm.

Liguori, Ana Luisa. 1994. "Más que un número" (More than a number). In *Mujer
y SIDA*, PIEM, pp. 73–81. México: El Colegio de México.

———. 1999. "Las mujeres y el SIDA en México" (Women and AIDS in Mexico).
In *México diverso y desigual. Enfoques sociodemográficos*, Beatriz Figueroa Campos, coord., pp. 31–37. México: El Colegio de México y Sociedad Mexicana
de Demografía.

Lozano, Alicia. 1994. "SIDA, aborto e ideología: Un análisis de prensa" (AIDS,
abortion and ideology: An analysis of the press). In *Mujer y SIDA*, El Programa Interdisciplinario de Estudios de la Mujer, pp. 59–72. México: El Colegio de México.

Magis, Carlos, Enrique Bravo, Luis Anaya, and Patricia Uribe. 1998. "La situación
del SIDA en México a Finales de 1998" (The situation regarding AIDS in
Mexico at the end of 1998). *Enfermedades Infecciosas y Microbiológicas* 18
(18): 226–244.

Magis, Carlos, Carlos del Río, and José Luis Valdespino. 1995. "Casos de SIDA en
el area rural de México" (AIDS cases in rural Mexico). *Salud Pública de México* 37 (6): 615–623.

Magis, Carlos, Raúl Ortíz, Armando Ruiz, Carmen Gómez, Carlos del Río, and
Mario Bronfman. 1995. "Participación de las ONG en la investigación sobre
VIH/SIDA en México" (Participation of NGOs in research about HIV/
AIDS in Mexico). Paper presented at the V National Congress on AIDS,
Mexico.

Márquez, A., and G. Licea. 1992. "Discriminación en México de mujeres seroposi-
tivas" (Discrimination in Mexico of HIV positive women). Paper presented
at the International Congress on AIDS, Amsterdam.

Martina, Rosa María. 1994. "SIDA: El riesgo de ignorar" (AIDS: The risk of not
knowing). In *Mujer y SIDA*, El Programa Interdisciplinario de Estudios de la
Mujer, pp. 41–58. México: El Colegio de México.

Monsiváis, Carlos. 1988. "Las plagas y el amarillismo: Notas sobre el SIDA en Méx-
ico" (Plagues and yellow journalism: News about AIDS in Mexico). In *El
SIDA en México: Los efectos sociales*, Francisco Galván Díaz ed., pp. 117–129.
México: Ediciones de Cultura Popular, S.A., and Universidad Autónoma
Metropolitana-Azcapotzalco.

Organista, K.C., P. Balls, J.E. García de Alba, M.A. Castillo, and L.E. Ureta. 1997. "Survey of Condom-Related Beliefs, Behaviors, and Perceived Social Norms in Mexican Migrant Laborers." *Journal of Community Health* 22 (3): 185–198.

Pamplona, Francisco. 1989. "El SIDA en la prensa en México: Análisis del discurso periodístico" (AIDS in the press in Mexico: An analysis of the journalistic discourse). *In SIDA, ciencia y sociedad en México,* Jaime Sepúlveda, Mario Bronfman, Guillermo Ruiz, and Estanislao Stanislawski, eds., pp. 391–411. México: Fondo de Cultura Económica.

Pérez, Hilda, Anuar Luna, and Juan Jacobo Hernńdez. 2000. *Fortaleciendo nuevos liderazgos y acrecentando las capacidades entre las organizaciones no gubernamentales con trabajo en VIH/SIDA menos favorecidas en los estados en México.* (Strengthening new leaderships and increasing capacities among the weakest nongovernmental organizations working with HIV/AIDS in the Mexican states). México City: Colectivo Sol A.C., The MacArthur Foundation, and the U.S. Embassy in Mexico.

Pescador, Juan Javier, and Mario Bronfman. 1989. "Sociedad y SIDA: Viejas reacciones frente a nuevos problemas" (Society and AIDS: Old reactions to new problems). In *SIDA, ciencia y sociedad en México,* Jaime Sepúlveda, Mario Bronfman, Guillermo Ruiz, and Estanislao Stanislawski, eds., pp. 375–390. México: Fondo de Cultura Económica.

Rico, Blanca, Mario Bronfman, and Carlos del Río. 1995. "Las campañas contra el SIDA en México: ¿Los sonidos del silencio o puentes sobre aguas turbulentas?" (Campaigns against AIDS in Mexico: The sounds of silence or a bridge over troubled waters?). *Salud Pública de México* 37 (6): 643–653.

Rico, Blanca, Patricia Uribe, Silvia Panebianco, and Carlos del Río. 1995. "SIDA y derechos humanos" (AIDS and human rights). *Salud Pública de México* 37(6): 661–668.

Rodríguez, Gabriela, Ana Amuchástegui, Martha Rivas, and Mario Bronfman. 1995. "Mitos y dilemas de los jóvenes en tiempos del SIDA" (Myths and dilemmas for youth in these times of AIDS). In *SIDA, adolescencia y género,* Mario Bronfman, Ana Amuchástegui, Rosa María Martina, Nelson Minello, Martha Rivas, and Gabriela Rodríguez, eds., pp. 91–200. México: Información Profesional Especialiazada, S.A. de C.V.

Saavedra, Jorge, Raúl Molina-Enríquez, Carlos Magis-Rodríguez, María Luisa Gontes-Ballesteros, Carlos Del Río-Chiriboga, and Mario Bronfman. 1997. "Costos de atención del paciente con VIH/SIDA en México" (The costs of caring for a patient with HIV/AIDS in Mexico). Paper presented at the VII National Congress of Research on Public Health, México.

Salgado, Nelly. 1998. "Migración, sexualidad y SIDA en mujeres de origen rural: Sus implicaciones psicosociales" (Immigration, sexuality and AIDS in women of rural origins: Its psychosocial implications). In *Sexualidades en México. Algunas aproximaciones desde la perspectiva de las ciencias sociales,* Ivonne Szasz and Susana Lerner, eds., pp. 155–171. México: El Colegio de México.

Secretaría de Salud. 1998. Available on the World Wide Web at: http://www.ssa.gob.mx/conasida.

Tapia-Conyer, Roberto, Jaime Sepúlveda, Blanca Maria de la Rosa-Montano, and

Arturo Revuelta-Herrera. 1992. "Direct Costs of the Treatment of AIDS in Mexico," *Salud Pública de México* 34 (4): 371–377.

Uribe-Zúñiga, Patricia. 1994. "Prostitución y SIDA" (Prostitution and AIDS). In *Mujer y SIDA*, El Programa Interdisciplinari de Estudios de la Mujer, pp. 113–137. México: El Colegio de México.

Uribe-Zúñiga, Patricia, Carlos Magis-Rodríguez, and Enrique Bravo-García. 1998. "AIDS in Mexico." *Journal of the International Association of Physicians in AIDS Care*. Available on the World Wide Web at: www.thebody.com/iapac/mexico/mexico.html.

Uribe-Zúñiga, Patricia, and Silvia Panebianco. 1997. "Situación de la mujer Mexicana ante la infección por VIH/SIDA" (The situation of the Mexican women with regard to infection with HIV/AIDS). In *Situación de las mujeres y el VIH/SIDA en América Latina*, Blanca Rico, Susana Vandale, Betania Allen, and Ana Luisa Liguori, eds., pp. 125–133. Cuernavaca: Instituto Nacional de Salud Pública.

9

THE NETHERLANDS

Johannes C. Jager and Wien C.M. Limburg

INTRODUCTION

Emerging as a new disease, AIDS was globally recognized as a serious health problem. From the beginning, it has been apparent that AIDS represented not just a biomedical problem but a complex and multidimensional one as well. A range of disciplines would be needed to find effective ways to curb the spread of the disease and to treat its victims. Next to basic research areas (virology, immunology), clinical and epidemiological aspects of HIV/AIDS would need to be considered alongside political, legal and ethical, socio-cultural, and economic aspects. Because it was a communicable disease that was not likely to stop at national borders, it also became clear that scientists, policymakers, caregivers, and patients should cooperate closely.

It was these three elements—multidisciplinarity, internationality, and plurality of people involved—that were explicitly present at the International AIDS Conferences organized by global organizations like the International AIDS Society, the World Health Organization (WHO), and the Joint United Nations Programme on HIV/AIDS (UNAIDS). Never before had a health problem had been approached from the start in such a cooperative and extensive way, facilitated by modern means of international transport and communication. People from the Netherlands figured prominently in the formulation of international coordination frames and brought their research and strategies to combat AIDS to the table. The Netherlands hosted the International AIDS Conference in Amsterdam in 1992 Dutch experts participated in the Working Party on AIDS-Research of the European Community. One soon realized that the HIV/AIDS pandemic was not a homogeneous process without differences between countries; on the contrary, it was composed of many subepidemics that depended on local circumstances and subcultures and required specific, targeted approaches. The Dutch response to HIV has recently been documented and found to be characterized by pragmatism and consensus of all parties involved (Sandfort 1998).

Next to the many specific studies of Dutch experts addressing basic, clinical, epidemiological, or sociocultural aspects, two multidisciplinary scenario studies were carried out, one at a national level (Van den Boom et al. 1992; referred to as the Dutch AIDS Scenario-Study [DAS])[1] and one at the European level. At the end of the first decade of the Dutch AIDS epidemic, the DAS was performed on the epidemiological, economic, and sociocultural impacts of AIDS in the Netherlands up to the year 2000. This scenario project was meant as a feasibility study for a similar one at the European level, the European Concerted Action (CA) on Multinational AIDS Scenarios (MAS).[2] The CA was organized around four Working Groups on Epidemiological Impact, Mathematical Modeling, Economic Impact, and Social Impact. By developing scenarios for the epidemic and its consequences at the national and international levels, both studies aimed to support policymaking (Jager and Van den Boom 1994). In view of the broad scope of these activities, the scenario studies will serve as a basis for structuring the present chapter on HIV/AIDS in the Netherlands. A concise overview on the main epidemiological developments of HIV/AIDS in the Netherlands will be followed by an outline of the economic and social impacts.

ISSUES RELATING TO HIV AND AIDS

Epidemiological Impact

Reported AIDS Cases

The first cases of AIDS in the Netherlands were reported in 1982. An AIDS case reporting system was set up by the Health Care Inspectorate (IGZ), which regularly published epidemiological data (since 1999 on the Web site: http://www.isis.rivm.nl/inf_fbul/). AIDS cases were reported on an anonymous and voluntary basis to the Inspectorate. The definition of AIDS was changed twice, in 1987 and 1994, by inclusion of more AIDS-defining conditions. The changes in definition slightly affected the incidences of reported patients. The reporting system worked rather well and generated regularly up-to-date information on the epidemic, despite underreporting (estimated at 10% to 20%) and a reporting delay. The system included for each case age, gender, and exposure group according to a standard risk groups breakdown in homo/bisexual men, injecting drug users, homo/bisexual men who also inject drugs, hemophiliacs, blood transfusion recipients, mother to child, heterosexual contact, and other or unknown. Mortality was registered by the Statistics Netherlands.

Up to the year 2000, 5,155 AIDS cases were diagnosed and reported (IGZ 2000). This number is substantially lower than the expected cumulative incidence as projected for the year 2000 from the AIDS data observed for the period 1982 up to and including 1990 and even lower than the expected cumulative incidence based on the assumption of no new HIV infections after 1988 (DAS). The majority of AIDS cases reported up to 1, January 2000 were male (88.7%) and adults 13+ (99.0%). The distribution over the risk groups was as follows: homo/bisexual men, 68.6%, injecting drug users, 10.8%; homo/bisexual men who also inject drugs, 0.8%; hemophiliacs, 1.3%; blood transfusion recipients, 1.0%; mother to child, 0.7%; heterosexual contact, 15.2%; and other or unknown, 1.5% (IGZ 2000). By 1999 about 3,500 AIDS patients had died (Hoogenboezem 1999). Until 2000 the most important trends were a decreasing proportion of homo/ bisexual men and slightly increasing proportions of heterosexuals and injecting drug users (IGZ 2000).[3] Since 1996 the course of the AIDS epidemic has been strongly affected by new treatments of HIV-infected persons delaying the onset of AIDS (Termorshuizen and Houweling 1997) and decreasing mortality (Hoogenboezem 1999). Whether the effect of these therapies on the life expectancy of HIV and AIDS patients will be sustained is as yet unknown.

Dutch AIDS figures have been regularly presented to the European Centre for the Epidemiological Monitoring of AIDS (Saint-Maurice, France), which adds a correction for reporting delay (Heisterkamp et al. 1989). Their reports on HIV/AIDS in European countries enable international comparisons. The Netherlands are typical for the north-south pattern. Transmission through homo/bisexual behavior has exceeded by far transmission through intravenous drug use. This pattern still exists, although the contribution of homo/bisexual men decreased steadily. Furthermore, the Netherlands showed a low incidence, like, for instance, Belgium, Denmark, and the United Kingdom (1998 incidence rate of AIDS cases diagnosed per million population adjusted for reporting delays was about 14), whereas Portugal and Spain showed high incidences (1998: about 89) (European Centre for the Epidemiological Monitoring of AIDS 1999).

HIV Epidemic

For epidemiological reasons the complementation of AIDS case reporting with observations on HIV by means of antibody testing (available since 1985) seemed indicated. However, this has not been realized for legal and ethical reasons (for HIV testing policy, see the section "Legislation," later in the chapter). Information was limited to specific HIV data such as from sexually transmitted disease (STD) clinics and local surveillance involving drug users, pregnant women, and homo/bisexual men. The occurrence of HIV in the general population remained hidden. As a consequence, much effort was directed at the theoretical estimation of HIV figures from the reported AIDS cases (tip of the iceberg of HIV infected). Within the framework of the MAS the development of back-calculation methods (from AIDS to HIV) was a major focus of attention (Downs et al. 1997, 2000; Heisterkamp 1995; Heisterkamp et al. 1989). The reconstruction of the HIV epidemic shows a peak in HIV incidence of 8 per 100,000 population in the Netherlands in 1983. A reliable estimation of the current HIV prevalence is lacking. Since HIV tests are available, the treatment of HIV infections has vastly improved; however, since AIDS case reporting does not reflect the hidden HIV epidemic, HIV surveillance is being reconsidered (Termorshuizen and Houweling 1997).

HIV and AIDS Modeling

During the first years of the AIDS epidemic, policymakers and health officials were highly interested in forecasting the future course of the AIDS epidemic, the related burden of disease, and the required health care resources. The early forecasts were subject to great uncertainty (wide confidence intervals) and, as was said above, in retrospect were rather high compared to the actual figures. These differences may have been the result of the extrapolation of an initially exponential trend in AIDS incidence and of effects of prevention. Eventually the course of the AIDS epidemic and its consequences proved far less serious than expected. However, the excessively high predictions inspired mathematical model building accounting for the dynamics of the epidemic (Jager, Heisterkamp, and Brookney 1993). The models have proven especially important for the identification of data needs and answering the what-if scenarios. They allow for medium-term predictions if sufficient data are available. The modeling support of AIDS policy has developed into an advanced field of research (see Kaplan and Brandeau 1994). These developments could be seen as an important spin-off effect of the AIDS epidemic, which might be useful in the emergence of new infectious diseases. In 1992 DAS concluded that although the epidemiological impact remained limited, there is a need for continued efforts in AIDS control. The recent rise in gonorrhea, an indicator of unsafe sexual behavior (Fennema, Cairo, and Coutinho 2000), and the unknown long-term effects of treatment, including resistance and effectiveness (Gezondheidsraad 1998), prove this conclusion to be still valid.

AIDS and the Public Health Forecasts

The Public Health Forecasts (PHF), published regularly, aim to describe the health status of the Dutch population. In the PHF 1997 it is estimated that for the year 1994 for AIDS the number of potential life years lost ranged between 10,000 and 30,000, the weights for seriousness between 0.50 and 1 (scale: 0, no loss of health; 1, maximal loss of health, equivalent to death), and DALYs (disability-adjusted life year) between 10,000 and 30,000. The disease-year equivalents were less than 1,000 (Ruwaard and Kramers 1998).

Economic Impact

Impact on Health Care Utilization

Studies on the economic impact of HIV/AIDS were motivated by the uncertain future development of the epidemic, the fear of a potentially high burden of disease with far-reaching consequences for the health care system, and the need of planning adequate resources. Again, early estimates of the impact were rather high and decreased with the availability of more data and a better understanding of the epidemic.

In the baseline, DAS tried to estimate the patient-related cost for the reference year 1990. For this year the total patient-related costs were estimated at at least DFL51.2 million (1990 U.S. $23.6 million)—86% for hospital care, 6% for out-of-hospital care (nursing home, district nurse, home help, intensive home care, and general practitioners [GP]), and 8% for AZT (azidothymidine) distributed outside the hospital. General program costs (prevention and information, HIV-antibody tests, and research) were estimated at DFL47.3 million (1990 U.S. $21.8 million). The total HIV/AIDS health care costs represented far less than 1% of the total health care costs. In DAS, future scenarios up to the year 2000 were developed, projecting the consequences of survival period, early intervention, and the development of AIDS as a chronic disorder, for the demand and organization of health care.

In MAS, in view of the large share of hospital costs in the total HIV/AIDS–related costs, attention focused on further scenario development concerning the impact on hospital resources in the European Union (EU) (Postma 1998; Postma et al. 1997). Data for individual countries were obtained from local/national databases on patient-related monitoring systems of care utilization and related costs. Dutch data came from the patient-related monitoring system set up for hospital care (Borleffs and Jager 1989; Dijkgraaf 1995). Dijkgraaf constructed longitudinal resource utilization profiles characterized by a pattern of a high use of resources immediately following AIDS diagnosis and just preceding death. In impact assessment and scenario analysis, it appeared to be important to discriminate between several stages in the disease progression (severity-staging concept; see Postma et al. 1997). Data for the so-called chronic stage and the late stage were linked with the outcomes of epidemiological models for the incidence and prevalence of HIV/AIDS (Downs et al. 1997) to construct impact scenarios. It was estimated that for the year 1995 about 8,100 hospital beds would be needed for AIDS patients in the EU (then 12 countries) as a whole, with 52% for the chronic stage and 48% of the late stage. The share for the Netherlands would be less than 2%. New medical treatment and technology will affect such estimates of health care utilization because of changes in disease progression (changing profiles of care utilization) and case mix. Danner (1996), in reflecting on the response of the Dutch health care system to HIV/AIDS over the period 1982 up to 1996, concluded that the health care system in the Netherlands coped adequately with the epidemic. Compared to the impact of a range of chronic diseases, it has been shown for a number of indicators (including direct health care costs) that the impact of AIDS in 1990 was relatively low (Jager et al. 1996). In the PHF 1997 the health care costs of AIDS and HIV infections for the year 1994 were estimated to be less than DFL100 million (1994 U.S.$47 million) (Post and Stokx 1997). The general picture is that HIV/AIDS has had no devastating effect on the health care system; economic aspects did not hamper an adequate response to AIDS. However, the current situation is not stable, as the impact of new therapies and their as yet hidden effects on the course of the HIV epidemic and care demands in later stages of HIV infection are unknown.

Cost-effectiveness of Prevention

In recent years the health economic methods for evaluation of interventions in care and prevention have been generally accepted and applied as a means to support health policy. Because of great differences between countries as to epidemiological patterns and the organization of the health care system, this type of evaluation is to be applied to the local situation. Also in the Netherlands the interest in this approach is growing, and AIDS has been subjected to it. A recent issue concerns screening pregnant women for HIV, which might result in considerable health gains (Coutinho, Hoogkamp-Konstanje, and Danner 1999). Analogous to a cost-effectiveness analysis of such a screening program in London (Postma et al. 1999), the situation in Amsterdam has been analyzed (Postma et al. 2000). The latter study showed a favorable cost-effectiveness with rather low costs per life-year gained through universal HIV screening of pregnant women. The evaluation of HIV screening activities in specific risk groups could make a valuable contribution to an adequate control of AIDS.

Social Impact

Introduction

Central to the understanding of the transmission and spread of HIV is the notion that next to biological determinants, behavioral (e.g., unsafe sex and intravenous drug use) and related social factors (e.g., legislation, ethics, discrimination, stigmatization, prevention, care) play an important role. These factors are to a large extent determined by local circumstances. The objective of this section is to present a brief description of those factors that are regarded as essential to HIV/AIDS control, prevention, and care in the Netherlands. The DAS baseline analysis of sociocultural aspects of AIDS will be used to structure this section. It starts out with an outline of the social context in which the Dutch response to AIDS took shape, to be followed by an overview of the major issues that featured in that response with regard to health care, prevention, policymaking, legislation, and the organizational structures dealing with HIV/AIDS.

Social Context

The DAS identified the following as the main background features of the social context in which AIDS emerged in the early 1980s:

- Sexual behavior of individuals during the various stages of their lives and liberal sexual morals including a generally tolerant attitude toward homosexuality and prostitution.
- Emancipation of gays and a strong and prolific gay movement.
- Increasing numbers of drug users.
- Prostitution becoming larger in scale and more commercial and attracting new groups of prostitutes like drug addicts and foreigners.
- Individualism with an emphasis on individual freedom, self-determination, personal responsibility, and respect for privacy.

At a more institutional level, these background features included the following:

- Health care with a high level of accessibility and already providing specific services for gay men, drug addicts, and prostitutes such as STD clinics, clinics for alcohol and drug abuse treatment, and outreach programs for prostitutes.
- Prevention already targeting gay men and drug addicts by STD campaigns and methadone and syringe exchange programs.
- Policymaking being very much an affair of all parties involved and based on principles like self-regulation, pragmatism, and seeking compromises.
- Legislation with the new constitution incorporating equality and nondiscrimination principles, elaborating the individual rights to privacy and bodily integrity, and obliging the government to promote public health.

Evidently, the features at an individual level affect those at an institutional level, and vice versa.

RESPONSES TO HIV AND AIDS

Health Care

Important principles underlying the Dutch health care system are solidarity and distributive justice; services should be available, accessible, and affordable to all. These principles constitute the backdrop against which governmental policy on AIDS care needs to be seen. From 1987 onward, governmental policy documents emphasize that AIDS care should be incorporated within existing health care and social services. Exclusively AIDS-related facilities were to be considered only if the existing services proved ineffective. AIDS appealed to a wide range of health care sectors including hospitals, nursing homes, district nurses, home help, intensive home care, GPs, and mental health care (DAS).

In line with the advice of the Standing Committee on AIDS of the Health Council (Gezondheidsraad 1987), in 1990, 11 hospitals were designated regional core hospitals, with the Amsterdam Medical Center (AMC) functioning as a national reference hospital (Kamerstuk 19218 nr. 38 1989). Their tasks include providing high-quality, specialized care to AIDS patients, formulating care protocols, acting as centers of experience and information for other hospitals, and conducting research and clinical trials. Regular hospitals can also care for AIDS patients but without receiving extra funds besides the usual rates for AIDS patient care. After 1993 the number of hospital days of AIDS patients showed a steady decline, which was reinforced by a shift to outpatient clinics due to the introduction of combination therapies in 1996.

The core hospitals employ nursing AIDS consultants. Over the years the tasks of the consultant shifted from providing information, psychosocial support, and terminal care to explaining about combination therapy and its consequences and promoting compliance.

Because of the growing need to monitor the rapid scientific advances in antiviral therapies and the importance of close interaction between clinicians, virologists, and immunologists for research and patient care, in 1990 the AMC received a subsidy to set up the National AIDS Therapy Evaluation Center (NATEC) and Virological Evaluation Unit (VEE). In 1998 NATEC/VEE started a national AIDS Therapy Evaluation project to evaluate the guidelines for and the effectiveness of HIV treatment. Twenty-two hospitals including the core hospitals and over 3,000 HIV patients are involved in this project (Lange, Jambroes, and Pakker 2000). The NATEC also participates in international trials, such as DELTA-9-Tetrahydrocannabinol. In 1999 NATEC established the International AIDS Therapy Evaluation Center (IATEC).

All nursing homes may care for AIDS patients, thus enabling the patients to remain nearby their place of residence. The nursing homes receive supplementary funds on a per patient per day basis. In addition, in 1990, 29 nursing homes all over the country were assigned the task to further expertise in nursing home care of AIDS patients. To this end they were awarded extra funds on a yearly basis. An evaluation study carried out in 1995 showed that the availability of nursing home care exceeded the demand with the exception of the nursing homes in the larger cities (Depla and de Lange 1996). As nursing home care for AIDS patients mainly concerns palliative, terminal care, the government considers incorporating it in regular terminal (nursing home) care (Terpstra 1997).

As the health of the HIV/AIDS patient deteriorates, the demand for home help and intensive home care rises. The latter combines professional home care, voluntary care, informal care, and self-help. It allows the patient to stay at home even if admission to a hospital or nursing home is indicated. This policy is in conformity with the government's intention to limit the AIDS patient's stay in hospital by empowering primary care and home care (Kamerstuk 19218 nrs. 8–9 1987).

A high-profile type of voluntary care in the Netherlands is buddy help. Buddies are trained volunteers who give practical, social, and emotional support to people with AIDS and, if needed, to informal caregivers (NCAB 1994). Initially, most buddies were homo/bisexual men caring for homo/bisexual men. The first buddy project was set up for homosexual men by the Schorer Foundation in 1984, to be followed in 1988 by the Rainbow Foundation with a project for drug addicts. In 1992 there existed a national network of about 22 buddy projects, and, because the epidemiological doom scenarios did not come true, with an oversupply in regional areas. With the exception of the exclusively homosexual buddy projects of the Schorer Foundation, the projects have been extended to include heterosexual patients with AIDS. The buddy help shifted from hectic crisis intervention in the 1980s to professionally organized, prolonged, intensive (terminal) care in the early 1990s, to short periods of practical support to promote quality of life in the late 1990s (Galesloot 1999). Approximately 1,700 individual AIDS patients have benefited from buddies, equaling one-third of the entire AIDS population up to 2000.

Patients in need of long-term home care, like HIV/AIDS patients, are entitled to a personal care budget. It allows them to purchase the care services they need from professional and voluntary agencies as well as informal caregivers of their choice.

As the gatekeeper to the health care system, the Dutch GP will often be the first to be consulted about HIV/AIDS and testing. However, most GPs have little experience with HIV/AIDS and tend to refer patients early to specialist services. Some GPs in Amsterdam, with a large population of homosexual men, are more or less specialized in HIV/AIDS care. To secure the care for other patients, they received a subsidy from the government to obtain increased coverage (Danner 1996). GPs may provide pre- and posttest counseling, monitor the patient to determine when to start treatment, and help the patient to comply with the treatment regimen and to cope with the side effects. The Dutch General Practitioners Association has formulated standards of care for HIV/AIDS patients. There is a network of GP experts on AIDS who may be called upon for education, peer consultation, and second opinions (Van Bergen and Wigersma 1998).

From the early days of the epidemic, an AIDS diagnosis has been recognized as a potential cause of severe psychosocial problems—particularly because it is an incurable and fatal disease that affected mainly younger people from socially vulnerable groups. Special services would be required to meet the demand for psychosocial care. Specific target group as well as regular organizations were to provide this care, but ultimately regular services were to be the principal providers (Kamerstuk 19218 nrs. 8–9 1987; nr. 48 1992). The Schorer Foundation, a (mental) health service for homosexual men and women, developed and executed programs for psychosocial care for HIV/AIDS patients and their informal caregivers. Such programs included buddy projects and discussion groups for patients and/ or their relatives. The Netherlands HIV Association (HIV-VN) organizes get-togethers for HIV/AIDS patients. Testing sites of STD clinics and municipal health services (GGDs) and GPs provide pre- and posttest counseling. Regular mental health care services include social services, consultative mental health care, and Regional Institutes for Mental Health Care. The National Committee for AIDS Control (NCAB 1995a) concluded that because of this wide variety of services continuity of care is a matter of concern.

Although not mentioned explicitly in the DAS, the GGDs occupy an important position in the health care for people with HIV/AIDS, in the research on epidemiology and care, and in implementing policy. Under the Law on Collective Prevention in Public Health (WCPV), which came into effect in 1990, health promotion and education activities, prevention interventions, and their funding are transferred from the national government to local governments. They are also in charge of STD clinics and test sites where people can be tested anonymously and receive pre- and posttest counseling.

With Amsterdam as the epicenter of the AIDS epidemic, the Amsterdam Municipal Health Service (GG&GD) has been involved from the start in the control of AIDS. It initiated the Amsterdam Cohort Studies on HIV infections and AIDS, one among homosexual men and one among intravenous drug users (IDUs). They provide data on the prevalence, incidence, and risk factors for HIV infection and AIDS, the natural history of HIV infection, and the effect of interventions and prevention programs. The Cohort Studies are a collaborative effort between the AMC, the Central Laboratory of the Netherlands Red Cross Blood Transfusion Service, and the GG&GD (Coutinho 1998).

The first drugs that really made a difference to people with HIV/AIDS were AZT (1986) and pentamidine (1987) as PCP-prophylaxis (medications to prevent pneumocystis infection). Many other drugs followed with varying success. In the Netherlands the registration of new drugs is bound by legal rules and regulations and may take quite some time. However, actions of the HIV-VN, the AIDS Fund, and Act Up led to early, accelerated introduction and compassionate use programs for a number of (unlicensed) AIDS/HIV drugs.

Prevention

From the start, prevention has been a major focus of attention in the fight against AIDS in the Netherlands.[4] DAS mentions the following target groups: homosexual men, young people, migrants, (customers of) prostitutes, drug addicts, health professionals, hemophiliacs, blood donors, people working/traveling in HIV high prevalence areas, tourists, and the general population. The first campaigns were directed exclusively at specific risk groups and organized by categorical organizations for homosexual men and drug addicts. Mass media campaigns initiated by the central government and targeted at the general population followed. Still later, mass media campaigns served as a so-called umbrella under which small-scale specifically targeted campaigns took place. Several campaigns address specific issues like AIDS and work, safe sex (on holiday), needle exchange, blood safety, and needle-stick accidents. The main objectives of the campaigns have been raising the level of knowledge, attaining behavioral change, preventing discrimination and stigmatization, and creating compassion. Initially the activities were HIV/AIDS specific, to be later incorporated in general STD campaigns. Major preventive activities are information and help lines, journals published by gay and HIV/AIDS organizations, television and radio advertisements, posters, leaflets, educational programs for secondary school pupils, outreach activities toward young people and prostitutes, availability of HIV tests, counseling, needle exchange programs, and hygiene measures for health professionals.

The first AIDS campaign in the Netherlands was executed in 1983 and targeted at homosexual men. The main objective was to make them refrain voluntarily from donating blood to warrant blood safety. The blood bank, the Ancillary Services Department (SAD), the Cultural Relaxation Center (COC) gay organization, and the GG&GD organized the campaign. It was followed by numerous prevention activities targeted at homosexual men. Initially, the message was dual in that it urged homosexual men to abstain from anal sex or to use a condom. This message was part of the Dutch policy from 1984 till 1992 (De Zwart, Sandfort, and van Kerkhof 1998). However, in time the abstinence message met with a lot of opposition and became untenable. In other European countries the message focused on the use of condoms only.

Small group activities included workshops on homosexual health issues and unsafe sex (the Safe Sex Video Shows, the Condom Workshop). Outreach activities took place in cruising areas and in gay bars and discos. Through semiprofessional shows and the distribution of safe sex kits, Safe Sex Promotion Teams sought to bring about and sustain behavioral changes in their homosexual audience.

An important source of information has been the periodical *AIDS-info* (1984–1993) and its successor *LUST for LIFE*. As an insert in gay journals, it informed their readers about the latest developments in AIDS policy, treatment, and prevention, and at times, it took a highly critical stand (Hospers and Bloem 1998). The periodicals *Aids, de stand van zaken*, and *Aids-Bestrijding*, published by the AIDS Fund, cover similar topics and address the general public and people professionally involved in AIDS policy, respectively. HIV/AIDS information helplines were set up by the National Committee for AIDS Control (NCAB), the AIDS Fund, and the HIV-VN. They offer their callers information and support on an anonymous basis.

The growing awareness that AIDS posed a potential threat to the public at large induced the government in 1987 to instigate a series of mass media campaigns on "safe sex." The first campaign was designed to inform the general public and to make condom use socially acceptable. This effort was followed by campaigns targeted at young people, like the "Safe Sex on Holidays" campaign, the "Excuses" campaign, which addressed the gap between intention and actual behavior, and the "Cupid" campaign in discos targeted at young people with a low educational level. Later campaigns under the heading of "Safe Sex or No Sex" explicitly promoted the use of condoms, thereby aiming to reinforce safe sex as the social norm and to improve practical and social skills for safe sex. They integrated AIDS prevention and STD prevention activities (Kok et al. 1998; Van Hasselt, de De Vroome, and Sandfort 1999).

Preventive activities targeted at IDUs include needle exchange programs and the supply of methadone, information leaflets, and outreach programs for drug-addicted prostitutes (Van Ameijden and van den Hoek 1998). The supply of methadone as an indirect form of STD control preceded the onset of the AIDS epidemic. The first needle exchange program was introduced in Amsterdam in 1984.

Prostitution is one of the sources of heterosexual HIV transmission. Preventive interventions targeted at drug addicts and migrants are relevant here. Small-scale activities included outreach programs for streetwalkers. Campaigns aimed to reinforce safe sex through condom use as the social norm (Vanwesenbeeck and de Graaf 1998).

In the late 1980s the NCAB initiated the first AIDS prevention program targeted at migrants. The program was not so much inspired by epidemiological data as by the fact that because of linguistic and cultural barriers Dutch campaigns were little known or even misunderstood by migrants and that many migrants originated from AIDS endemic countries (Singels 1998). Its objectives were similar to those of the Dutch campaigns, that is, raising awareness, increasing knowledge, and bringing about behavioral changes. Later prevention activities were targeted at all migrants, not just those at risk, and migrant organizations participated to promote social acceptability and accessibility of the campaigns. To maximize the impact of the activities the cultural background of the different migrant populations was taken into account, native languages were used, and information was disseminated through migrant information channels (Van Haastrecht 1999).

Partner notification as an HIV/AIDS prevention strategy has never been actively promoted in the Netherlands (NCAB 1995b). As with testing, the absence of an effective treatment and the potentially adverse consequences of the knowledge of having HIV/AIDS led to a restrictive policy. New, early treatment modalities have loosened that policy but only to the extent that during posttest counseling partner notification is discussed and may be offered as a service. Without the patient's consent, partner notification is both practically and legally hardly feasible. Health care professionals are bound by professional secrecy and may only breach this secrecy under the strictest conditions.

Thus, the Dutch prevention campaigns involved a wide range of activities targeted at the general population and numerous risk groups, with a variety of objectives and with a great number of organizations engaged in their design and execution. Over the past two decades, preventive efforts have been huge and highly intensive. Undoubtedly, they will have had an effect—but to what extent is hard to estimate, as evaluation of prevention activities is not common practice and methodologically extremely complicated. They certainly raised the levels of awareness and knowledge of their target groups concerning AIDS and HIV and preventive behavior. However, bringing about and sustaining behavioral changes will need constant attention.

Policy

During the first years of the AIDS epidemic the Dutch government refrained from any active involvement in developing and implementing a policy regarding AIDS. Because of a growing awareness that AIDS might pose a serious threat to public health, the government decided in 1987 to adopt a more active role (Kamerstuk 19218 nrs. 8–9 1987). Key issues pertain to information and prevention, care, AIDS and drugs policy, research, legal and ethical aspects, international cooperation, and finance. The AIDS policy has been characterized as aiming for normalization; that is, AIDS is to be considered a serious and difficult but ultimately not exceptional problem that should be dealt with within the framework of existing institutions (Van den Boom and Schnabel 1998). By 1991 it had become clear that AIDS was not going to be the epidemic that had been feared. The *AIDS Policy in the Netherlands; Progress Report* (Kamerstuk 19218 nr. 48 1992) presents a program of action for the next few years. Central to this program is the role of the government as setting out the main lines and creating general conditions for societal organizations and local authorities to work out the practical details of effective action against AIDS.

Since the introduction of new therapies in 1996 the prognosis of persons infected with HIV or AIDS has changed dramatically. AIDS is said to have become a chronic disease. But there is still no cure, and AIDS is still a lethal disease. In its factsheet (Ministerie 1997), the Ministry of Health points out that the main goals of AIDS policy still stand: to prevent the spread of AIDS, to offer good care to persons with HIV/AIDS, to fight against discrimination and stigmatization, and to promote scientific research. The role of the Ministry remains the same: to integrate the contribution of the various actors in the field.

Legislation

In the Netherlands the legal and ethical debate about HIV/AIDS has been influenced by various simultaneous developments. From the 1960s onward the role of the patient in health care has changed. Relevant changes are the emancipation of the patient, the increasingly important role of patient organizations in health care (policy), and the social position of ill people. In addition, health care became very much a focus of ethical and legal attention (Markenstein 1999). HIV/AIDS relevant issues include the balance between social and individual rights in decisions on, for example, surveillance and testing, the doctor-patient relationship, informed consent, and the ownership of medical data and bodily material. Although these issues have played a prominent role in the debate preceding the adoption of various laws in the 1980s and 1990s, HIV and AIDS are governed by the same laws and regulations as other diseases.

The adoption of the new constitution in 1983 was an important feat in the recognition of individual rights. The equality and nondiscrimination principles are elaborated in Article 1, and the individual rights to privacy and bodily integrity in Articles 10 and 11, respectively (DAS; Veenker 1998). These rights were subsequently incorporated in the Medical Contract Act (WGBO), the Medical Examination Act (WMK), the Personal Data Protection Act (WPR), the Population Screening Act (WBO), and the Medical Research Involving Human Subjects Act (WMO). These acts are relevant to HIV/AIDS. The WGBO, put into effect in 1995, covers all voluntary relationships between patient and health professional regarding medical and obstetric treatment, including medical examination. Under the WGBO, treatment requires the patient's informed consent; the doctor has the duty to inform; the patient has the right not to know; the patient has the right to confidentiality; and regarding scientific research, the patient has the right to the protection of privacy. The WMK, put into effect in 1998, regulates medical examinations in other than voluntary situations, for example, when applying for a job or insurance. The WPR protects the individual from unduly disclosure and use of personal data for purposes other than consented to and collected for. The WBO, put into effect in 1996, aims to protect individuals against potential dangers of population screening. If there is a risk of inducing physical or mental harm, for example, screening for a serious, incurable illness, it requires the permission of the Health Council. The WMO, put into effect in 1999, regulates the review of planned medical research involving human subjects by a recognized review committee to protect the legal position of the subjects (Ministerie 2000).

HIV/AIDS has not been included in the Infectious Diseases Act (IZW). This law allows the government to enforce measures to prevent or curtail the spread of an infectious disease in the interest of public health even if it involves taking actions that impinge on the constitutional rights of individuals. It contains a list of diseases that doctors and laboratories are obliged to report to the authorities (Dute and van Wijngaarden 1999). The decision not to include HIV/AIDS in the list (1983) was based on the considerations that in the absence of a cure the only way to curtail the spread of the disease was prevention and that since AIDS then seemed to be a gay disease, discrimination and stigmatization needed to be avoided.

From the beginning of the epidemic, one of the major ethical, legal, and political issues has been testing, whether for scientific purposes, taking out an insurance policy, or as part of a job assessment procedure. Until the introduction of the combination therapy in the late 1990s, the policy regarding testing was restrictive in nature. In the absence of an effective treatment, the cons of testing were thought to prevail over the pros. At a personal level, knowing that one is HIV-positive or has AIDS may cause severe mental stress; at a social level, it may lead to discrimination and stigmatization and affect the accessibility of insurance or work. Moreover, since a negative test result is valid only at a particular moment, it may give a false sense of security and make people become less cautious (Kamerstuk 19218 nrs. 8–9 1987). In the Netherlands, informed consent, privacy protection, and a medical indication are prerequisites to testing (WGBO, WMK). The person tested has the right not to know the outcome of the test. Blood donation is the only exception to the right not to know. When a blood bank finds a donor to be HIV-infected, the donor will be informed (Van den Boom and Schnabel 1998).

In the Netherlands, epidemiological research on HIV/AIDS is considered of great importance, but its execution has been hampered by the restrictive testing policy (Van den Boom et al. 1990). In the discussion about the individual versus social interests, the former prevailed. Anonymous screening of blood samples was refused (Akveld et al. 1990). As a result, mathematical modeling of the epidemic did become a focus of attention, and research based on HIV surveillance is presently being reconsidered.

The debate on insurance and testing concerned in particular life and supplementary work disability insurance. Health insurance is in principle accessible to everybody. Because of a short life expectancy, insurance companies considered people with HIV/AIDS too big a financial risk with consequently too high a premium to be feasible and too little opportunity for spreading the risk by underwriting. They also feared for autoselection. The government appreciated the considerations of the insurance companies (Kamerstuk 19218 nr. 10 1987; Kamerstuk 19218 nr. 41 1990; Kamerstuk 19218 nr. 49 1992). Eventually a code of conduct was adopted, stating when a medical examination and an HIV test are warranted (Kamerstuk 19128 nr. 54 1992). This code of conduct was later incorporated into the WMK. In practice, people with HIV/AIDS are still virtually excluded from life insurance and, if self-employed, from work disability insurance.

When testing as part of a job selection procedure became a public topic in the 1980s, there was more or less consensus on procedural matters concerning medical examination and its goal, the applicant's privacy and medical secrecy, and a person's past diseases or possible future absenteeism. Being HIV-positive was no ground for rejecting an applicant, and an HIV test was not allowed (Kamerstuk 19218 nrs. 15–16 1988; Kamerstuk 19218 nr. 40 1990; Kamerstuk 19218 nr. 45 1991). The WMK provides a legal basis to that consensus. It stipulates that medical examinations are limited in their character, contents, and size by the goal they serve and that data obtained by examinations may be used for that goal only. A medical examination of a job applicant is allowed only if the job makes special demands on the medical suitability, and the employer already intends to take on the applicant.

Since the introduction of combination therapy, there has been a lot of debate about changing testing policy. If starting as soon as possible with the therapy was to postpone the onset of AIDS, it no longer holds that the cons always prevail over the pros. According to the AIDS Fund, from a medical point of view, testing on HIV antibodies is to be promoted actively (Van der Kroef 1998). The Health Council is also in favor of a less restrictive testing policy, especially when it concerns pregnant women with an (un)certain risk status and people who belong to high-risk groups. Testing for insurance purposes should be as restrictive as possible (Gezondheidsraad 1999).

Organizations

Local initiatives of the GG&GD, gay organizations, health information and education organizations, blood bank, and the Netherlands Association of Hemophiliacs (NVHP) led in 1983 to the establishment of the National AIDS Policy Coordination Team. The IGZ and the National Institute of Public Health and the Environment (RIVM) also participated on the team. The main tasks of the Coordination Team were to provide adequate information and education to risk groups and interested parties, to develop AIDS policy, to maintain consensus regarding an integrated policy by optimum communication, and to coordinate the provision of information to the general public.

The Coordination Team strongly promoted the development of AIDS Platforms. The Platforms are consultative structures in which local and regional groups, organizations, and establishments involved in action against AIDS work closely together (Ministry 1994). Their main aim is to implement national policies at a local and regional level. In doing so, they focus primarily on coordinating activities, social care, and psychosocial counseling. Under the WCPV, the GGDs are responsible for the Platforms. There are about 40 local and regional AIDS Platforms.

By 1987 it had become clear that AIDS posed a potential threat to society at large and that a national policy was required. The government established the NCAB to succeed the Coordination Team. Its tasks were twofold: to advise the government, solicited or unsolicited, on policy matters regarding AIDS and to perform tasks assigned to them by the government. It consisted of experts rather than representatives of interest groups, thus limiting the influence of gay groups (Van den Boom and Schnabel 1998). The NCAB was a network organization that cooperated closely with local, regional, and national organizations, thus assuring a broad basis for policy implementation.

When the NCAB's mandate came to an end in 1994, its tasks were taken over by the AIDS Fund and regular organizations like the Netherlands Institute for Alcohol and Drugs (NIAD) and the Foundation for STD Control (SOA-stichting). The AIDS Fund was set up in 1985 to raise funds for scientific research and to provide financial support to affected persons. Its present goals are to support and promote politically, financially, and organizationally activities to prevent and control HIV infection and AIDS and all related physical, psychological, and social consequences and to support international cooperation. It also manages government funds for AIDS-related research and projects.

Established in 1984, the Program Committee AIDS (PCA) of the National Health Council was assigned the task of advising the government on scientific and medical matters concerning AIDS.

The Program coordination committee on AIDS-research (PccAo) was established by the Health Research Council (RGO) (1988) in answer to the intention to promote AIDS research as formulated in the Memorandum on AIDS Control of 1987 (Kamerstuk 19218 nr. 48 1992). Its tasks were to design a sound multidisciplinary research program thereby ensuring an efficient use of resources, and to promote close cooperation between the different researchers and between researchers and consumers of research. With government funds it instigated the Stimulating Program AIDS-Research, which included the Amsterdam Cohort Studies. After being housed with the AIDS Fund, their tasks were taken over by the Scientific Advisory Board of the AIDS Fund in 1998. Funding and programming of AIDS research is also taken care of by general institutions for health services research (Health Services Research the Netherlands [ZON]) and fundamental research (Netherlands Organisation for Scientific Research [NWO]).

The HIV-VN is an interest organization of HIV-infected persons. It organizes self-help groups, parents' evenings, and opportunities to meet fellow patients to enhance the quality of life of infected persons.

Next to the specific HIV and AIDS organizations, there have been a considerable number of organizations involved in the fight against AIDS. Just to name a few: the Foundation for STD Control (SOA-stichting), the SAD-Schorer Foundation, the Rutgers Foundation, the National and Amsterdam Centers for Health Education, the Dutch Society for the Integration of Homosexuality/Cultural Relaxation Center (NVIH/COC), Netherlands Institute for Social Sexological Research (NISSO), Netherlands Institute for Care and Welfare (NIZW), and the National Association of General Practitioners (LHV).

CONCLUSION

In the Netherlands the HIV/AIDS epidemic has had a limited epidemiological impact and lagged behind the grim projections. The dynamics of the HIV epidemic can no longer be derived from the AIDS incidence, due to the effects of new therapeutic interventions and preventive activities. An adequate control of the AIDS epidemic continues to require detailed research and sustained vigilance.

From an economic point of view, the HIV/AIDS epidemic did not have a disrupting effect on the care system. The demand for care could be met in a satisfactory way, and care was accessible to all. Still, there is no clear picture of the exact costs involved in out-of-hospital care and prevention. The study of the cost-effectiveness of health care interventions needs to be extended to ensure a sound budget allocation and effective HIV/AIDS control.

AIDS prompted an extensive response in the fields of health care, prevention, and related legislation and policymaking, involving a large number of organizations. In time, the initially AIDS-specific approach has been brought in line with general practices. Important aspects in this process have been identified such as personal versus social rights. HIV/AIDS has contributed to the emancipation of the patient and patient organizations, it has added to the diversification of health care and prevention, and it has played an important role in the debate preceding new health legislation.

NOTES

1. DAS was commissioned by the Steering Committee on Future Health Scenarios (STG), an advisory committee of the Dutch Ministry of Health, and supervised by a multidisciplinary committee chaired by E.J. Ruitenberg. A summary of DAS was included in the government Memorandum on AIDS (Kamerstuk 19218 nr. 48 1992).

2. MAS was funded by the European Commission (contract BMH1-CT-1723) and coordinated by the National Institute of Public Health and the Environment. Papers resulting from the activities are listed in the final report by Jager and Ruitenberg (1997).

3. For a detailed discussion of AIDS surveillance in the Netherlands, see Houweling (1997: 88–105).

4. For an overview of the prevention campaigns see Sandfort (1998).

BIBLIOGRAPHY

Akveld, J.E.M., H.E.G. Hermans, L.H. Lumey, H. Houweling, J.C. Jager, and L. Wan. 1990. *AIDS en anoniem onderzoek: Juridische en epidemiologische aspecten* (AIDS and anonymous research: Legal and epidemiological aspects). Lelystad: Vermande BV.

Borleffs, J.C.C., and J.C. Jager. 1989. "Registratie en kostenschatting van klinische en poliklinische werkzaamheden voor patiënten met HIV-infectie" (Registration and estimation of costs of clinical and outpatient clinical activities for HIV-infected patients). *Nederlands Tijdschrift voor Geneeskunde* 133: 767–772.

Borst-Eilers, E. 1999. "Herziening HIV-testbeleid" (Revision of HIV testing policy). Brief aan de voorzitter van de Gezondheidsraad. *GZB/GZ* 1.002.028.

Coutinho, Roel A. 1998. "The Amsterdam Cohort Studies on HIV Infection and AIDS." *Journal of AIDS and Human Retrovirology* 17 (Supp. 1): S4–S8.

Coutinho, R.A., J.A.A. Hoogkamp-Korstanje, and S.A. Danner. 1999. "Therapeutische mogelijkheden bij HIV-infectie nopen tot verruiming van het HIV-testbeleid" (Therapeutic possibilities of HIV infection induce a liberalization of HIV testing policy). *Nederlands Tijdschrift voor Geneeskunde* 143(12): 598–599.

Danner, Sven A. 1996. "Health Care System in Transition: The Netherlands. Part II: The Response of the Dutch Health Care System to HIV-AIDS." *Journal of Public Health Medicine* 18 (3): 285–288.

Depla, Marja, and Jacomine de Lange. 1996. "Verpleeghuiszorg voor mensen met AIDS" (Nursing home care for people with AIDS). *Tijdschrift voor Sociale Gezondheidszorg* 74 (6): 341–346.

De Zwart, Onno, Theo Sandfort, and Marty van Kerkhof. 1998. "No Anal Sex Please: We're Dutch. A Dilemma in HIV Prevention Directed at Gay Men."

In *The Dutch Response to HIV Pragmatism and Consensus*, Theo Sandfort, ed., pp. 135–152. London: UCL Press.

Dijkgraaf, Marcel G.W. 1995. *Utilization of Hospital Resources and the Costs Related to HIV Infection*. Amsterdam: Thesis Publishers. (Thesis)

Downs, Angela M., Siem H. Heisterkamp, Jean-Baptiste Brunet, and Françoise F. Hamers. 1997. "Reconstruction and Prediction of the HIV/AIDS Epidemic among Adults in the European Union and in the Low Prevalence Countries of Central and Eastern Europe." *AIDS* 11: 649–662.

Downs, Angela M., Siem H. Heisterkamp, Lucilla Ravà, Hans Houweling, Johannes C. Jager, and Françoise F. Hamers for the European Union Concerted Action on Multinational AIDS Scenarios. 2000. "Back-Calculation by Birth Cohort, Incorporating Age-Specific Disease Progression, Pre-AIDS Mortality and Change in European AIDS Case Definition." *AIDS* 14: 2179–2189.

Dute, J.C.J., and J.K. van Wijngaarden. 1999. "Infectieziektenwet: Nieuwe wetgeving voor infectieziektenbestrijding" (Infectious Diseases Act: New legislation for infectious diseases control). *Nederlands Tijdschrift voor Geneeskunde* 143: 1049–1053.

European Centre for the Epidemiological Monitoring of AIDS. 1999. "HIV/AIDS Surveillance in Europe." *Report* 61: 8–9.

Fennema, J.S.A., I. Cairo, and R.A. Coutinho. 2000. "Sterke toename van gonorroe en syfilis onder bezoekers van de Amsterdamse SOA-polikliniek" (Strong increase in gonorrhea and syphilis among visitors of the Amsterdam STD-outpatient clinic). *Nederlands Tijdschrift voor Geneeskunde* 144: 602–603.

Galesloot, Hansje. 1999. *Vriendschap voor een vreemde; vijftien jaar buddyzorg aan mensen met HIV en AIDS* (Friendship for a stranger; fifteen years of buddy care for people with HIV and AIDS). Amsterdam: Schorer Boeken.

Gezondheidsraad: Beraadsgroep Infectie en Immuniteit. 1998. *Resistentievorming bij het gebruik van HIV-remmende geneesmiddelen* (Development of resistance with the use of HIV-inhibiting drugs). Den Haag: Gezondheidsraad.

———. 1999. *Herziening van het HIV-testbeleid* (Reconsidering the policy on HIV testing). Den Haag: Gezondheidsraad.

Gezondheidsraad: Permanente Commissie AIDS. 1987. *Zorg voor AIDS-patiënten: De zorg voor patiënten met AIDS en andere ziekteverschijnselen als gevolg van infectie met het humaan-immunodeficiëtievirus* (Care for AIDS-patients: Care for patients with AIDS and other symptoms as a consequence of infection with the human immunodeficiency virus). Den Haag: Gezondheidsraad.

Heisterkamp, Siem H. 1995. *Quantitative Analysis of AIDS/HIV: Development of Methods to Support Policy Making for Infectious Disease Control*. Utrecht: Elinkwijk BV. (Thesis)

Heisterkamp, S.H., J.C. Jager, A.M. Downs, J.A.M. van Druten, and E.J. Ruitenberg. 1989. "Correcting Reported AIDS Incidence: A Statistical Approach." *Statistics in Medicine* 8: 963–976.

Hoogenboezem, Jan. 1999. "Forse afname aidssterfte. Nieuwe therapie betekent uitstel van executie" (Dramatic fall in AIDS mortality. New therapy means a temporary reprieve). *Index* 6: 26.

Hospers, Harm, and Cor Bloem. 1998. "HIV Prevention Activities for Gay Men in the Netherlands 1983–93." In *The Dutch Response to HIV Pragmatism and Consensus*, Theo Sandfort, ed., pp. 40–60. London: UCL Press.

Houweling, Hans. 1997. *Public Health Surveillance of AIDS and HIV Infections in the Netherlands and Europe.* Delft: Eburon Publishers. (Thesis)

IGZ. 2000. *AIDS in Nederland per 31 december 1999* (AIDS in the Netherlands by 31 December 1999). Den Haag: Inspectie voor de Gezondheidszorg.

Jager, J.C., and E.J. Ruitenberg for the European Union Concorted Action on Multinational AIDS Scenarios. 1997. "Multinational Scenario Analysis Concerning Epidemiological Social and Economic Impact of HIV/AIDS on Society." Final Report. Bilthoven: National Institute of Public Health and the Environment; Amsterdam: Central Laboratory of the Netherlands Red Cross Blood Transfusion Service.

Jager, J.C., P.W. Achterberg, M.J. Postma, and H. Houweling. 1996. "Comparative Impact Assessment of AIDS: Between Doomsday and Complacency." *AIDS* 10: 238–240.

Jager, Johannes C., Siem H. Heisterkamp, and Ron Brookmeyer. 1993. "AIDS Surveillance and Prediction of the HIV and AIDS Epidemic: Methodological Developments." *AIDS* 7: (Supp. 1): S67–S71.

Jager, Johannes C., and Frans M.L.G. van den Boom. 1994. "Scenario Analysis, Health Policy and Decision Making." In *Modelling the Epidemic. Planning, Policy and Prediction*, Edward H. Kaplan and Margaret L. Brandeau, eds., pp. 237–252. New York: Raven Press.

Kamerstuk 19218 nrs. 8–9. 1987. Het verworven immuum deficiëtiesyndroom (AIDS). *Brief en Nota inzake aids-beleid* (AIDS policy in the Netherlands). Den Haag: SDU.

Kamerstuk 19218 nr. 10. 1987. Het verworven immuum deficiëntiesyndroom (AIDS). *Notitie over de juridische aspecten van verzekering in geval van Aids-risico* (Note on the legal aspects of insurance in case of AIDS risk). Den Haag: SDU.

Kamerstuk 19218 nrs. 15–16. 1988. Het verworven immuum deficiëntiesyndroom (AIDS). *Brief en notitie AIDS en aanstellingskeuring* (Letter and note on AIDS and medical examination for a job). Den Haag: SDU.

Kamerstuk 19218 nr. 38. 1989. Het verworven immuum deficiëntiesyndroom (AIDS). *Brief van de Staatssecretaris inzake centrumziekenhuizen* (Letter of the Secretary of State on core hospitals). Den Haag: SDU.

Kamerstuk 19218 nr. 40. 1990. Het verworven immuum deficiëntiesyndroom (AIDS). *Kabinetsstandpunt met betrekking tot de medische keuring bij aanstelling* (Cabinet's point of view on medical examination for a job). Den Haag: SDU.

Kamerstuk 19218 nr. 41. 1990. Het verworven immuum deficiëntiesyndroom (AIDS). *Notitie AIDS/seropositiviteit, erfelijkheidsonderzoek en verzekeringen* (Note on AIDS/seropositivity, genetic research and insurance). Den Haag: SDU.

Kamerstuk 19218 nr. 45. 1991. Het verworven immuum deficiëntiesyndroom (AIDS). *Brief inzake militaire aanstellingskeuringen* (Letter on medical examination for a job in the military). Den Haag: SDU.

Kamerstuk 19218 nr. 48. 1992. Het verworven immuum deficiëntiesyndroom (AIDS). *Voortgangsnotitie inzake AIDS-Beleid* (AIDS policy in the Netherlands; progress report). Den Haag: SDU.

Kamerstuk 19218 nr. 49. 1992. Het verworven immuum deficiëntiesyndroom

(AIDS). *Aids/seropositiviteit, hemofilie, erfelijkheidsonderzoek en verzekeringen* (AIDS/seropositivity, hemophilia, genetic research and insurance). Den Haag: SDU.

Kamerstuk 19218 nr. 54. 1992. Het verworven immuum deficiëntiesyndroom (AIDS). *Brief van de Minister van Justitie over verzekeringen* (Letter of the Minister of Justice on insurance). Den Haag: SDU.

Kaplan, E.H., and M.L. Brandeau, eds. 1994. *Modelling the Epidemic. Planning, Policy and Prediction.* New York: Raven Press.

Kok, Gerjo, Lilian Kolker, Ernest de Vroome, and Anton Dijker. 1998. " 'Safe Sex' and 'Compassion': Public Campaigns on AIDS in the Netherlands." In *The Dutch Response to HIV Pragmatism and Consensus*, Theo Sandfort, ed., pp. 19–39. London: UCL Press.

Lange, Joep, Mariëlle Jambroes, and Nadine Pakker. 2000. "ATHENA: Evaluatie van de behandeling van HIV- en AIDS-patiënten in Nederland" (ATHENA: Evaluation of the treatment of HIV- en and AIDS-patients in the Netherlands). *Aids-Bestrijding* (48): 13–16.

Markenstein, L.F. 1999. "Juridische eisen voor wijziging van het HIV-testbeleid" (Legal requirements for the revision of HIV testing policy). *Aids-Bestrijding* (47): 6–7.

Ministerie van Volksgezondheid, Welzijn en Sport. 1997. *Het Nederlandse aids-beleid* (Dutch AIDS-policy). Documentatie 10. Den Haag: Ministerie van Volksgezondheid, Welzijn en Sport.

———. 2000. *The Medical Research Involving Human Subjects Act (WMO).* The Hague: Ministry of Health, Welfare and Sport. International Publication Series Health, Welfare and Sport nr. 2.

Ministry of Health, Welfare and Sport. 1994. *Aids Policy in the Netherlands.* Factsheet V-3-E. The Hague: Ministry of Health, Welfare and Sport.

NCAB. 1994. *Toekomst van de buddyzorg in Nederland. Advies aan de Staatssecretaris van Welzijn, Volksgezondheid en Cultuur* (Future of buddy care in the Netherlands. Advice to the State Secretary of Welfare, Health and Cultural Affairs). Amsterdam: NCAB.

———. 1995a. *Het AIDS-beleid geactualiseerd. Eindadvies van de Nationale Commissie AIDS-bestrijding* (AIDS policy updated. Final advice of the National Committee on AIDS Control). Amsterdam: NCAB.

———. 1995b. *Hulpverlening in verband met partnernotificatie in het geval van HIV/AIDS* (Assistance with partner notification in case of HIV/AIDS). Amsterdam: NCAB.

Post, D., and L.J. Stokx, eds. 1997. *Volksgezondheid Toekomst Verkenningen 1997. VI Zorgbehoefte en zorggebruik* (Public Health Forecasts 1997. VI Care needs and care utilization). Bilthoven: Rijksinstituut voor Volksgezondheid en Milieu; Utrecht: Elsevier/De Tijdstroom.

Postma, Maarten Jacobus. 1998. *Assessment of the Economic Impact of AIDS at National and Multinational Level: Development of a Scenario-Analytic Approach to Support Health-Care Policy.* Zutphen: Koninklijke Wöhrmann bv. (Thesis)

Postma, M.J., E.J. Beck, S. Mandalia, L. Sherr, M.D.S. Walters, H. Houweling, and J.C. Jager. 1999. "Universal HIV Screening of Pregnant Women in England: Cost Effectiveness Analysis." *British Medical Journal* 318: 1656–1660.

Postma, Maarten J., Keith Tolley, Reiner M. Leidl, Angela M. Downs, Edward J.

Beck, Andrea M. Tramarin, Yves A. Flori, Miguel Santin, Fernando Antoñ-anzas, Helen Kornarou, Vasili C.C. Paparizos, Marcel G.W. Dijkgraaf, Jan Borleffs, August J.P. Luijben, and Johannes C. Jager, for the European Research Team on AIDS Scenarios. 1997. "Hospital Care for Persons with AIDS in the European Union." *Health Policy* 41: 157–176.

Postma, M.J., J.A.R. van den Hoek, E.J. Beck, B. Heeg, J.C. Jager, and R.A. Coutinho. 2000. "Farmaco-economische evaluatie van universele HIV screening in de zwangerschap; een kosten-effectiviteits analyse voor Amsterdam" (Farmaco-economic evaluation of universal HIV screening of pregnant women; a cost-effectiveness analysis for Amsterdam). *Nederlands Tijdschrift voor Geneeskunde* 144: 749–754.

Ruwaard, D., and P.G.N. Kramers, eds. 1998. *Public Health Forecasts 1997. Health, Prevention and Health Care in the Netherlands until 2015.* Bilthoven: Rijksinstituut voor Volksgezondheid en Milieu; Utrecht: Elsevier/De Tijdstroom.

Sandfort, Theo, ed. 1998. *The Dutch Response to HIV Pragmatism and Consensus.* London: UCL Press.

Singels, Loes. 1998. "AIDS Prevention for Migrants in the Netherlands." In *The Dutch Response to HIV Pragmatism and Consensus*, Theo Sandfort, ed., pp. 107–120. London: UCL Press.

Termorshuizen, F., and H. Houweling. 1997. "HIV/AIDS in Nederland: Betere behandelingsmogelijkheden maken HIV-in plaats van AIDS-surveillance noodzakelijk" (HIV/AIDS in the Netherlands: Better treatment modalities necessitate HIV surveillance instead of AIDS surveillance). *Nederlands Tijdschrift voor Geneeskunde* 141: 1928–1929.

Terpstra, Erica. 1997. "Aidsbeleid in verpleeghuizen." Brief aan de Voorzitter van de Vaste Commissie voor Volksgezondheid, Welzijn & Sport van de Tweede Kamer der Staten Generaal (AIDS policy in nursing homes. Letter to the chairman of the Standing Committee on Public Health, Welfare & Sport of the Lower House). *DOB/ZO-U-977443.*

Van Ameijden, Erik, and Anneke van den Hoek. 1998. "AIDS among Injecting Drug Users in the Netherlands: The Epidemic and the Response." In *The Dutch Response to HIV Pragmatism and Consensus*, Theo Sandfort, ed., pp. 61–80. London: UCL Press.

Van Bergen, J.E.A.M., and L. Wigersma, eds. 1998. *De HIV-wijzer voor huisartsen en andere hulpverleners* (HIV guide for general practitioners and other caregivers). Amsterdam: Schorer Boeken.

Van den Boom, F.M.L.G., J.C. Jager, L.H. Lumey, and E.J. Ruitenberg. 1990. "Het wetenschappelijk Aids-onderzoek: Randvoorwaarden van de onderzoeksprogrammering" (Scientific AIDS-research: Constraints of research planning). In *Aids Instellingen, individu, samenleving* (AIDS organization, individual, society), I. Ravenschlag, M.A.M. de Wachter, and H.A.E. Zwart, eds., pp. 155–179. Baarn: Ambo.

Van den Boom, F.M.L.G., D.P. Reinking, M.J. Postma, C.E.S. Albers, and J.C. Jager. 1992. *AIDS Up to the Year 2000. Epidemiological, Sociocultural and Economic Scenario Analysis for the Netherlands.* Scenario Committee on AIDS. Dordrecht: Kluwer Academic Publishers.

Van den Boom, Frans, and Paul Schnabel. 1998. "The Impact of AIDS on the Dutch

Health Care System." In *The Dutch Response to HIV Pragmatism and Consensus*, Theo Sandfort, ed., pp. 153–174. London: UCL Press.

Van der Kroef, Moniek A. 1998. Aids-bestrijding: "Confectie of maatpak? Integrale aanpak gepresenteerd" (AIDS control: Off the peg or made to measure? Presentation of integral approach). *Aids-Bestrijding* (42): 2–3.

Van Haastrecht, P. 1999. "Aids-voorlichting in de eigen taal en cultuur; een onmisbare strategie" (AIDS education adapted to native language and culture; an essential strategy). *SOA Bulletin* 20: 24–27 (Jubileumnummer).

Van Hasselt, N., M. de De Vroome, and Th.G.M. Sandfort. 1999. "Het publieke gezicht van de aids- en soa-bestrijding; vrij veilig campagnes 1987–1999" (The public appearance of AIDS and STD control; safe sex campaigns 1987–1999). *SOA Bulletin* 20: 8–12 (Jubileumnummer).

Vanwesenbeeck, Ine, and Ron de Graaf. 1998. "Sex Work and HIV in the Netherlands: Policy, Research and Prevention." In *The Dutch Response to HIV Pragmatism and Consensus*, Theo Sandfort, ed., pp. 86–106. London: UCL Press.

Veenker, Janherman. 1998. "The Decisive Role of Politics: AIDS Control in the Netherlands." In *The Dutch Response to HIV Pragmatism and Consensus*, Theo Sandfort, ed., pp. 121–134. London: UCL Press.

10

SPAIN

Jesús Castilla, Ángela Bolea, Mónica Suárez,
and Luis de la Fuente

INTRODUCTION

Spain is a country of some 39 million inhabitants, situated in the southwest of Europe and forming part of the European Union since 1986. Like other countries, it has witnessed a progressive concentration of the population in urban centers and a corresponding move away from rural areas in the interior. The economy is predominated by the service sector, with large-scale tourist activity, particularly along the country's coasts and on its islands.

With the introduction of the democratic 1978 Constitution, the administrative structure, which until then had been very centralized, began to undergo a progressive, though uneven, process of decentralization of competence to the 17 so-called Autonomous Regions (*Comunidades Autónomas*). During the first few years, public health competence was thus transferred to the respective regional authorities, with the Ministry of Health & Consumer Affairs retaining the functions of basic regulation, coordination, and international relations.

In 1986, the National Health System was set up, thereby extending free medical and hospital health care coverage to the entire population. Drugs administered in hospitals are available free of charge, whereas those dispensed in pharmacies are subsidized (60% reduction), except in the case of pensioners and the chronically sick who receive all such medication costfree. The public sector prevails, both in primary health care and the nation's hospital network, although a growing percentage of persons also tend to carry private medical insurance.

Education is both compulsory and free until the age of 16 years. Competence in education has been gradually transferred to the regions in recent years. Since 1990, teaching programs have included health education, including sex education. Approximately 30% of all nonuniversity students attend private schools, which in the main are linked to the Catholic Church. There is no official state religion in Spain, yet Catholicism remains predominant and maintains an important—albeit steadily waning—influence in political and social spheres. In comparison with other European Union countries, nongovernmental organizations (NGOs) have enjoyed less tradition and development but have nonetheless received great impetus in recent decades and are gradually acquiring an ever greater role in social life.

The first HIV infections occurred in Spain around 1980. At that time, there were a series of demographic, social, and political circumstances that had a marked influence on the spread of HIV and in shaping the epidemic. The 1960s saw a baby boom, which coincided with a mass migratory movement to the industrial belts surrounding the country's major towns and cities, as well as to other countries. As a result, in the outlying working-class suburbs of the larger cities, these same birth cohorts were to reach adolescence and young adulthood just at a time when injecting heroin use and HIV were beginning to burgeon. The large-scale social movements that marked the 1960s elsewhere met with a somewhat attenuated public repercussion in Spain, owing to the then-prevailing political system. Yet when the dictatorship came to an end in 1975, there was an accelerated expression of sweeping political and social change, with any elements regarded as rebellious or innovative being consequently overvalued. At times, the sheer pace of this change exceeded the capacity of the social structures to adapt. This process coincided with a period of pronounced economic recession and rising unemployment as a consequence of the "oil crisis." In these years—with a lag vis-à-vis other European countries—use of illegal drugs began to spread; Initially this drug use involved cannabis, amphetamines, and LSD and subsequently heroin and cocaine. Drugs were seen as appealing and attractive by the youth, and the associated risks were not well known. Consumption of heroin acquired a special relevance and was distributed nationwide, particularly in the working-class suburbs of large cities and in industrial areas. Due to delinquency on the part of addicts seeking funds to maintain the habit, an atmosphere of insecurity grew up around heroin, and this in turn led to the drug being perceived by society as a problem second only in importance to unemployment and to many heroin addicts being frequently sentenced to prison. The exact number of regular heroin users was never accurately ascertained, but all the evidence points to Spain as having one of the highest prevalence rates in Europe (EMCDDA 1997). Heroin users evolve rapidly toward the injected route, with needle sharing being commonplace. Unlike other countries, in Spain it is still unusual to find injecting drug users (IDUs) that do not consume heroin, regardless of whether or not they also inject other substances (de la Fuente et al. 1994).

ISSUES RELATING TO HIV AND AIDS

Sources of Epidemiological Information

To date, the principal epidemiological information system has been the National AIDS Registry. The Registry is based on the reporting of AIDS cases in accordance with the definition currently in force in Europe (Ancelle-Park 1993). Reporting is mandatory for all medical practitioners and is completed by professionals who carry out active case searching. The completeness of the system has gradually improved and is estimated at 90%. The Registry also records deaths, though with a lesser degree of completeness. Complementary information is furnished by national mortality statistics, but these are published with several years' delay. Population-based reporting systems covering new HIV diagnoses are currently in place in three regions, with plans to extend these to the remainder of the country.

Numerous surveys have been conducted on HIV prevalence and risk behaviors in IDUs, men who have sex with men (MSM), prostitutes, and the general adult and adolescent population. Some of these surveys have been repeated, thus making it possible to analyze the trend over time. Special mention should be made of two large-scale surveys undertaken under the aegis of the National Drug Plan in 1989 and 1996, with national representativeness of heroin addicts attended at drug detoxification centers (DGPNSD 1997). Some centers follow up seronegative persons who indulge in risk practices, thus enabling the incidence of seroconversion to be monitored. The first unlinked anonymous HIV seroprevalence surveys date back to 1994. Since then, this procedure has been used to analyze newborns in various regions; more recently, it has been extended to include sexually transmitted disease (STD) patients. Analysis and modeling based on the above-described epidemiological information have allowed for other epidemiological indicators to be estimated (Castilla and de la Fuente 2000).

Evolution of the HIV/AIDS Epidemic

The Spread of the Epidemic (1980–1989)

Although the first AIDS cases in Spain were officially confirmed in 1983, retrospective investigation revealed a first diagnosis in 1981. From this information it was deduced that HIV probably began to spread in Spain somewhat later than in other Western European countries (European Centre for the Epidemiological Monitoring of AIDS 1995). At that juncture, Spain had a large population of heroin users, the majority of whom favored the intravenous route and frequently indulged in needle sharing. HIV spread rapidly among this group, which from the mid-1980s onward registered seroprevalence rates close to 50% (Fernández-Sierra et al. 1990). In the years that followed, seroprevalence remained stable, probably indicating a saturation effect as regards infection in this population. This stability does not mean that HIV transmission was halted but rather that a point was reached where it was balanced by the rate of incorporation of new heroin injectors. This transmission mechanism came to account for two out of every three cases of infection.

Simultaneously, infection was spreading among MSM, though propagation was less abrupt among this group than among IDUs. The few seroprevalence studies conducted on MSM at the time reflected that, both in Madrid and in Barcelona, HIV propagation continued increasing until the early 1990s, by which time a third of this community had become HIV infected (CEESCAT 1998; del Romero et al. 1998).

In the early 1980s cases of infection were reported in hemophiliacs and blood transfusion recipients, until in 1985 it was made compulsory for all blood products to undergo heat treatment for inactivation of HIV, and analysis of donations became generalized. Transfusion-related infection levels never rose very high, possibly because of the prohibition on payment for blood donations.

In the early years of the epidemic, infections due to heterosexual transmission accounted for a small percentage of the total. On occasion, seroprevalence among female prostitutes exceeded the 10% mark. However, while IDUs registered rates of 50%, non-IDUs rarely attained 4% (Estébanez et al. 1992; Hernández-Aguado et al. 1992). In the second half of the 1980s, there were already considerable numbers of IDUs infected with HIV—mostly young, sexually active adults—which led to a secondary rise in heterosexual transmission in circles close to injectors principally among the latter's sexual partners. The proportion of AIDS cases in the immigrant population was low, in contrast to other Western European countries having a more active exchange with sub-Saharan Africa (Parras Vázquez 2000). Dating from the first half of the 1980s, cases of perinatal HIV transmission began to be detected, with practically all of these involving children of mothers who were either IDUs or sexual partners of IDUs.

The situation described above has been known retrospectively, but at the time its true dimension could not be appreciated. Seroprevalence studies targeting high-risk populations only provided a quantification in relative terms, and it took some time before reported AIDS case figures raised the alert as to the special magnitude of the epidemic in Spain. The jump in the number of cases took place slightly later than in other countries, and this pattern, in tandem with certain reporting deficiencies in the initial years, placed Spain at a comfortable level, occupying a middle ranking among the countries of Western Europe (European Centre for the Epidemiological

Monitoring of AIDS 1995). These events contributed to the fact that society's and the public health authorities' response to this epidemic was late
and irresolute.

Acknowledgment of the Problem and Attempts at Control (1990–1995)

By the beginning of its second decade, the epidemic had already given
rise to over 100,000 HIV infections. The first reliable estimates of living
HIV-infected persons reflected a rate of 3 per 1,000 population, rising to 6
per 1,000 among adults aged 20 to 39 years (Downs et al. 1997). Epidemiological surveillance became more complete and revealed the true gravity
of the situation. AIDS case reporting showed a rapid increase in the number
of new diagnoses. The 1994 expanded AIDS case definition, which included
pulmonary tuberculosis among other diseases (Ancelle-Park 1993), led to a
rise of 20% in the number of cases (Castilla, Gútíerrez, and Sánchez, 1994).
Since 1990, Spain has come to have the highest AIDS rates in Europe, well
ahead of all the remaining countries. Warranting attention here are the remarkably high rates among IDUs and in cases of mother-to-child transmission and the fact that, since 1994, Spain has also come to have the highest
AIDS rates in respect of heterosexual transmission (European Centre for the
Epidemiological Monitoring of AIDS 1995). AIDS has been steadily rising
in the rankings of the main causes of death among young adults. In 1993,
it had become the leading cause of death in the population aged 25 to 44
years (Castilla et al. 1997), and in 1995, the leading cause of years of potential life lost.

A breakdown by sex of the HIV-affected population revealed a proportion
of four men to every one woman, with a mean age of around 30 years. Two
out of every three persons infected were IDUs, over 10% were MSM, and
a percentage that rose to 20% had become infected through heterosexual
relations. The geographical distribution of those affected proved very uneven, with some regions registering AIDS rates five times higher than those
of others. The highest rates were found in Madrid, Barcelona, the Basque
Country, and the Balearic Isles, with IDUs being the most affected group
in all four sites.

The seriousness of the situation placed the local authorities on the alert,
with the result that they reacted by intensifying their prevention programs.
Society came to feel the presence of AIDS as something frequent and close
to home, and attitudes began to spread that were more evenhanded and
effective for the purposes of fighting the infection. The sensation of vulnerability to and fear of HIV infection became ever more intense among populations with high-risk behaviors, and this in turn contributed to a reduction
in the frequency of such risk practices. As a consequence of the response of
society itself and of activities undertaken in the fight against AIDS, the occurrence of new HIV infections began to decline (Figure 10.1), as has been

Figure 10.1
Estimated Time Trends in the HIV Epidemic in Spain, 1981–1999

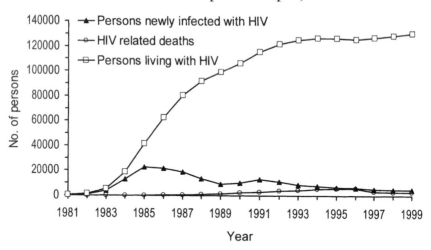

Source: Adapted from Castilla and de la Fuente 2000. Used by permission.

demonstrated by a series of seroprevalence studies targeting IDUs, MSM, and prostitution. However, the results of these studies did not become known until some years later.

Certain changes took place among heroin addicts that were to prove crucial in the control of HIV transmission. Successive generations of young adults joined the ranks of heroin users in declining numbers, a trend that manifested itself in the gradual aging of the heroin addict population. Added to this change was a progressive shift in the principal route of consumption, which moved away from being predominantly injection based toward smoking (de la Fuente et al. 1998). Indeed, this shift was in evidence earlier in the southwest of Spain and then moved gradually northward (de la Fuente et al. 1996). An important role in this process would appear to have been played by increased market availability of brown heroin, a substance better suited to smoking-based consumption ("chasing the dragon").

Era of Highly Active Antiretroviral Therapy (1996–2000)

By the mid-1990s, the consequences of the AIDS epidemic had attained extremely worrying dimensions. Approximately 120,000 persons were living with HIV infection (Figure 10.1), and more than 6,000 AIDS cases and 5,000 deaths happened annually, without any signs of remission in the short term. Subsequently, however, the introduction of new advances in the treatment of HIV infection led to a spectacular about-turn in this situation. In 1994, zidovudine began to be applied, in an effort to reduce HIV transmission from infected pregnant women to their offspring. This measure brought about an 80% reduction in the number of new perinatal AIDS cases over the following four years. In 1996, viral-load quantification techniques and protease inhibiting drugs became available at a number of public hospitals. The following year, these advances were incorporated into standard clinical practice and led to substantial decreases in the number of new AIDS diagnoses and deaths. From 1996 to 1999, AIDS incidence and AIDS-related mortality declined to less than half, though the most spectacular advance took place in 1997, with falls of 27% in AIDS incidence and 48% in associated mortality. It is estimated that in the period 1996–1998 development of full-blown AIDS in approximately 4,000 to 6,000 HIV-infected persons and a similar number of deaths were successfully prevented.

Data on HIV transmission in this period reflect levels that were clearly lower than in the past. All sources of information on heroin addicts coincide in showing a continuous decline in the number of new infections, particularly since ever fewer young adults were becoming initiated into injecting drug use (Hernández-Aguado et al. 1999). Among female prostitutes followed up in sexually transmitted disease clinics, HIV seroprevalence remains under 2%, with injecting drug use having become an infrequent practice (Ballesteros et al. 1999; Vioque et al. 1998). However, in marginal groups, mainly immigrants, that are engaged in prostitution and do not have regular medical checkups, higher rates of infection have been reported. Sexual partners of HIV-infected persons (mostly IDUs) are the one population group that seems to register a worse trend, with seroprevalence levels still moving upward (SPNS 1999). Available seroprevalence data would not appear to support the hypothesis of any important degree of HIV propagation affecting wide sectors of the heterosexual population outside the confines of IDU-related circles. These data are in line with the relatively low frequency of sexual risk behaviors found in the Spanish population versus those of other countries (Castilla et al. 1998).

In the three regions having population-based HIV reporting systems, the number of new diagnoses has fallen by over 50% since the early 1990s. Notwithstanding, for the three regions as a whole, 16.4 new HIV infections per 100,000 population were diagnosed in 1998, a figure that is still very high in comparison with other countries and regions of Europe (European Centre for the Epidemiological Monitoring of AIDS 2000; Moreno et al. 2000).

An overall assessment shows a predominant pattern of declining HIV transmission, particularly among those populations with the greatest relative weight in the epidemic. Nevertheless, the spectacular improvement in survival of HIV-infected persons has meant that the number of living persons with this infection has been maintained and is even increasing (Figure 10.1). At year-end 1999 the total figure was put at 110,000 to 150,000 persons, and it is estimated that over 30% had not yet been diagnosed.

RESPONSES TO HIV/AIDS

Coordination and Resources

The decentralized structure of Spain has had a significant impact on the organizational response to HIV/AIDS. Regions enjoy a large degree of autonomy in domains central to management of HIV/AIDS, namely, public health and education. Local responsibilities are very limited. The central government plays a crucial role as coordinator of the different policies at a national and regional level.

The first political reaction to AIDS dates back to 1983. This year saw the creation of a National AIDS Commission for the purpose of coordinating sectorial (Public Health, Social Affairs, Education, Justice, Interior) and regional interventions, in which professional medical, dentistry, and retail pharmacist associations and—since 1987—NGOs also took part. The National AIDS Plan Secretariat, which comes under the Ministry of Health, is the Commission's standing body, tasked with drawing up proposals for the prevention and control of infection and compiling all the information required for the taking of decisions in matters pertaining to HIV and AIDS.

In the fight against AIDS, the health authorities initially had very limited human and financial resources and scant political backing. At the time, social concern was focused on the problem of drugs, to which substantial resources were devoted. In recent years, new impetus has been lent to the AIDS program in the form of an increasingly generous fund allocation, a factor that has in turn enabled innovative strategies to be given a boost and wider commitment secured from the different sectors involved at both an official and social level. The "1997–2000 HIV/AIDS Multisectorial Plan" has proved to be a genuine driving force for prevention, with an increase of over 300% in the central government's budget for the fight against AIDS being matched by increases in the budgets of other public administrations, both sectorial and regional (SPNS 1998).

Funds allocated to HIV prevention are difficult to quantify, given that these are managed by different administrative authorities, as well as by citizen associations. It is estimated, however, that in 1998 public health authorities as a whole made a joint budget allocation of over U.S. $18 million to HIV prevention, despite the fact that this figure accounts for only 1% of the amount spent on health care for HIV-affected persons.

Until 1999, public funds allocated to AIDS research had been scant in proportion to the dimension of the epidemic. Research was basically undertaken in hospitals, was focused on clinical and immunological aspects, and was financed by private corporate funding. In the last two years, however, research into HIV prevention has received a considerable boost, with the setting up of a mixed research foundation that enjoys public and private participation and is financed with funds from pharmaceutical companies.

Evolution of Prevention Policies

Initial measures concentrated on transfusion safety and information campaigns. Little by little, epidemiological information began to guide prevention activities, and programs were implemented to address the issue of prevention of HIV transmission via injecting drug use and sex, principally among young adults and populations most vulnerable to infection.

In 1986, the Ministry of Health launched the first of a series of nationwide mass media campaigns, which sought to create a social climate that was favorable both to prevention and "normalization" of the disease, as a point of departure for other strategies. Designated campaign goals have gradually evolved over time: The first campaigns sought to enhance the level of information on HIV transmission and prevent discrimination against infected persons. In 1992, for the first time ever, the Ministry of Health promoted the use of condoms as an HIV prevention measure, in a campaign (using the slogan "Póntelo, pónselo," loosely translatable as "Wear it, share it") that marked a watershed in its day and unleashed a lively controversy with the Church authorities, who eventually succeeded in having it withdrawn. This did not manage to prevent the same goal from being maintained as the linchpin of most of the ensuing campaigns, yet the social impact and debate generated by the original campaign has never been surpassed.

Currently, prevention in IDUs is based on extending and diversifying harm reduction programs, promoting safe sex, and fostering peer education. For many years, however, there was no clear HIV prevention policy for IDUs, nor was there adequate coordination among the relevant authorities. The debate that prevailed in Spain in the mid-1980s surrounding the issue of drug use was dealt with as a problem of public safety, with considerations of any possible impact on public health being relegated to a secondary plane. Treatments were geared to eliminating drug abuse, whereas harm reduction programs were rejected by society, including NGOs active in the sector, and were applied with enormously restrictive criteria. This focus meant a considerable lag with respect to other European countries, such as the United Kingdom or the Netherlands (Stimson 1995), despite the fact that rates of infection in the latter were lower than in Spain.

Only when the public health consequences of this policy became patently evident did the authorities begin to rely on harm reduction programs. Since then, the number of centers offering and persons enrolled in methadone maintenance programs, financed by the drug administration, have grown steadily (Figure 10.2). Most of these therapies are administered in public drug-addiction centers. Needle exchange programs (NEPs) experienced a similar evolution, though in this case the impetus came from AIDS programs. There have never been any legal restrictions in Spain on the sale of hypodermic needles in pharmacies, but until relatively recently these establishments have solely seen IDUs as a threat to their safety and their business,

Figure 10.2
Evolution of Two Harm Reduction Programs Directed to Injecting Drug Users, 1985–1998

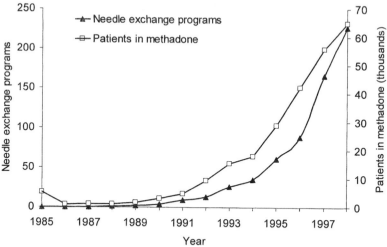

Source: DGPNSD 1997.

an attitude that has greatly limited the latter's possibilities of access to sterile injection material. Although the first NEP was introduced in 1987 with the backing of the Basque Regional Authority, the Spanish government did not fully support such programs until the mid-1990s, when they began to spread throughout the country (Figure 10.2). From the start, NGOs played a decisive role in the development of these programs, participating via mobile units or based at their own premises. However, almost all the programs have been financed by health administrations.

Harm reduction programs have likewise become generalized in prisons. In the late 1980s, AIDS had also become a public health problem of the first order in the country's jails, with close to 30% of inmates infected with HIV. It was at this time that the State Prison Service embarked upon an in-depth reform of its health care policy. In 1989, a number of health programs were implemented, in the shape of generally available HIV testing and the first harm reduction measures, that is, distribution of condoms and bleach to all inmates. Some years later—and not without difficulty—methadone maintenance programs were introduced. By 1997 these were already in place in all prisons (Dirección General de Instituciones Penitenciarias 1999). Needle exchange was, however, systematically rejected by the prison authorities on the basis of the alleged illegality of the measure and problems of security. Nonetheless, in 1997, at the insistence of the Basque Regional Parliament, the first prison-based needle exchange program was introduced as a pilot scheme. Subsequent evaluation showed its feasibility and the absence of any ensuing tension. As a result, in 1999 there were already four prisons with NEPs, and their extension to others is being actively promoted, a unique situation without equal in any other country.

Different indicators highlight the advances achieved over the last three years, namely: NEPs in health care centers (drug addiction centers, primary health care centers, or pharmacies) have doubled (SPNS 2000); attitudes held by pharmacists toward harm reduction programs have undergone a radical change—that is, in 1998, almost 15% of all 20,000 pharmacy outlets supplied anti-AIDS kits and methadone or exchanged needles, and over 60% were willing to do so (Menoyo et al. 2000); the year 2000 has witnessed the opening of Spain's first safe injection facility in Madrid, and there is a scheme for controlled distribution of heroin currently pending approval in Andalusia; moreover, drug-user associations have been set up in several cities around Spain. Coordination between AIDS and drug programs has made it possible for a training plan to be implemented at a national level. Aimed at professionals and NGOs that work with drug addicts, it will enable prevention of sexual transmission of HIV among IDUs to be introduced at drug addiction centers.

Another of the foremost prevention priorities has been the country's youth. Strategies targeting this population have been clear from the start, namely, school sex education and promotion of condom use. Insofar as school-based sex education is concerned, while Spanish legislation is progressive in this respect and includes the topic as a general-interest subject in the education syllabus, in practice the prejudices of the educational authorities and teachers have not yet been overcome when it comes to tackling the issue in schools, to the extent that there have even been periods of unequivocal retreat, coinciding with governments of a more conservative persuasion. By and large, parents' associations have maintained a more open-minded attitude. Rejection, though more evident in Church schools, also exists at the state school level. This resistance has in no way prevented numerous projects and educational activities from being undertaken in schools, by both NGOs and the public health authorities themselves, albeit on a one-time only basis. Greater acceptance of these activities has gradually become apparent, enabling sex education and HIV and other STD prevention programs to be introduced in a number of regions.

Condoms are sold without restriction in pharmacies and, to a lesser extent, in shops and supermarkets. Promotion of condom use has been based on publicity campaigns and other measures aimed at making them more accessible to young adults, such as a reduction in the price or distribution free of charge in places where youngsters tend to gather. Condoms are being increasingly used, especially among the youth. Nevertheless, there continue to be cultural limitations that call for more specific educational action.

The special characteristics of the epidemic—that is, its concentration above all in IDUs—had the effect of relegating institutional sex prevention interventions aimed at MSM to a secondary plane, despite the latter's being the second-most-affected group. Homosexuality in Spain is little accepted socially and raises problems for prevention peculiar to a partially hidden population. In this case, the response to the epidemic did not come from the administration but rather from the gay organizations themselves, which swiftly mobilized to draw up their own prevention strategies and create specific prevention and counseling resources that have since demonstrated their effectiveness in achieving change in risk behaviors in this community. From the very outset, the authorities supported these organizations' programs. These NGOs have been particularly active in bigger cities, yet their programs have seen far less development in the smaller towns. Citizen associations have likewise been the principal promoters of HIV prevention programs in other population groups, such as sex workers or, much more recently, immigrants.

The prevention of mother-to-child transmission is based on early diagnosis through the offer of HIV testing to all pregnant women (SPNS 1996). HIV infection is one of the statutory cases in which voluntary interruption of pregnancy has been legally permissible since 1985. Moreover, since 1994, all infected women wishing to continue their pregnancy are put on antiretroviral therapy.

As with many other countries, save in the case of pregnant women, there had been no active policy of promoting HIV testing as a prevention strategy. Now, however, highly effective treatments have made it essential for this approach to be subjected to an in-depth review, and a range of measures to encourage testing is currently being considered. On the other hand, postoccupational exposure prophylaxis is recommended to all health care staff after individual risk assessment.

Antidiscriminatory Policy

The Spanish Constitution ensures the right of all citizens to protection of health and safeguards the fundamental rights of the individual, without discrimination as to sex, age, or disease. Confidentiality of personal data is guaranteed by law, in the context of health care and of epidemiological surveillance systems.

In the first few years, ignorance of the transmission mechanisms and identification of the epidemic with given "risk groups," IDUs in particular, generated attitudes of rejection and discrimination, even in health care circles. Accordingly, public health authorities and citizen organizations initially devoted their efforts to informing the population about transmission mechanisms and HIV prevention and seeking to prevent discrimination against infected persons. Nowadays a climate of tolerance prevails.

Legislation governing the matter stipulates that both treatment and detection of HIV are to be voluntary and prohibits any type of discrimination on these grounds. HIV testing is performed on a voluntary and confidential basis. In the cities there are centers where diagnosis of infection may be made anonymously, though this is not the case in rural areas. Under Spanish law, HIV analysis is mandatory only in the case of blood, semen, or organ donations made voluntarily by the donor (Sánchez Caro and Giménez Cabezón 1995).

Social and Health Care for Persons Living with HIV/AIDS

The response of the public health system came far earlier and was far more intense in the area of health care than in that of prevention. Assistance is based on the general principle of ensuring quality health care for all, including cost-free access to antiretroviral therapy in line with currently recommended guidelines. The self-same principle was applied in prisons. Patient follow-up was conducted by specialized units at public hospitals, which have been quick to incorporate the newest advances, whether technological (e.g., by 1997, 92% of all public hospitals had viral load–determination capability, with resistance testing to be introduced over the course of the year 2000) or therapeutic in nature (e.g., the introduction of the first AZT [azidothymidine] antiretroviral treatments in 1987, combined treatments in 1990, and protease inhibitors since 1996). Since 1995, AIDS patients have also been entitled to access, on a practically cost-free basis, to any medication that they may require. In this respect, AIDS in Spain can be said to enjoy a privileged situation vis-à-vis other diseases. These conditions have probably led to all HIV patients being treated in the public sector. The cost of antiretroviral therapy to the National Health System in 1999 totaled U.S.$253 million, approximately 5% of the total annual expenditure on medical drugs.

The great challenge now confronting patient care is compliance with treatment. On the part of both the public health system and certain NGOs, there is a move to develop programs for health care professionals and information campaigns targeted at persons in treatment, with the aim of enhancing therapy-compliance levels.

The magnitude of the epidemic and the characteristic traits of the hardest-hit population—IDU with serious work-, family-, and marginalization-related problems—had the effect of immediately rendering the social services inadequate to the task. It has been the NGOs that have contributed to mitigating existing shortfalls, setting up hospices for terminal patients without resources, and delivering home-based attention, with funds furnished by the Administration. AIDS patients receive a pension calculated in accordance with preestablished criteria. In addition, in 1993 official recognition was given to the right of HIV-infected persons to compensation for actions undertaken by the public health system.

The life expectancy of HIV-infected persons has embarked upon a process of ongoing improvement. Advances in therapy have also been reflected in a reduction in hospital admissions and a better quality of life for patients, who have recovered their autonomy in activities of daily living. These changes pose new challenges and call for strategies to be sought, which will ensure the social integration and reincorporation of such persons.

NGOs Active in AIDS

In Spain there has traditionally been scant development of the social fabric. As a result of a reaction to the emergence of HIV/AIDS, a widespread network of citizen organizations was developed, little by little. As in other countries (Kenis and Marin 1997), these organizations emerged progressively, with the first appearing in 1984. Initially, there was a rapid growth in the number of NGOs, but from the mid-1990s onward, it seems that they then entered a phase of consolidation. Parallel to the creation of new organizations, others traditionally present in the field of social welfare (Caritas, Red Cross, and others) intensified their activities in the HIV/AIDS field. There is no homogeneity in the territorial distribution of these associations. Though concentrated in the largest Spanish towns and in those regions hardest hit by HIV, they are nevertheless present throughout the country.

NGOs have been of special importance, not only in fighting the stigmatization of and discrimination against persons living with HIV/AIDS but also in the prevention of infection among MSM and prostitutes and in psychological and social support for persons living with AIDS. In the case of IDUs, however, until the epidemic was already very advanced, sector-specific NGOs maintained a stance geared to strategies that were aimed at abstinence and so not favorable to the prevention of HIV.

During the initial stage, networks were not integrated, working parallel to public services without any coordination among themselves. In recent years, improvement has been observable, both as to coordination between the respective HIV/AIDS players and in the shape of better integration of networks. In 1989, the Ministry of Health introduced a policy of subsidies to promote the management of HIV/AIDS programs by NGOs active in the field, a policy that has remained in place until today. Regional authorities and town and city councils also contribute to financing these organizations. Indeed, NGO funding comes almost entirely from the Administration. Nevertheless, this excessive financial dependence has not prevented such organizations from playing an important role as activists, a factor that has proved decisive in getting the authorities to furnish financial support for HIV-affected persons, ensure patients rapid, cost-free access to new therapies, and extend harm reduction programs throughout the prison system. By the end-1990s, the implementation of the new HIV reporting system was a bone of contention between the two sides. NGOs sit on AIDS policy decision-making bodies solely as observers. Nonetheless, relations with the public health authorities are fluid, exchange of points of view is, in general, active, and a large number of joint activities are undertaken.

CONCLUSION

Spain is the Western European country in which the HIV epidemic has acquired its greatest dimension, with a prevalence rate estimated at 3 infected persons per 1,000 population. The principal mechanism of spread has been injecting drug use, which at a secondary level has given rise to a considerable degree of heterosexual and perinatal transmission. Despite the fact that the number of new diagnoses of infection has been markedly reduced, such diagnoses are nonetheless still frequent. Moreover, the extremely sharp fall in mortality—achieved through generalized access to new treatments—means that the number of persons now living with the infection remains high. Patients enjoy free access to health care, which has steadily incorporated successive therapeutic advances, despite the enormous cost that this inevitably entails to the health care system.

The initial response that came from drug programs (aimed at abstinence and control of social conflict) proved substantially ineffective in halting HIV transmission, and it was only when harm reduction programs were incorporated that any real progress was ultimately achieved. Recent years have witnessed the rapid rise of programs targeting the most vulnerable groups, including particularly delicate areas, such as prisons.

In the medium term, it is envisaged that HIV infection will continue to require substantially greater investment than in other countries around Europe, both in prevention activities, so as to ensure an ongoing reduction in the rate of new infections, and in healthcare delivery to the large numbers of persons infected with the disease. Prevention programs will have to lay greater stress on sexual transmission and allow for regular evaluations of and improvements to their effectiveness.

BIBLIOGRAPHY

Ancelle-Park, R.M. 1993. "Expanded European AIDS Case Definition." *Lancet* 341: 441.

Ballesteros, Juan, Petunia Clavo, Jesús Castilla, Carmen Rodríguez, M. José Belza, Natividad Jerez, Santos Sanz, and Jorge del Romero. 1999. "Low Seroincidence and Decrease in Seroprevalence of HIV among Female Prostitutes in Madrid." *AIDS* 13: 1143–1144.

Castilla, Jesús, Gregorio Barrio, Luis de la Fuente, and María José Belza. 1998. "Sexual Behaviour and Condom Use in the General Population of Spain, 1996." *AIDS Care* 10: 667–676.

Castilla, Jesús, and Luis de la Fuente. 2000. "Trends in the Number of HIV Infected Persons and AIDS Cases in Spain: 1980–1998" (in Spanish). *Medicina Clinica (Barcelona)* 115: 85–89.

Castilla, Jesús, M. Victoria Martínez de Aragón, Angeles Gutiérrez, Alicia Llácer, M. José Belza, Cristina Ruiz, Julio Perez dela Paz, and Isabel Noguer. 1997. "Impact of HIV Mortality among Young Men and Women in Spain." *International Journal of Epidemiology* 26: 1346–1351.

Castilla, J., A. Gutiérrez, and M.F. Sánchez. 1994. "Marked Impact of the Expanded AIDS Case Definition in Spain." *AIDS* 8: 1632–1633.

CEESCAT (Centre d'Estudis Epidemiològics sobre la Sida de Catalunya). 1998. *Sistema integrat de vigilància epidemiològica del VIH/Sida a Catalunya (SIVES). Informe anual 1997.* Barcelona: Departament de Sanitat i Seguretat Social.

De la Fuente, Luis, Gregorio Barrio, María J. Bravo, and Luis Royuela. 1998. "Heroin Smoking by 'Chasing the Dragon': Its Evolution in Spain." *Addiction* 93: 444–446.

De la Fuente, Luis, Gregorio Barrio, Luis Vicente, María José Bravo, and Pablo Lardelli. 1994. "Prevalence of Intravenous Route of Administration among Heroin Users in Treatment in Spain. Geographical Variations and Other Related Factors." *International Journal of Epidemiology* 23: 805–811.

De la Fuente, Luis, Paloma Saavedra, Gregorio Barrio, Luis Royuela, Julián Vicente, and the Spanish Group for the Study of the Purity of Seized Drugs. 1996. "Temporal and Geographic Variations in the Characteristics of Heroin Seized in Spain and Their Relation with the Route of Administration." *Drug & Alcohol Dependence* 40: 185–194.

Del Romero, Jorge, Jesús Castilla, Soledad García, Carmen Rodíguez, Cruz Ayerbe, Dulce Carrió, Maria José Belza, José Luis Aparicio, Maria Angeles Neila, Antonio Quintana, Sonsoles del Corral, and Montserrat Raposo. 1998. "Trends in HIV Seroprevalence in Homosexual or Bisexual Men from Madrid (Spain), 1986–1995" (in Spanish). *Medicina Clinica (Barcelona)* 110: 209–212.

DGPNSD (Delegación del Gobierno para el Plan Nacional sobre Drogas). 1997. *Memoria 1996.* Madrid: Author.

Dirección General de Instituciones Penitenciarias. 1999. *Memoria de actividades de la Subdirección General de Sanidad Penitenciaria de 1998.* Madrid: Ministerio del Interior.

Downs, Angela M., Siem H. Heisterkamp, Jean-Baptiste Brunet, and Françoise F. Hamers. 1997. "Reconstruction and Prediction of the HIV/AIDS Epidemic among Adults in European Union and Low Prevalence Countries of Central and Eastern Europe." *AIDS* 11: 649–662.

EMCDDA (European Monitoring Centre for Drugs and Drug Addiction). 1997. *Annual Report on the State of the Drugs Problem in the European Union.* Lisbon: Author.

Estébanez, P., C. Sarasqueta, K. Fitch, V. Zunzunegui, G. Contreras, J.M. Valera, V. Palacios, and R. Nájera. 1992. "Prevalence of HIV-1 and Other Sexually Transmitted Disease in Spanish Prostitutes" (in Spanish). *Medicina Clinica (Barcelona)* 99: 161–167.

European Centre for the Epidemiological Monitoring of AIDS. 1995. *AIDS Surveillance in Europe.* Quarterly Report no. 46. Saint Maurice, France: Author.

———. 2000. *HIV/AIDS Surveillance in Europe.* End-year Report no. 62. Saint Maurice, France: Author.

Fernández-Sierra, M.A., M. Gómez Olmedo, M. Delgado Rodríguez, and R. Gálvez Vargas. 1990. "Infection by the Human Immunodeficiency Virus in the Spanish Population (II). A Meta-Analysis of the Time and Geographic Trends" (in Spanish). *Medicina Clínica (Barcelona)* 95: 366–371.

Hernández-Aguado, I., M.J. Aviñó, S. Pérez-Hoyos, J. González-Aracil, I. Ruiz-Pérez, A. Torrella, M. Garcia de la Hera, F. Belda, E. Fernández, C. Santos, J. Trullen, and A. Fenosa for the Valencian Epidemiology and Prevention of HIV Disease Study Group. 1999. "Human Immunodeficiency Virus (HIV) Infection in Parenteral Drug Users: Evolution of the Epidemic over 10 Years." *International Journal of Epidemiology* 28: 335–340.

Hernández-Aguado, I., E. Fernández García, M. García de la Hera, and C. Alvarez Dardet. 1992. "Infection by the Human Immunodeficiency Virus-1 in Prostitutes and Risk Factors" (in Spanish). *Medicina Clínica (Barcelona)* 99: 406–409.

Kenis, Patrick, and Bernd Marin, eds. 1997. *Managing AIDS. Organizational Responses in Six European Countries.* European Centre Vienna. Aldershot: Ashgate Publishing Limited.

Menoyo, Cristina, Ángela Bolea, Mónica Suárez, and María J. Bravo. 2000. "HIV/ AIDS Prevention Programme and Risk Reduction through Community Pharmacists in Spain." 11th International Conference on the Reduction of Drug Related Harm, Jersey, United Kingdom. (Abstract 61)

Moreno, Conchi, Ismael Huerta, María Eugenia Lezaun, Amelia González, Julio Sola, and Jesús Castilla. 2000. "Time-Trend in the Number of People Diagnosed with HIV Infection in Asturias, Navarra and La Rioja (Spain)" (in Spanish). *Medicina Clínica (Barcelona)* 114: 653–655.

Parras Vázquez, Francisco. 2000. "Spain." In *HIV/AIDS Care and Support for Migrant and Ethnic Minority Communities in Europe*, Kris Clarke and Georg Bröring, eds., pp. 135–144. Woerden, The Netherlands: Netherlands Institute for Health Promotion and Disease Prevention.

Sánchez Caro, Javier, and José Ramón Giménez Cabezón. 1995. *Derecho y Sida.* Madrid: Editorial MAPFRE.

SPNS (Secretaría del Plan Nacional sobre el Sida). 1996. *Recomendaciones para la atención a la mujer embarazada.* Madrid: Ministerio de Sanidad y Consumo.

———. 1998. *Plan de movilización multisectorial contra el VIH/sida, 1997–2000.* Madrid: Ministerio de Sanidad y Consumo.

———. 1999. "Vigilancia de la infección por VIH en centros y consultas de VIH, ETS y planificación familiar. Resultados de las pruebas voluntarias, 1995–1997." *Boletín Epidemiológico Semanal* 7: 13–16.

———. 2000. *Informe sobre actividades de prevención en las comunidades autónomas.* Madrid: Ministerio de Sanidad y Consumo.

Stimson, Gerry V. 1995. "AIDS and Injecting Drug Use in the United Kingdom, 1987–1993: The Policy Response and the Prevention of the Epidemic." *Social Science & Medicine* 41: 699–716.

Vioque, J., I. Hernández-Aguado, E. Fernández García, M. García de la Hera, and C. Álvarez-Dardet. 1998. "Prospective Cohort Study of Female Sex Workers and Risk of HIV Infection in Alicante, Spain (1986–1996)." *Sexually Transmitted Infections* 74: 264–288.

11

SUB-SAHARAN AFRICA

Helen Jackson and Tim Lee

INTRODUCTION

Of all regions in the world, the HIV/AIDS epidemic took hold first and with greatest impact in sub-Saharan Africa. The areas most affected early on were central and eastern Africa, but today the southern part of the continent has the highest infection levels and AIDS-related mortality.

The pandemic is unfolding in sub-Saharan Africa at a difficult historical period. Most countries have had to implement International Monetary Fund—and World Bank—approved structural adjustment programs, which have often been to the detriment of health, education, and welfare services, as well as formal employment. Many countries have faced corruption and inappropriate government expenditures; political upheaval and change; the legacies of colonialism; civil wars and other forms of conflict; population movement; and environmental difficulties, including severe drought and, more recently, floods. These factors have all made it more difficult for countries to mount adequate responses to the epidemic while, at the same time, they have tended to exacerbate HIV spread and the ultimate levels of infection, morbidity, and death.

This chapter explores the scale and nature of the HIV/AIDS pandemic in sub-Saharan Africa in general, giving particular emphasis to the southern Africa subregion (the epicenter) in particular. It discusses the broad context of the epidemic in the region, methods of data collection, and the impact of HIV/AIDS on human development. Finally, the chapter outlines and analyzes the main responses of government and nongovernment sectors with regard to HIV prevention, care, and long-term mitigation.

Figure 11.1
Adults and Children Living with HIV/AIDS as of End of 1999

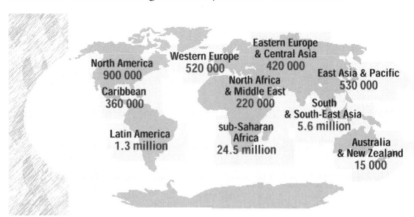

Source: UNAIDS 2000.

ISSUES RELATING TO HIV AND AIDS

HIV Prevalence in Sub-Saharan Africa

The first AIDS cases in the sub-Saharan region were identified in the early 1980s in central and eastern Africa, but there must already have been widespread HIV infection in other parts. Zimbabwe was first in the region (indeed in the entire developing world) to begin routine screening of donated blood in 1985. The results provided the first clear evidence of a widespread epidemic: 2% of the 70,000 blood samples were infected. Ironically, Zimbabwe was also one of the last countries in the region to publicly acknowledge having a serous epidemic (in early 1990).

UNAIDS (2000) estimates that sub-Saharan Africa accounts for 71% of the global total of 34.3 million adults and children living with HIV/AIDS (Figure 11.1).

The region also accounts for the bulk of new infections (3.8 million of the global total of 5.6 million for 1999). Africa constitutes around 10% of the global population, and given that the population of Asia is far higher, the relative severity of the epidemic in sub-Saharan Africa is even starker (Figure 11.2).

Infection levels vary greatly between countries in sub-Saharan Africa. Over time, the pandemic has spread along trade routes, and now the southern countries have the highest infection rates. HIV prevalence is estimated at 1 in 5 adults in South Africa and Zambia, and 1 in 4 adults in Botswana and Zimbabwe. Currently, Swaziland is thought to have the highest adult prevalence rate, at 33%. South Africa, on the other hand, has one of the fastest-

Figure 11.2
HIV and AIDS Estimates, Global and Sub-Saharan Africa

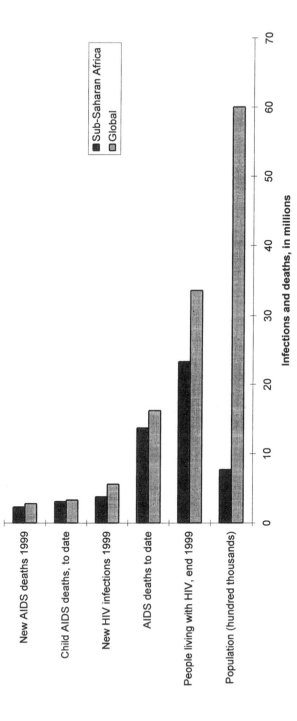

Source: Pisani 1999: 5.

growing epidemics in the world. Between 1990 and 1998, HIV prevalence increased from under 1% to nearly 23%; there are 5 million adults and children living with HIV in South Africa (Wilson 2000). Ethiopia also comes close to this total, with an estimated 3 million people living with HIV at the end of 1999.

At the other extreme, Mauritius has an extremely low prevalence rate of between 0 to 0.2%. Countries such as Angola, Democratic Republic of the Congo, Gabon, and Ghana also seem to provide a contrast to the high figures for southern Africa, with reported HIV prevalence at a much lower level, of 1 to 5%. However, practical difficulties in data collection and differences in methodologies must be acknowledged; the accuracy of some of these data is questionable.

The epidemics experienced in west Africa seem to develop more slowly and plateau at lower levels than those in southern Africa. In sub-Saharan Africa, Uganda is the only country reporting a decline in HIV infection rates, at least in urban areas (see, e.g., Caraël et al. 1997; also see Chapter 7 in this volume).

HIV prevalence varies considerably within countries (as well as from country to country). In Zambia, for example, provincial HIV prevalence rates vary from under 12% in North-Western province to over 26% in the Copperbelt and over 27% in Lusaka (Zambian Ministry of Health/Central Board of Health 1999).

In sub-Saharan Africa, roughly equal numbers of males and females are infected with HIV, but there are clear age differences between the sexes. Females tend to be infected younger and die younger. The age group at greatest risk is women aged 15 to 25, but it is critical to reach youth of both sexes with awareness and prevention efforts before the establishment of risky sexual behavior. The proportion of women infected has possibly overtaken that of men: The Joint United Nation Programme on HIV/AIDS (UNAIDS) estimates that 55% of infections in sub-Saharan Africa are in women, far higher than anywhere else in the world. This means that the region also has the highest risk of transmission to infants. In terms of children infected with HIV during 1999, sub-Saharan Africa accounted for over 460,000, or over 80% of the global total.

In some countries, such as Zambia and Zimbabwe, HIV prevalence may be leveling off except in more remote areas. However, it will nonetheless be many years before AIDS cases begin to decline.

HIV Transmission

Sexual Behavior

In sub-Saharan Africa, HIV transmission is predominantly heterosexual. Although the extent to which men have sex with men is without doubt underestimated and as yet inadequately researched, there is probably relatively little male homosexual transmission. In South Africa, HIV infections were first seen among the predominantly white gay male community in the late 1980s, and a network for people living with HIV/AIDS was initiated; this pattern has not been observed elsewhere in the region. Gay men have become seen as a minority of those with HIV infection in South Africa itself, although still contributing significantly to human rights issues of treatment access and discrimination.

Mother-to-Child Transmission

Mother-to-child transmission, the second most common cause of HIV infection in the region, is exacerbated by a number of factors. These factors include the long period of breastfeeding typical of much of the region and the lack of options for women that know their serostatus. There is little access through the public health sector to cheap antiretroviral drugs, such as nevirapine, and the majority of women do not even know their HIV status anyway, as counseling and testing facilities are unavailable or underutilized.

Other Infection Routes

Blood transfusion and infection through infected needles and other sharps are believed to be low because of relatively effective sterilization, although standards vary considerably between and within countries; in rural and poor settings, some infection by this route is likely. Injecting drug use is probably underestimated but nonetheless thought to be relatively low throughout the sub-Saharan region.

Factors Facilitating Transmission

Social and Cultural Issues

Despite high levels of HIV infection and mounting deaths in the region, HIV/AIDS remains a difficult focus for discussion within families and communities, by governments and churches, and in most public forums. This difficulty is partly because HIV/AIDS is closely associated with the taboo subjects of sex and death. It is also due to a pervasive and virulent stigma against those infected and affected. These cultural factors limit prevention opportunities and hamper efforts that are made; it also means that very few people in any country in the sub-Saharan region have publicly disclosed that they are living with HIV. One woman in Durban, South Africa, who did so in December 1998 was beaten to death in her local community.

Gender Issues

Transmission is facilitated to varying degrees throughout the region by high levels of sexual violence and gender inequality. In most of the region, rape is not a legal offense within marriage, and husbands are deemed to have complete conjugal rights on their own terms.

For married women it is usually their husband's behavior that determines their risk of HIV, and, paradoxically, sex within marriage is, for many women, their biggest risk factor for infection. A huge contrast between public and private morality exists. Extramarital sex is widespread, and men are largely condoned having multiple sexual partners (see, e.g., Aliro, Ochieng, and Fiedler 1999, discussing Uganda). In Zambia, at least 1 in 5 men are thought to engage in commercial sex, and 1 in 10 to engage in casual relationships. When combined with unsafe sexual practices, particularly reticence to use condoms, such behavior puts married women at great risk from their husbands. For example, HIV infection rates of close to 100% have been found among commercial sex workers in Abidjan, Côte d'Ivoire, and in Nairobi, Kenya. In many other cities in the sub-Saharan region, over half of sex workers are living with HIV (cited in Roseberry and Paul 1998). Gender inequalities in power and risk of HIV infection are exacerbated by the pattern of men taking younger female partners (hence the high infection levels in young women).

Poverty and Development Issues

There is a complex relationship between HIV/AIDS transmission and social development factors. In the early days of the pandemic, more infection was documented among higher economic groups. Indeed, the association between higher socioeconomic status or education levels and higher rates of HIV infection has been documented in Malawi, Rwanda, Tanzania, Zaire (Democratic Republic of Congo), and Zimbabwe (cited in Roseberry and Paul 1998).

Typically across the region, HIV infection levels are highest along trade routes, in cities, ports, and border towns, and in rural growth points. Ironically, risk of HIV transmission is higher in some respects in more developed areas where good roads and transport systems allow increased population movement. As far back as 1992, 27% of truckers plying the Mombassa to Nairobi highway were found to be HIV-positive (Bwayo et al. 1992). Infection is generally higher among the armed forces, sex workers, prison populations, migrant laborers, and the long-distance transport sector. For example, several countries in the region are thought to have infection rates of 50% or more among armed forces personnel (Roseberry and Paul 1998).

Furthermore, development projects themselves, through generating higher incomes, can promote increased alcohol and increased numbers of commercial or casual sex partners (see, e.g., Welbourn 1995: 58–59).

In general, however, it is the poorest communities that are at enhanced risk and experience the greatest impact. The link between lower socioeconomic status or education levels and higher rates of HIV infection has been documented in Ethiopia, Nigeria, and Tanzania, for example (Roseberry and Paul 1998).

Many low-income communities depend on the earnings of laborers working away from home in the towns, in mines, and on commercial farms. This institutionalized separation of spouses, an enduring legacy of colonial economic systems, is a major risk factor for HIV transmission (Wilson 2000). The end results of these factors can be seen in high HIV and AIDS rates in deep rural communities in KwaZulu Natal in South Africa, for example. It is also illustrated by an HIV infection rate of 70% found by antenatal testing of women in Chiredzi, Zimbabwe. These women work seasonally on the sugar plantations and supplement inadequate annual earnings with commercial sex work.

Access to Prevention and Health Services

The lack or inadequacy of prevention campaigns, condom use, and treatment for sexually transmitted infections (STIs) is also a major contributing factor to HIV transmission in the region. In many rural communities, access to condoms remains poor. Lack of access to condoms in a high-risk environment is vividly illustrated by Wilson's (2000) study of border points on the Lusaka to Durban trade route (Table 11.1).

An additional problem is that even when supplies are available, whether free or for sale, many in need of condoms may not be able to access supplies due to embarrassment or fear of being seen procuring them. This problem is particularly true for young and unmarried people, that is, those who "should not need them."

Conflict

Although countries such as Mozambique and Angola may have been partly protected from infection for a while because of civil war impeding population movement (and hence viral spread), this "protection" disappears once refugees return home and the process of rebuilding the economy begins. The involvement of multiple armies from neighboring countries in the Democratic Republic of the Congo is a major concern in relation to HIV infection in that country and the region; and fears are also developing around the possibility of new recombinant strains of HIV emerging.

Data Collection

Data collection in the region remains problematic and incomplete, although it provides sufficient information to confirm the existence of a pandemic and highlights the main areas and population groups affected. The main data come from unlinked screening studies of pregnant women without their knowledge or consent. Selected sites screen all clinic attendees for

Table 11.1

Condom Availability at Key Border Points in South Africa, Zambia, and Zimbabwe

	Messina (South Africa)	Beitbridge (Zimbabwe)	Chirundu (Zimbabwe)	Chirundu (Zambia)
Sex workers	400-700	500-700	100-300	300-500
Truckers staying overnight per month	3000	3000	1000	1000
Public condom outlets	4	3	2	3
Private condom outlets	4	4	1	2
Availability of public or socially marketed condoms	Not easily obtainable	Generally available	Generally available	Short supply

Source: Wilson 2000: 4.

a given period of time or until they reach a target sample size, utilizing a portion of the blood drawn for syphilis and other tests.

The limitations to the quality of the data relate mainly to the representativeness of sites selected; small sample size; lack of sufficient repeat surveillance to show trends; and lack of comparability across sites within and between countries. By definition, such antenatal surveillance only covers females and is skewed toward younger and sexually active women. However, recent research suggests that, if anything, antenatal data tend to underestimate HIV prevalence in the general adult population when controlled for age (UNAIDS 1999).

Countries also sporadically obtain data from public health service patients and from men (typically) receiving treatment for STIs. These data tend to overestimate infection levels in the general population, but they provide important information for health sector planning and cost assessment. Finally, blood donors are also screened throughout the region. These data are significantly affected by the donor selection policy and reveal little of relevance to monitoring the epidemic. In Zimbabwe, for instance, blood donor

HIV seroprevalence has remained stable and low (under 2%) during the 1990s despite antenatal seroprevalence rising to an estimated 25%.

National notification is being considered in some countries (such as Namibia, Zimbabwe, and South Africa), but this strategy is unlikely to add much to the accuracy of statistics if it is ever implemented. The proportion of AIDS deaths actually reported is estimated to be low, perhaps one-third in the more optimistic assessments. Several countries do not even try to provide annual or cumulative figures, knowing that accurate data do not exist and that mathematical models are only as reliable as the inputted data and the assumptions made.

Impact

The central impact of the epidemic is increased morbidity and mortality in what is normally the healthiest adult age cohort, the productive and re-productive age group. Overall, it is estimated that nearly 14 million of the 16.3 cumulative total of AIDS deaths so far have occurred in sub-Saharan Africa. In 1999, nearly 80% of AIDS deaths worldwide were in sub-Saharan Africa (UNAIDS/WHO 2000). In countries such as Botswana, Zimbabwe, and Zambia, life expectancy has declined significantly since 1990; in each case, around 10 years of life expectancy have been lost. By 2010, life expectancy is predicted to be a mere 33 years in Zambia and 40 years in Zimbabwe, for example (U.S. Bureau of the Census, cited in Wilson 2000). Already in Zimbabwe, population 12 million, over 1,000 people die of AIDS each week.

Life expectancy calculations are greatly influenced by infant and child mortality rates. Figure 11.3 shows the projected impact of AIDS on under-five child mortality rates in selected countries in east and southern Africa by the year 2010. The expected impact is worst in those countries that had already reduced child mortality, showing clearly in these countries how AIDS wipes out the development gains in child survival of the previous decades.

What primarily appears to be a health problem gradually becomes a major risk for human development itself, even though many working in develop-ment have been slow to realize this risk. Most countries in sub-Saharan Africa are characterized by high levels of poverty, shortages of skilled pro-fessional, managerial, and technical labor, high unemployment, and heavy reliance of large sectors of the population on subsistence farming and in-formal sector activities.

The impact of HIV and AIDS is to worsen poverty and mitigate against development at all levels, but particularly among the poorest sectors of the population. Families lose their breadwinners and caregivers; rural families lose remittances from workers living in the towns, mines, and farms; house-

Figure 11.3
Estimated Impact of AIDS on Under-Five Child Mortality Rates in Selected African Countries by 2010

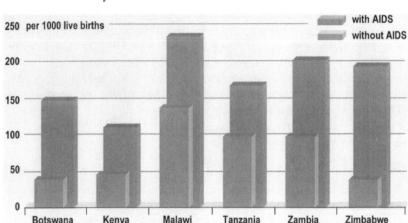

Source: U.S. Bureau of the Census, cited by UNAIDS 1999.

hold expenditures on health care and funerals, and care-related travel, increase enormously.

AIDS deaths often have a greater impact on livelihoods than deaths by other causes because they usually occur earlier and after a long period of illness and decline and because they are often associated with illness or death of the spouse. Households typically respond by reducing expenditures on nonessentials and shortening their planning horizons (UNAIDS 1999), including the withdrawal of girls from school to provide care for the sick and siblings. In addition, new sources of income are required, which may include girls and single women selling sex and thereby increasing their own HIV risk.

A tragic consequence of high deaths among young-middle-aged adults is the escalating number of orphans. By the end of 1999, UNAIDS estimated that 10.7 million African children aged 15 or younger had been orphaned by AIDS, i.e., had lost their mother or both parents. Several southern African societies are experiencing the most severe demographic changes due to AIDS. By 1996, 13% of all Zambian children were orphans, and by 2014, orphans will account for roughly 1 in every 12 in the population (Joint USAID/UNICEF/SIDA Study Fund Project 1999; Zambian Ministry of Health/Central Board of Health 1999).

Orphaned children risk poor socialization, poverty, and lack of education, as well as sexual and physical abuse. The majority are still absorbed into their extended families; however, the strains are beginning to show in many communities (Foster 2000a). Inevitably, many orphaned children will grow up at high risk of HIV themselves, especially girls, who are more likely to be withdrawn from education when household resources are squeezed. Direct evidence from orphaned children in Zimbabwe suggests that both sexes may experience low self-esteem, isolation, stigma, and discrimination (Lee et al. 1999).

The long-term impact of HIV/AIDS—sickness, death, and orphaning—on social and economic functioning and development is difficult to determine with accuracy but will include reduced productivity; pressure on managerial, professional, and technical expertise; greatly increased demand on health and welfare services; and reduced capacity to deliver. AIDS exacerbates poverty, hinders development, and radically changes dependency ratios.

RESPONSES TO HIV/AIDS

This section describes the response to HIV/AIDS by governments and the nongovernmental sector. Of necessity, what follows is a generalized summary of the activities of many thousands of different organizational and institutional actors across the sub-Saharan region.

The Governmental Response

Throughout the region, the main governmental response has been from the health sector, with relatively low levels of engagement of other departments and ministries. National AIDS Programs tend to be based in health ministries, with a primary focus on HIV prevention, enhancing care through mainstream health services and in the community, and trying to promote a multisectoral response. The latter activity has proved an uphill battle, with other ministries tending to view AIDS as primarily a health issue. Nonetheless, some progress has been made. For example, the Southern Africa Development Community (SADC) has endorsed a progressive employment code on HIV/AIDS, which enshrines the rights of HIV-positive employees to confidentiality and equal treatment, while people with AIDS should be treated the same as others with different life-threatening conditions. The code also prohibits preemployment HIV screening and discrimination. At the same time, it acknowledges the rights and responsibilities of employers. Several countries in the region have developed national codes on employment practice in line with the regional code, Zimbabwe being one example.

Given their lead role on HIV/AIDS, it is a great concern that health ministries are seriously underfunded in most of the region and struggle to provide primary health care and basic treatments for opportunistic or sexually transmitted infections. Antiretroviral drugs are generally available only to the elite who can afford them through private health care and, in some countries, to pregnant mothers enrolled in trials to reduce mother-to-child HIV transmission.

Overall, there is little serious evidence of governments taking on board the implications of HIV/AIDS for itself as a major employer, never mind the broader, critical development issues associated with the pandemic that affects all sectors. For instance, not one African president attended the International Conference on AIDS and STIs in Africa held in Lusaka, Zambia, in 1999. Furthermore, in early 2000, President Thabo Mbeki of South Africa publicly questioned the link between HIV and AIDS and curbed policies around distribution of antiretroviral drugs to pregnant mothers and the armed forces. Nonetheless, a start is being made. For instance, the Ministry of Agriculture in Malawi began to explore the impact of AIDS in early 1999, looking both internally (i.e., implications as an employer) and externally (e.g., impact on production and livelihoods).

For long-term mitigation of the epidemic, a clear sense of the likely pattern and scale of the epidemic is essential, with a good understanding of long-term impacts. Policies, planning, and programs are required to address current needs but also to prepare for changes in production patterns and household structures, challenges to community functioning, and the depletion of human capital and its impact on the economy. Governments cannot achieve all these goals alone and need to explore how best to foster and work with nongovernmental organizations (NGOs), the private sector, international agencies, and communities and civic society to meet the urgent challenges facing them.

Support is also increasing from international and other donors, particularly from the United States of America, and the UNAIDS-led International Partnership against HIV/AIDS in Africa. The Partnership is developing on the premise of greatly enhanced government involvement and leadership. This integrated effort aims to strengthen national programs through encouraging visible and sustained political support; helping to develop nationally negotiated joint plans of action; increasing financial resources; and strengthening national and regional technical capacity.

Positively, some departments and ministries—for instance, in South Africa, Zambia, and Zimbabwe—have endorsed community care approaches, for example, in the care of children. New mechanisms are beginning to be developed to promote more effective working between the NGO and government sectors to meet welfare and other needs in the community, particularly around child care, home-based care, and voluntary counseling and testing.

The Broader Response

Welfare needs are clearly growing around AIDS and poverty in general, and governments are heavily reliant on the nongovernment sector to augment their own insufficient resources. The NGO sector in the region is diverse and sometimes vibrant. It comprises AIDS service organizations, that is, local NGOs that have developed in response to the epidemic; existing development organizations that integrate AIDS into their work or have developed additional "HIV/AIDS projects"; international NGOs; diverse community-based organizations and support groups for people living with HIV/AIDS; and churches and other civic society bodies. In addition, there is a strong presence of bilateral and multilateral agencies throughout the region.

AIDS service organizations (ASOs) have mushroomed in most countries, providing counseling and testing, awareness and prevention services, home-based care, orphan care, and support for people living with HIV/AIDS. Many have a religious orientation, which brings the added advantage of spiritual support in a region characterized by widespread religious belief. The extent of ASO development is uneven across the region, but it is increasing throughout.

Development NGOs have tended to be slow to incorporate AIDS into their mandates. The primary reasons for this pattern appear to be the following:

- They do not have a specific "health brief" (and view AIDS as primarily a health issue).
- They do not consider that they have the right expertise, particularly to deal with sensitive issues such as sexuality and death.
- Communities may not directly raise AIDS as a felt concern (although indirectly it undoubtedly is, as morbidity and mortality increase).
- They consider ASOs to be experts in the field whose job it is to respond to the epidemic.
- They are already overloaded with work and wish to narrow rather than widen their mandate.
- They have not sufficiently recognized how AIDS impacts on their own constituents and programs or on themselves as employers in high-prevalence countries.

These reasons all have an internal logic but must be challenged. Mainstreaming AIDS in the development process is not optional. In high-prevalence countries, AIDS impacts increasingly severely on both organizations and the communities they serve. In low prevalence countries, integrating AIDS into development is a way of operationalizing the development process as prevention, rather than cure for social and economic problems. By early 2000, some development NGOs in the region such as ActionAid, Oxfam, Plan International, and Save the Children USA and UK had begun the mainstreaming process or established responses specific to the changing demands of the epidemic.

Services

HIV testing services are not widely available throughout the region, although increasing numbers of voluntary counseling and testing centers are being established, often through donor funding from international agencies and through partnerships with NGOs rather than government. The great majority of people do not know their HIV status. Furthermore, in the absence of adequate follow-on services, such as health care and counseling, many see no advantage in knowing their status even when testing services are available. A great deal still needs to be done to reduce stigma and risks of discrimination and to ensure that people with HIV gain better access to the counseling, support, and medical care they need.

Basic general awareness about AIDS and HIV transmission does appear to have been achieved in much of the region, but this knowledge has not been widely translated into appropriate behavior change, and various myths and a degree of disbelief still abound. The continued high prevalence of HIV among antenatal women is warning enough that campaigns and prevention programs must be massively scaled up and become far more effective than at present, requiring solid linkages and collaboration between government and all other sectors.

Prevention efforts have tended to focus on condom distribution, STI treatment, and information, education, and communication campaigns. In many parts of the region, "abstinence and faithfulness" still constitutes the principal prevention message, especially for youth and the clients of church-based groups, although safer sex messages are increasingly common. Most effective prevention and awareness programs employ peer education techniques, whether worker to worker, youth to youth, ex-commercial sex worker to practicing commercial sex worker, or church member to church member.

Peer support is also advocated, hence the proliferation of support groups and networks for people living with HIV. At community level, support groups offer invaluable support, advice, peer counseling, and "safe space" for people living with HIV. Often, these groups have an income generation or training dimension, usually with the goal of promoting self-sufficiency for individuals, rather than the sustainability of the organization or group itself.

Networks exist at national and regional levels, such as the Zimbabwe National Network of People Living with HIV/AIDS (ZNNP+) or the Network of African People Living with HIV/AIDS (NAP+). These structures have great potential to contribute to stigma reduction and advocacy around the rights and needs of those infected and affected by HIV/AIDS. However, their effectiveness so far is limited by lack of capacity, funds, and in many cases, lack of clearly defined objectives that link to tangible outputs and outcomes.

In sub-Saharan Africa, the great majority of people with AIDS die within 10 years of infection. Most die at home, having had little or no access to effective treatments or palliative care to reduce suffering. Traditional healers are utilized by large numbers of people with varied results in medical terms but with the added potential to contribute to mental and spiritual coping with the disease.

One particular area of need is for home care. Zambia had the first widely acclaimed AIDS home care service as a mobile outreach program based at the Salvation Army's Chikankata Hospital in Kitwe in the mid-1980s. This service was influential for many other programs, as it developed a regional home care training service; nonetheless, as a model to emulate it remained problematic, requiring high expenditure per home visit and intensive use of professional expertise. Other programs have had to try to reduce costs and also to provide integrated services to reduce the stigma attached to AIDS home care.

A wide range of home care services have been developed. In rural areas, these services are primarily based in mission and district hospitals, whereas in urban areas they are mainly AIDS NGOs or church based. The main services provided are nursing and basic medical care, counseling and family support, and varying degrees of material provision including food. The more effective home care programs integrate prevention and awareness into their work and link families of the sick with local orphan support providers.

A survey in Zimbabwe (Woelk et al. 1997) found that although the home care services were greatly appreciated, the quality of service was usually quite low and costs were relatively high. Major expenditures, particularly in rural schemes, tended to go on transport and salaries, rather than direct services to patients and families.

Models of home care with the greatest potential value are those that strongly involve community members in the direct provision of services and strong referral networks between the formal health services and the community. They are also linked with a broad range of community-based HIV/AIDS–related services and even legal advisory services.

Despite the number of organizations and groups active in home care, coverage remains patchy. The numbers of people progressing to AIDS and needing home care continue to wildly outstrip the provision of services.

The spread and growth of orphan care programs is much more recent than other, predominantly adult-oriented services around HIV/AIDS. Responses to this "third wave" in the region do include institutional care; however, the overwhelming emphasis is on community-based approaches. In the front line of the response is the extended family, and the most effective orphan programs build on this through supportive visiting, often by neighbors acting as community volunteers (see, e.g., Lee et al. 1999). On this basic model, many alternatives are built, including the CINDI (Countrywide Integrated Noncommunicable Diseases Intervention) program in

Zambia, the COPE (Community-Based Options for Protection and Empowerment) and the FOCUS (Families, Orphans, and Children under Stress) program in Zimbabwe. Core activities of such programs include identifying and monitoring the most vulnerable children, supporting community coping mechanisms, keeping children in school, income generation, practical help, and child-minding facilities (Foster 2000b).

In recent years, there has been increasing interest by international donors and development agencies in the development or funding of orphan programs. This support is welcome, though there are many challenges and unknowns associated with how to effectively channel funds to household level without swamping, subverting, or undermining community-based initiatives.

Overall, across all dimensions of the response to HIV/AIDS, there is a pressing need to move toward a better awareness and understanding of cost-effectiveness issues, which will necessitate closer attention to measures of service quality. At present, most clients receive what they are given and are very grateful for it. However, this is an inadequate rationale for continuation of ill-targeted and overly expensive programs that cannot, in any case, be sustained long term and scaled up.

CONCLUSION

The scale of the HIV/AIDS pandemic south of the Sahara is such that a massive commitment at all levels and from all sectors is required to promote prevention, ensure care, and work toward effective and appropriate mitigation. The relative silence on HIV/AIDS issues and continuing stigma must be resolved. Crucially, the underlying driving forces of the pandemic—gender inequality, human rights abuse, and poverty—must be tackled.

Some changes can be swiftly implemented and are directly targeted on HIV/AIDS, such as increasing access to and use of condoms. Others require long-term measures and link to a much broader development agenda, for example, improved education or employment opportunities and changes in gender relations. Nevertheless, all require a supportive conceptual policy framework—or enabling environment—endorsed from the top.

Given the myriad other issues facing the region, it will be difficult to gain the priority that the pandemic requires and the energy required in our response. However, communities, organizations, and institutions across the region are beginning to stir from slumber, and many others have already demonstrated their commitment to the process. It is on this foundation that sub-Saharan Africa will build its response to HIV/AIDS.

BIBLIOGRAPHY

AIDS Analysis Africa. (bimonthly newsletter on HIV/AIDS in Africa). HEARD, Durban, South Africa.

Aliro, Ogen, H. Ochieng, and A. Fiedler. 1999. "Male Adolescence and Sex Education in Uganda." In *AIDS and Men: Taking Risks or Taking Responsibility*, Martin Foreman, ed., pp. 99–109. London: Panos.

Bwayo, Job, M. Omari, A. Mutere, F. Plummer, S. Moses, J. Ndinya-Achola, and J. Kreiss. 1992. "HIV Infection in Long Distance Truck Drivers in Kenya: Seroprevalence, Seroincidence and Health Factors." Paper presented at the Eighth International Conference on AIDS, Amsterdam.

Caraël, M., A. Opio, J. Musinguzi, E. Madraa, G. Tembo, and G. Asiimwe-Okiror. 1997. "Change in Sexual Behaviour and Decline in HIV Infection among Young Pregnant Women in Urban Uganda." *AIDS* 11(14): 1757–1763.

Foster, Geoff. 2000a. "The Capacity of the Extended Family Safety Net for Orphans in Africa." *Psychology, Health and Medicine* 5(1): 55–62.

———. 2000b. "Responses in Zimbabwe to Children Affected by AIDS." *SAfAIDS News* 8 (1): 2–7.

Jackson, Helen, R. Kerkhoven, D. Lindsey, G. Mutangadura, and F. Nhara. 1999. *HIV/AIDS in Southern Africa: The Threat to Development*. London: CIIR Comment.

Joint USAID/UNICEF/SIDA Study Fund Project. 1999. *Orphans and Vulnerable Children: A Situational Analysis, Zambia 1999*. Lusaka: Author.

Lee, Tim, S. Kagoro, S. Muzanya, C. Makufa, G. Foster, and R. Gonyora. 1999. *FOCUS Evaluation Report: Report of a Participatory, Self-Evaluation of the FACT Families Orphans and Children under Stress (FOCUS) Program*. Mutare: FACT.

Pisani, Elizabeth. 1999. "AIDS into the 21st Century: Some Critical Considerations." *SAfAIDS News* 7 (4): 2–10.

Roseberry, Wendy, and R. Paul. 1998. *The Impact of AIDS on Capacity Building*. Washington, D.C.: World Bank.

SAfAIDS News (quarterly newsletter on HIV/AIDS in southern Africa). SAfAIDS, Harare, Zimbabwe.

Sexual Health Exchange (quarterly newsletter on programs, policy, research around AIDS and other aspects of sexual health, global focus). KIT and SAfAIDS, Amsterdam, Netherlands, and Harare, Zimbabwe.

UNAIDS. 1999. *A Review of Household and Community Responses to the HIV/AIDS Epidemic in the Rural Areas of Sub-Saharan Africa*. Best Practice Collection. Geneva: Author.

UNAIDS/WHO. 2000. *Report on the Global HIV/AIDS Epidemic*. Geneva: Author.

Welbourn, Alice. 1995. "Participatory Approaches to HIV/AIDS Programs: Introduction." *PLA Notes* 23: 57–61.

Wilson, David. 2000. *Corridors of Hope in Southern Africa: HIV Prevention Needs and Opportunities in Four Border Towns*. Arlington, VA: Family Health International.

Woelk, Godfrey, H. Jackson, R. Kerkhoven, K. Hansen, N. Manjonjori, P. Maramba, J. Mutambirwa, E. Ndimande, and E. Vera. 1997. *Do We Care? The Cost and Quality of Community Home Based Care for HIV/AIDS Patients and Their Communities in Zimbabwe*. Harare: University of Zimbabwe, SAfAIDS, and Ministry of Health and Child Welfare.

Zambian Ministry of Health/Central Board of Health. 1999. *HIV/AIDS in Zambia: Background Projections, Impacts, Interventions*. Lusaka: Author.

12

SWITZERLAND

Thomas Steffen

INTRODUCTION

In June 1982, the Swiss Federal Office of Public Health (SFOPH) received its first medical report of Kaposi's sarcoma. The patient had recently returned to Switzerland from the United States. From September 1982, the SFOPH received additional case reports about this disease (AHS/SFOPH 1993), and the number of diagnoses increased rapidly. In March 1983, the SFOPH recorded 18 similar cases of the disease, of which 16 persons had died. In 1984, the total reached 40 cases. A total of 100 cases of Kaposi's sarcoma were reported by 1985; however, several unreported cases were estimated. As a consequence, Switzerland saw itself facing one of the greatest public health challenges in recent decades.

Compared to other European countries, the number of new HIV and AIDS cases had increased substantially. Hence by the end of 1994, Switzerland had the second highest AIDS prevalence in Europe, with 61 AIDS cases (cumulative) per 100,000 inhabitants versus 75 cases per 100,000 in Spain (Schneider 1996).

This rapid appearance of a new and dangerous infectious disease triggered a multitiered process, which went far beyond the development of individual prevention and therapy measures. In keeping with the complex disease picture, which appeared frequently in social fringe groups, it was necessary to create differentiated health care and intervention structures. The authorities and the public health experts had to consider total social development as well as the constantly changing state-of-the-art strategies for prevention and therapy.

ISSUES RELATING TO HIV AND AIDS

History of HIV and AIDS

AIDS was first described in 1981 as an independent disease of the immune system. During the following years, HIV/AIDS spread dramatically world-wide. In 1997 Switzerland still remained in the category of European countries with the highest AIDS prevalence (8.1 AIDS cases per 100,000 inhabitants). By comparison, the prevalence in neighboring countries was clearly much lower: Italy (6.6 per 100,000), France (4.7 per 100,000), Germany (1.7 per 100,000), Austria (1.5 per 100,000) (European Centre for the Epidemiological Monitoring of AIDS 1997).

Differentiated data analyses gained great importance for assessing the epidemiological situation. Data on the HIV/AIDS epidemic in Switzerland are based largely on reports of AIDS cases from attending physicians, AIDS fatalities, and laboratory reports of new HIV infections. The absolute number of initial HIV diagnoses is projected from lab reports and other supplementary reports by physicians (Table 12.1).

Table 12.1 shows the number of positive HIV test results between 1986 and 1999 in Switzerland. Mainly infections resulting from drug injections and sex between men were determined during the first years. New infections from heterosexual contacts became a third category (Gebhardt 1997; SFOPH 2000; UNAIDS/WHO 2000). Thus for men in 1989, for example, 45% of all new cases were transmitted through injecting drug use (IDU) and 36% through sex between men. Among women that year, 53% of new infections were related to injecting drug use and 40% in connection with heterosexual contact. Other categories of transmission were much more rare. Hence up to June 2000 a total of 92 AIDS cases in Switzerland were caused by mother-child transmission, 80 cases by blood transfusions, and 37 cases involving hemophiliac patients (SFOPH 2000).

Since 1992 the number of newly diagnosed HIV infections has declined. This development owes above all to the decrease in infections through IDU and sex between men. Since the beginning of the 1990s, heterosexual infections represent the largest portion of newly diagnosed cases. The reasons for HIV infections in this group are mainly sexual contacts with people from countries with mainly heterosexual HIV transmission, with people who inject drugs, as well as with known HIV-positive people.

The portion of women with new infections in Switzerland during 1999 was above 36%. Since the mid-1990s there has been a related increase in the portion of women with new HIV infections. The increase among women is explained by the rise in portion of heterosexual infections with a high

Table 12.1
HIV in Switzerland: Positive HIV Test Results as Reported by Confirmation
Laboratories, According to Gender, Year, and Three Major Groups

Gender	1986	1989	1992	1995	1996	1997	1998	1999
Men								
Number of positive results	2,128	1,161	1,179	611	561	484	381	377
Homosexual men		36%	44%	42%	36%	39%	42%	38%
Injecting drug users		45%	31%	23%	23%	19%	15%	16%
Heterosexuals		14%	21%	28%	34%	35%	39%	40%
Others		5%	4%	7%	7%	7%	5%	6%
Women								
Number of positive results	830	578	516	324	293	283	219	216
Injecting drug users		53%	32%	23%	18%	14%	10%	13%
Heterosexuals		40%	61%	67%	73%	77%	77%	78%
Others		7%	8%	10%	9%	9%	13%	9%
Gender unknown	294	217	214	84	69	67	57	10
Total	3,252	1,956	1,909	1,019	923	834	657	603

Source: SFOPH 2000.

portion of women and the reduction in infections involving IDUs, which
indicate a high portion of men. On the other hand, there was no evidence
that more women than men were infected in the same manner (SFOPH
2000). Approximately three-fourths of the persons living with AIDS or HIV
are residents of the cantons of Zurich, Geneva, Vaud, Berne, or Basel, all

of which have large urban agglomerations. Current epidemiological trends are also published regularly on the home page of the Swiss Federal Office of Public Health (http://www.admin.ch/bag).

An increase in fatalities owing to HIV infection has been observed in Switzerland since 1982, largely all in the age group 25–44. By the mid-1990s AIDS-related illnesses were the second-highest cause of death in this age group for both men and women. HIV-related mortality in Switzerland has declined again since 1995 (Figure 12.1). Thus, 686 fatalities due to AIDS were registered in Switzerland in 1994 (10 death cases per 100,000 inhabitants), and in 1998 the figure had declined to 136 (2 death cases per 100,000 inhabitants). The decline in fatalities since 1995 owes largely to the use of antiretroviral combination therapies (Gebhardt, Rickenbach, and Egger 1998).

In summary, it can be stated that a substantial increase in newly reported HIV infections appeared during the mid-1980s, but it should be noted that the HIV test only came into widespread use beginning in 1985. For this reason the number of positive test results in the mid-1980s was particularly high. Since 1992 the number of newly established HIV infections has declined, which is assessed as an effect of the interventions to be described later. AIDS-related mortality has also declined, and this is attributed mainly to new antiretroviral combination therapies. Especially striking is the decrease in new HIV infections among IDUs. In the late 1980s, half of all new infections among men were linked to injection drug use. That portion dropped to below 20% by the end of the 1990s (Steffen and Gutzwiller 1999). The same pattern was found among women. Thanks to a well-structured recording system, the trends found in recent years have been consistently integrated into ongoing planning and monitoring of preventive measures. Examples of this process are discussed in the following pages.

The Social, Political, and Medical Context of HIV and AIDS

The appearance of the HIV epidemic posed the greatest public health challenge to Switzerland's health care system of the twentieth century. The challenge did not result from the epidemic alone but also from the complex and historically evolved structure of Swiss public health services. Compared to other industrialized nations, Switzerland has one of the most complicated public health services for its roughly 7 million citizens. Thus, the main authority for Switzerland's public health care is not a central federal office but one decentralized among 26 Swiss cantons that share public health decision making with the federal government and various other federal and nongovernmental organizations (Gutzwiller and Jeanneret 1999). Such a structure has the advantage of decisions being taken near the areas affected. Alternatively, there is a danger that urgently needed decisions cannot be carried out promptly or consistently.

Figure 12.1
Death Cases AIDS/HIV in Switzerland, by Gender and Year, 1985–1999

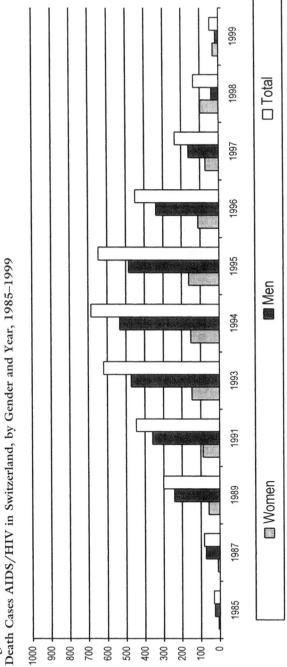

Source: SFOPH 2000.

Table 12.2
AIDS Prevention Strategy in Switzerland: A Three-Tier Campaign

1. Measures addressed to the general public, for example, the "Stop AIDS" campaigns. These campaigns use nationwide media coverage to give accurate information on HIV and condom use, and encourage solidarity with people living with HIV/AIDS, and so on.
2. Measures aimed at specific target groups, for example, specific information for homosexuals, drug users, and adolescents.
3. Specific support based on individual interactions. Use of prevention "multipliers" such as parents, teachers, doctors, and peer counselors.

Source: AHS/SFOPH 1993.

Yet in the case of HIV, the possibility arose that the federal government in cooperation with cantons could launch comprehensive measures to combat communicable diseases based on the epidemic law of 1970. The SFOPH drafted the guidelines for political decision making, monitoring of the epidemic, intervention, and information. Table 12.2 shows the three main points of the Swiss prevention strategy, and Table 12.3 describes the concept of the Swiss global evaluation of the national AIDS prevention strategy. The SFOPH is also responsible for national and international coordination. On the other hand, the current Swiss concept makes local authorities responsible for implementing and coordinating measures within their areas, while nongovernmental organizations (NGOs) often assume specific tasks in close direct contact with those affected.

During the course of this intervention process, special coordination committees were created. Experts from the various specialties belong to these committees. Among the committees' tasks are information exchange, working out solutions to current problems, and initiating and coordinating new projects in combating AIDS. This interdisciplinary development made it possible to reach a broad consensus on appropriate intervention measures (SFOPH 1991). It also had a substantial impact on other problem areas. Hence at the beginning of the 1990s an innovative measures package to combat drugs was launched that provided harm reduction measures such as widespread dispensing of syringes and new therapy options including heroin-supported treatment (Klingemann 1999; Rihs-Middel 1996; Uchtenhagen et al. 1999).

Compared with other major public health problems, a very efficient organizational structure was created in the HIV/AIDS sphere. Such an efficient organizational structure is still partially lacking in Switzerland, for example, in the area of legal drugs such as alcohol and tobacco and in the case of various other health care concerns. But intensified efforts have been under way during recent years to make use of positive experiences in combating AIDS in other fields of public health intervention.

Table 12.3
**Long-Term Global Evaluation of the Swiss National AIDS Prevention
Strategy: Examples of Indicators**

Process Indicators

1. Prevention activities such as number of campaign posters, syringes distributed, press and radio coverage.
2. Mediators working with risk population.
3. Acceptance of prevention activities.

Outcome Indicators

1. AIDS/HIV knowledge such as information on means of transmission and methods for protection.
2. Risk behavior such as number of sexual partners, injecting drug use.
3. Protective behavior such as use of condoms, reported HIV testing, condom sales.
4. Possible unwanted side effects of prevention strategy such as sexual promiscuity.
5. Epidemiological surveillance of new HIV cases.

Source: Dubois-Arber et al. 1999.

Medical care for people who are HIV-positive or AIDS victims has changed considerably during the last 20 years. During the early years, only symptomatic or palliative treatment was available for patients. This situation was changed substantially during the 1990s with the availability of antiviral substances (highly active antiretroviral therapy [HAART]). Besides the effect on mortality already described, a notable improvement in the health status was achieved in many HIV-positive people in recent years. However, since the outset of the HIV/AIDS epidemic, medical and health care support have placed high demands on the public health system. Various adaptations were necessary in the outpatient as well as inpatient clinical care system. Today a broad network of specialized outpatient clinics as well as hospital departments, in addition to the well-developed family-doctor system, is available to patients. Medical treatment costs are covered by medical insurance, which is mandatory for all residents of Switzerland. Yet various social issues that have arisen from the improved medical situation still remain open. For example, in this context, during recent years the impact of an HIV infection on job performance has also been discussed more frequently. Due to the disease's expected rapid progress in the past, a prompt appearance of permanent incapacity on the job was also anticipated. Hence differentiated assessment systems must be found today. At present this question is being discussed increasingly in Switzerland.

Besides medical treatment, high priority was placed very early on building up a well-documented cohort treatment system so as to contribute to further development of HIV/AIDS therapy. This Swiss HIV-Positive Cohort Study gained importance in clinical as well as medical research. The Study is a multicentric research project initiated in 1987 by the SFOPH, among others. Leading Swiss university clinics are involved in the study. In total, 10,000 volunteer study participants have been recruited to date, of which 4,400 are given regular checkups (Lebergerber et al. 1994; Opravil, Rickenbach, and Ledergerber 1998; SFOPH 1999b). Owing to the broad database, a wide variety of studies based on the Swiss HIV Cohort Study have been conducted in the areas of epidemiology, clinical research, laboratory methods, patient care, and public health. Selected study results have been published in international specialist journals (e.g., Furrer et al. 1999; Lebergerber et al. 1999; Phillips et al. 1999; SFOPH 1999a).

As the AIDS prevention campaigns for general population in Switzerland began in 1986, they had the character of a crisis intervention during a period when there were still no therapeutic measures available. The campaigns aimed at behavioral changes and focused on the social aspect of the AIDS problem. The "combat AIDS" strategy pursued three major goals:

• Preventing new HIV infections
• Reducing the negative impact of the epidemic on those affected and
• Promoting solidarity.

Three campaign levels were determined for the primary preventive strategy that has been carried out in Switzerland since 1986.

• General measures to inform and motivate the entire population;
• Specific interventions for special target groups using suitable channels and messages; and
• Interventions with in-depth and long-term impact that were based on individual interactions such as counseling.

The strategies mentioned used an integration model based on the conviction that people can be motivated toward preventive behavior by a learning process (Dubois-Arber et al. 1996). Moreover, a pragmatic procedure was often selected that placed high value on free choice. Thus condom use was broadly urged in campaigns as part of sexual behavior with a potential HIV infection risk, as was use of sterilized syringes for those who inject drugs. Maintaining behavior with no risk of infection—for example, sexual monogamy and abstinence from injecting drugs—was recommended especially.

Evaluation data showed that public knowledge regarding methods of HIV transmission and the possible steps to prevent it clearly improved during the course of the campaign. Hence, only 23% of 20- to 69-year-olds surveyed in an initial public opinion poll indicated the correct response to an item relating to HIV risk through exchanging needles. One year following introduction of the public campaign, 95% responded correctly with regard to this issue. The knowledge level among the general public also remained high in the succeeding years, perhaps due to additional reinforcement campaigns (AHS/SFOPH 1993). Increased use of condoms in situations with potential risk of HIV infection is one of the most important changes to be mentioned since the start-up of AIDS prevention campaigns began. Among 17- to 30-year-olds, consistent use of condoms with occasional partners rose from 8% in 1987 to 56% in 1994. AIDS prevention seems to have had no great impact on sexual activity; however, the number of people with multiple partners appears to have decreased, and the trend toward changing partners seems to occur less often (Dubois-Arber, Jeannin, and Spencer 1999; Dubois-Arber et al. 1996, 1999).

Due to the high rate of infection through injecting drug use, special importance has been placed on informing this group since the start of AIDS prevention campaigns. Harm reduction and therapeutic measures for IDUs were expanded considerably in the context of AIDS prevention. Today 1,700 inpatient abstinence-oriented therapy slots are available for the roughly 30,000 IDUs. Some 15,000 drug addicts are in methadone-supported treatment, and 1,000 are in heroin-supported treatment. Heroin-supported treatment was developed at the outset of the 1990s due to the sharp outbreak of the AIDS epidemic, among other reasons (Steffen et al. forthcoming).

Dispensing injection materials through low-threshold facilities has also gained importance in connection with AIDS prevention. For instance, about 7 million syringes were provided at such institutions during 1993. Fortunately the initiative brought about a sharp decline in new HIV infections through injecting drugs. This positive development has stabilized during recent years (Table 12.1).

A broad consensus supporting the AIDS prevention strategy selected could be determined in the population. For example, Swiss drug policy has been directly or indirectly accepted in public voting. A plebiscite that would have made substantial changes in the drug policy described was clearly rejected with 71% "No" votes in September 1997.

Beside IDUs, the group of homosexual men has gained special importance because of the epidemiological situation. The gay community was severely affected by the AIDS epidemic in Switzerland. A survey among 1,195 homosexual men in 1994 showed that 76% knew an HIV/AIDS–positive person. This clearly lay above the average of 25% among the Swiss population (Moreau-Gruet and Dubois-Arber 1995). About half of all new AIDS cases in Switzerland before 1990 involved homosexual men (SFOPH 2000).

It was possible to introduce necessary protective measures even during the epidemic's early years through a specific and broad-based prevention campaign carried out in connection with those affected. Thus 89% of those surveyed in the study mentioned above indicated that they always used protection during sexual contact. However, that study also showed that neglect of protective measures often occurred in emotional situations (e.g., a problem in the partnership, lack of communication between partners). At present, it is vital to maintain good protective behavior through other targeted preventive measures. This issue presents a special challenge particularly among young men who have not experienced the earlier development.

In summary, it can be determined that the AIDS prevention strategy pursued is broadly accepted as appropriate in Switzerland today. Quite within the sense of the Ottawa Charter, the World Health Organization (WHO) has succeeded at least partially in initiating structural and individual changes in its overall procedure. Evidence of favorable effects can also be noted at the process and outcome levels.

RESPONSES TO HIV/AIDS

Governmental Efforts

Combating AIDS in Switzerland is a national and cantonal task. As already pointed out briefly, the national government has to work on the following priority tasks:

1. Monitoring the epidemic
2. Information and prevention
3. Coordination of AIDS prevention measures
4. Assistance in training specialists
5. Support for research

The cantonal governments need to support patient care, direct information, and public education as well as preventive efforts in the drug sphere. The federal government offers special programs to support the cantonal governments in these tasks.

As presented, Swiss health care policy in the HIV and AIDS sphere is today based on a broad consensus among federal centers, cantons, communities, and NGOs. These measures were supported with resources made available by the federal government. In 1997 the SFOPH made available about U.S. $11 million for AIDS prevention and $5 million for AIDS research. Despite the positive development overall, the effort to date must be maintained in order to stabilize the outcome over the long term. The forces on hand must be transformed into a continuing process, and the experience gained needs to be used for other non-AIDS-specific public health processes. Accordingly, innovative goals for the coming years have been formulated that should support this process (Table 12.4). This clear formulation of

Table 12.4
HIV and AIDS: National Program Goals, 1999–2003

Health Promotion

1. State authorities take coordinated steps to ensure that existing inequalities relative to diseases, work, and social security are systematically eliminated from the law.
2. Self-determination, self-responsibility, and collective responsibility with respect to health are discussed and dealt with at the national level.
3. A survey on the needs of people living with HIV is conducted to improve their quality of life.

Prevention

1. Adolescents and adults continue to receive adequate information on risk situations and necessary preventive behavior. Established modes of preventive behavior are maintained; long-term prevention is improved.
2. By the end of 2001, HIV should form an integral part of the discussion of love, relationships, and sexuality in primary vocational and secondary schools. Sexually transmitted diseases and substance abuse will also be included in this educational process.
3. Vulnerable groups or individuals are addressed more frequently and reached more sustainably with proposals for prevention.
4. As of 2001, 9 of 10 people living with HIV will have integrated preventive behavior into their lifestyle.
5. The importance of diagnostic and therapeutic measures and their relationship to prevention are communicated regularly.

Therapy and Diagnostics

1. As of 2002 almost all people living with HIV will be sufficiently competent to decide on a therapy adapted to their personal lifestyle.
2. By the end of 2001, 9 of 10 HIV-positive individuals will be in a position to obtain the counseling or support they require for HIV-related problems.

Development of Knowledge and Transfer of Skills

1. Organizations or other services are mandated to coordinate HIV/AIDS-related activities and to inform cantonal and local structures.
2. The AIDS research program will continue to be financed as before.
3. International cooperation relative to HIV and AIDS is adapted to current and future requirements at multinational and bilateral levels.

Quality

1. By the end of 2001, all organizations and institutions active in the areas of HIV and AIDS that are financed by the public sector will have introduced quality management.

Source: SFOPH 1999b.

goals for the years ahead should provide an effective approach toward combating AIDS in Switzerland that can be developed successfully in the future.

Nongovernment Efforts

As described, the federal government is largely responsible for carrying out measures for monitoring the epidemic, for disseminating information on prevention, and for coordinating research and training in Switzerland. Various committees were formed for specialized tasks (e.g., for global AIDS issues or for Swiss AIDS research). These national committees coordinate activities in the research, prevention, epidemiology, therapy, and social sectors.

Moreover, other important organizations in the AIDS relief area emerged during the 1980s and have taken on central importance. Three organizations are described briefly.

AIDS Help Switzerland (AHS)

AHS was founded as a national association in 1985 by representatives of various organizations that catered to gay men and women. Today 18 cantonal centers in Switzerland and the principality of Liechtenstein are linked to it. About 80% of the budget is provided by the federal government (Federal Office of Public Health [FOPH]). Among the most important AHS goals are information directed toward the public and various population groups (e.g., homosexuals, prostitutes, their clients, and drug consumers) on HIV and AIDS risks and combating discrimination against people affected by them. Information and prevention campaigns are considered to be major objectives of the organization. AIDS Help Switzerland also helps affected patients with professional, insurance, and social policy issues.

AIDS Info Docu Switzerland

The AIDS Info Docu Foundation of Switzerland was founded in 1988. It is financed in part by the federal government. The major goal of this documentation center is to distribute information for multipliers (i.e., people who concern themselves with AIDS for professional reasons, e.g., teachers, physicians, social workers). Since 1998 the AIDS-Info-Docu database has been accessible via the Internet (http://www.hivnet.ch).

People with HIV/AIDS (PWA) Switzerland

PWA Switzerland was founded in 1991 and is the national umbrella organization of people with HIV/AIDS (various independent regional organizations had existed previously). The organization is committed to a better quality of life for those directly affected. It looks out for their interests and works to prevent them from being discriminated against and excluded.

Besides those organizations involved specifically in AIDS matters, various traditional relief agencies (e.g., Swiss Red Cross) and specialist associations (e.g., Swiss Medical Association) have committed themselves. Moreover, the cantons' own AIDS help centers are active at the regional level, and there is a well-developed network of sociomedical assistance (e.g., housing and nursing).

CONCLUSION

After a very rapid initial rise in HIV/AIDS incidence in Switzerland, targeted public health measures were able to reduce the spread of HIV during the 1980s and 1990s. Previous success is attributed to an innovative and nationally coordinated strategy that could mobilize the necessary financial resources. At present, this process, which was triggered by a crisis situation, must be transformed into ongoing sustainable development. This represents a special challenge and especially at a time when the cost situation in health care is being discussed more intensively in many industrialized countries. As already mentioned, clear formulation of future goals here should enable the best possible and most visible development. Precisely from this vantage point, the positive prevention and intervention measures that have been implemented should be adapted broadly in other areas. This developmental process in other regions, however, remains in the initial phases.

BIBLIOGRAPHY

AHS/SFOPH (AIDS Help Switzerland and Swiss Federal Office of Public Health), eds. 1993. *Stop AIDS—Die Stop AIDS—Story, 1987–1992.* Berne: Author.

Dubois-Arber, Françoise, André Jeannin, Giovanna Meystre-Agustoni, Florence Moreau-Gruet, Mary Haour-Knipe, Brenda Spencer, and Fred Paccaud. 1996. *Evaluation of the AIDS Prevention Strategy in Switzerland Mandated by the Federal Office of Public Health: Fifth Synthesis Report 1993–1995.* Lausanne: Institute universitaire de médecine sociale et préventive.

Dubois-Arber, Françoise, André Jeannin, and Brenda Spencer. 1999. "Long Term Global Evaluation of a National AIDS Prevention Strategy: The Case of Switzerland." *AIDS* 13: 2571–2582.

Dubois-Arber, Françoise, André Jeannin, Brenda Spencer, Giovanna Meystre-Agustoni, Mary Haour-Knipe, Florence Moreau-Gruet, Fabienne Benninghoff, and Fred Paccaud. 1999. *Evaluation of the AIDS Prevention Strategy in Switzerland Mandated by the Federal Office of Public Health: Sixth Synthesis Report 1996–1998.* Lausanne: Institute universitaire de médecine sociale et préventive.

European Centre for the Epidemiological Monitoring of AIDS. 1997. *HIV/AIDS Surveillance in Europe.* Quarterly Report no. 56. Saint Maurice, France: Author.

Furrer, Hansjakob, Matthias Egger, Milos Opravil, Enos Bernasconi, Bernard Hirschel, Manuel Battegay, Amalio Telenti, Pietro L. Vernazza, Marin Rickenbach, Markus Flepp, and Raffaele Malinverni. 1999. "Discontinuation of Primary Prophylaxis against *Pneumocystis carinii pneumonia* in HIV-1 Infected Adults Treated with Combination Antiretroviral Therapy. Swiss HIV Cohort Study." *New England Journal of Medicine* 340: 1301–1306.

Gebhardt, Martin. 1997. *Aids und HIV in der Schweiz—Epidemiologische Situation Ende 1996*. Berne: EDMZ.

Gebhardt, Martin, Martin Rickenbach, and Matthias Egger. 1998. "Impact of Antiretroviral Combination Therapies on AIDS." *AIDS* 12: 1195–1201.

Gutzwiller, Felix, and Jeanneret Olivier, eds. 1999. *Sozial- und Präventivmedizin Public Health*. Berne: Hans Huber Verlag.

Klingemann, Harald. 1999. "Harm Reduction and Abstinence: Swiss Drug Policy at a Time of Transition." In *Drug Treatment Systems in an International Perspective*, Harald Klingemann and Geoffrey Hunt, eds., pp. 94–111. Thousand Oaks, CA: Sage Publications.

Lebergerber, Bruno, Matthias Egger, Véronique Erard, Rainer Weber, Bernard Hirschel, Hansjakob Furrer, Manuel Battegay, Pietro Vernazza, Enos Bernasconi, Milos Opravil, Daniel Kaufmann, Philippe Sudre, Patrick Francioli, and Amalio Telenti. 1999. "AIDS-Related Opportunistic Illness Occurring after Initiation of Potent Antiretroviral Therapy: The Swiss HIV Cohort Study." *JAMA* 282: 2220–2226.

Lebergerber, Bruno, Jan von Oberbeck, Matthias Egger, Ruedi Lüthy, and the Swiss HIV Cohort Study. 1994. "The Swiss HIV Cohort Study: Rationale, Organization and Selected Baseline Characteristic." *Soz Praeventivmed* 39: 387–394.

Moreau-Gruet, Florence, and Françoise Dubois-Arber. 1995. *Evaluation de la Stratégie de prévention du Sida en Suisse*. Lausanne: Institute universitaire de médecine sociale et préventive.

Opravil, Milos, Martin Rickenbach, and Bruno Ledergerber. 1998. "Die Schweizerische HIV-Kohortenstudie—Verbindung Zwischen Klinischer Forschung und ärztlicher Praxis." *Therapeutische Umschau* 55: 329–334.

Phillips, N. Andrew, Sophie Grabar, Jean-Michel Tassie, Dominique Costagliola, Jens D. Lundgren, and Matthias Egger. 1999. "Use of Observational Databases to Evaluate the Effectiveness of Antiretroviral Therapy for HIV Infection: Comparison of Cohort Studies with Randomized Trials. EuroSIDA, the French Hospital Database on HIV and the Swiss HIV Cohort Study Groups." *AIDS* 13: 2075–2082.

Rihs-Middel, Margret. 1996. "The Swiss Federal Office of Public Health's Research Strategy and the Prescription of Narcotics" In *The Medical Prescription of Narcotics*, Margret Rihs-Middel, ed., pp. 16–25. Berne: Hogrefe & Huber Publisher.

Schneider, Richard E. 1996. "HIV-Infektionen in der Schweiz." *Internist* 37: 419–421.

Steffen, Thomas, and Felix Gutzwiller. 1999. "Hepatitis B und C bei Intravenös Drogenkonsumierenden in der Schweiz." *Medizinische Rundschau Praxis* 88: 1937–1944.

Steffen, Thomas, Stephan Christen, Richard Blättler, Felix Gutzwiller, and PROVE Team. Forthcoming. "Infectious Diseases and Public Health: Risk Taking Behaviour during Participation in the Swiss Programme for a Medical Prescription of Narcotics (PROVE)." *Substance Use and Misuse*.

Swiss Federal Office of Public Health (SFOPH), ed. 1991. *Aids in der Schweiz 1991.* Berne: EDMZ.

———. 1999a. *Aids-Forschung Schweiz No. 2.* Zollikofen: GEWA.

———. 1999b. *HIV and AIDS—National Program 1999–2003.* Berne: EDMZ.

———. 2000. "Aids-Statistik." *BAG-Bulletin* 31: 624–625.

Uchtenhagen, Ambros, Anja Dobler-Mikola, Thomas Steffen, Felix Gutzwiller, Richard Blättler, and Silvie Pfeifer. 1999. *Prescription of Narcotics for Heroin Addicts—Main Results of the Swiss National Cohort Study.* Basel: Karger Verlag.

UNAIDS/WHO. 2000. *Epidemiological Fact Sheet on HIV/AIDS and Sexually Transmitted Infections Switzerland Update 2000.* Geneva: Author.

13

UNITED KINGDOM

Kathryn Higgins and Sally Haw

INTRODUCTION

The United Kingdom, a member state of the European Community, is made up of the four countries of England, Scotland, Wales, and Northern Ireland. It has a combined population of almost 60 million. With a population of 50 million, England is the largest, followed by Scotland with 5 million, Northern Ireland with about 1.6 million and Wales with a population of 1 million. The United Kingdom is a major trading and financial center and has the fourth largest economy in Western Europe. Service industries, particularly banking, insurance, and business, account for the largest proportion of the gross domestic product. In contrast, manufacturing industry has declined in importance and currently employs only 18% of the workforce. In fact, the widespread closure of traditional industries such as coal mining, shipbuilding, and other large-scale manufacturing over the recent decades has meant that many regions, particularly those in Northern England, Scotland, and Wales, have been characterized by high and long-term unemployment. In many communities in these areas, people are dependent on state benefits, and the social security budget currently accounts for over one-third of all public expenditure in the United Kingdom. Social exclusion is a major issue for many localities in Northern England, Scotland, and Northern Ireland.

There are a number of different black and ethnic minority groups in the United Kingdom including African, Caribbean, Indian, Pakistani, Bangladeshi, and Chinese. They tend to be concentrated in particular communities mainly in the Southeast and Northwest of England and the West Midlands. Within these regions ethnic minorities consist largely of people of Indian, Pakistani, and Chinese origin. There are comparatively fewer people from black and ethnic minorities resident in Scotland and Northern Ireland.

Following 18 years of Conservative government, a Labour government was elected to power in the United Kingdom in 1997. Significant political issues include debate surrounding monetary and political integration with continental Europe. Northern Ireland has seen the signing of the historic peace agreement in April 1998, which ended almost 30 years of political upheaval and extreme sectarian violence. In addition, there has been major constitutional reform, with the establishment of a separate Parliament in Scotland and Assemblies in Wales and Northern Ireland.

In this chapter we describe the historical background to policy responses, current levels and patterns of HIV in the United Kingdom, and the development of prevention, harm reduction, and treatment and care responses to the HIV epidemic. While overall HIV and AIDS policy is dictated by central government, its implementation is dependent on statutory agencies and nongovernment organizations (NGOs), and the pivotal but changing role of the NGOs is discussed. We also address the changing public attitudes toward HIV and AIDS. The chapter concludes by looking to the future and identifies key issues to be addressed by the new HIV and AIDS strategies, currently under development in the United Kingdom.

The chapter considers issues from an overall United Kingdom perspective. However, it is important to note that there are significant structural and organizational differences among the four countries within the United Kingdom, and these differences affect both the organization and delivery of services. These differences and their implications are not discussed in detail.

ISSUES RELATING TO HIV AND AIDS

History of HIV and AIDS in the United Kingdom

The first *official* report on AIDS appeared in 1983 (Communicable Diseases Surveillance Centre 1983). By that time the number of people affected by the disease was growing rapidly, and three had already died. An alliance of gay organizations, clinicians, and scientists began to exert pressure on the government to respond to the problem. In 1985 an Expert Advisory Group on AIDS (EAGA), chaired by then Chief Medical Officer Donald Acheson, was set up to provide guidance on policy. Later that year, funding of £6.5 million ($10 million) was announced by central government for the development of treatment services and a national information campaign. In 1986, a special government cabinet committee was also set up, the first of its kind to deal with a specific disease. At that time, scientists had an incomplete understanding of the mechanisms of HIV transmission and predicted exponential growth in the number of new infections. The lack of information caused considerable alarm in political circles not only because of the cost in human terms but also because of the potential costs of treatment and care. Subsequently, significant downward revision of these estimates was made.

With new funding, a network of services was beginning to develop, and in 1987 AIDS Liaison Officers were appointed in all health authorities and health boards throughout the United Kingdom to coordinate activity at a local level. In addition, the AIDS Control Act (1987) was enacted, which required health authorities and health boards throughout the United Kingdom to give annual reports on AIDS work. It also encouraged more coherent joint working across agencies involved in service provision. In the same year the Social Services Committee on AIDS succeeded in setting HIV and AIDS as a one-nation issue.

By the end of the 1980s significant funding was available to support HIV and AIDS services. In 1992, the English White Paper on Public Health, *Health of the Nation* (1992), set HIV/AIDS clearly within the context of sexual health. It provided guidance on the range of services required and set a framework for development in the 1990s. In the second half of the 1990s, there were significant advances in the development of new drug therapies, but these placed considerable strain on budgets. In 1997, an additional £23 million ($35 million) funding was announced to support drug treatment costs because of new drug treatments that took the 1998–1999 spent on treatment and care for HIV and AIDS in England to £228 ($342 million).

Prevalence of HIV and AIDS

Routine data on the prevalence of HIV infection in the United Kingdom are available from two separate but complementary monitoring programs. Data on all named HIV tests in the United Kingdom (testing is available free of charge from Genito-Urinary Medicine [GUM], drug treatment centers, and general practitioners) are collected by the Public Health Laboratory Service (PHLS) and the Scottish Centre for Infection and Environmental Health (SCIEH). There is also an Unlinked Anonymous Prevalence Monitoring Program, which has been in operation since 1990. This program monitors the prevalence of HIV infection in accessible groups of adults whose behavior is deemed to make them vulnerable to infection. These include attendees at GUM clinics and injecting drug users (IDUs). The program also monitors the prevalence of HIV infection in blood donors and pregnant women. These combined monitoring systems provide high-quality HIV and AIDS surveillance information, which have been consistent both over time and in their coverage throughout the United Kingdom. However, as with any reporting systems, there are issues about the extent to which these monitoring systems provide data that are *wholly* representative of either the high-risk or general populations.

Table 13.1
HIV Infection in the United Kingdom: Cumulative Data to
End December 1999

	Males	Females	Total
Likely Exposure Category			
Sex between men[a]	13,031	---	13,031
Sex between men and women	3.003	4,383	7,386
Injecting drug use	1,417	705	2,122
Blood factor	426	4	430
Blood/tissue transfer	57	57	114
Mother to infant	157	147	304
Undetermined	689	251	940
Total	18,780	5,547	24,327

[a]Includes 647 persons who were exposed through both sex between men and IDU.

Source: Public Health Laboratory Service 2001.

Data on named HIV tests indicate that by the end of 1999, 40,312 people had been diagnosed with HIV in the United Kingdom. Table 13.1 shows that over half of HIV cases are attributed to sex between men, whereas 23% are to sex between men and women, and 9% to injecting drug use. Approximately 7% of infections are attributed to blood tissue/blood transfer and/or undetermined means. The ratio of male to female cases is about 5 to 1.

There is considerable variation in the geographical distribution of HIV infection more generally. England accounts for over 90% of known infections, with 68% of those coming from the London area. In sharp contrast, in Northern Ireland there are only 192 known cases of HIV-infected individuals, which represents 0.5% of the total infection of the United Kingdom. Data from Figure 13.1 show the pattern of new cases over time and by transmission category. Regional differences are not shown in Figure 13.1; however, data from Figure 13.2 suggest that the proportion of cases within transmission categories is similar in England, Wales, and Northern Ireland. The exception is Scotland, where 41% of cases have been attributed to injecting drug use, 20% to sex between men and women, and only 32% to sex between men. Also in Scotland the number of hemophiliacs infected

Figure 13.1
New Cases of HIV Infection in the United Kingdom, by Year and Transmission Category

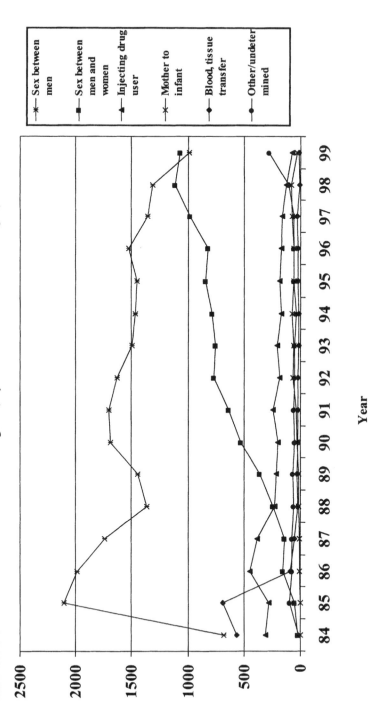

Year

Source: Public Health Laboratory Service 2000.

Figure 13.2
Comparison of Patterns of New HIV Transmissions within the UK
Cumulative Data to End December 1999

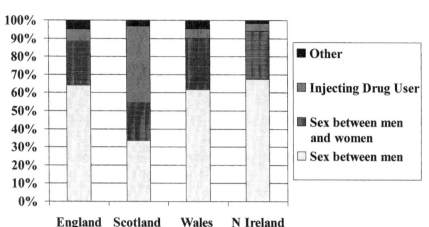

Source: Public Health Laboratory Service 2000.

with HIV by contaminated blood products is very small, as Scotland has been self-sufficient in artificial blood factor from the early 1980s.

Analysis of the number of new infections by year (Figure 13.1) indicates a stabilization of spread of infection among homosexual and bisexual men. There is also evidence of a decline in new cases of infection attributed to injection drug use. However, the number of new diagnoses of HIV infection attributed to heterosexual transmission has risen steadily since the early 1980s, and in 1999, the number of new infections attributed to this transmission category exceeded those attributed to sex between men for the first time.

Most heterosexual HIV infections in the United Kingdom are thought to have been acquired abroad, mainly in Africa by people from there or who have spent time there (Department of Health 1999). Most have also been reported from the London areas. Brown (2000), reporting on a national conference for the *British Medical Journal*, highlighted the fact that Africans in Britain represent the group most often infected with HIV, second only to homosexual men. They are also less likely to be aware that they have the virus and less likely to seek treatment, with the result that they die more quickly from the disease.

As a result of increasing heterosexual transmission, the number of babies born to HIV-positive mothers has increased. In 1999, around 300 births took place to HIV-positive women, resulting in around 31 infected babies. Mother-to-baby transmissions between 1988 and 1997 revealed that 84%

of children born with HIV in London were black African compared with 38% of HIV-positive babies born elsewhere in the United Kingdom (Department of Health 1999).

Paradoxically, although the number of new cases of HIV infection in the United Kingdom has stabilized, the total number of people who are living with HIV has increased by about 45% since 1996. This change has been attributed largely to improved survival of those diagnosed with HIV and receiving highly active antiretroviral treatment (HAART), although the most recent data suggests a leveling out of this effect. It is also estimated that about one-third of people who are infected with HIV are unaware that they are positive for HIV infection (Department of Health 1999).

Figure 13.3 provides indexed trends in AIDS cases by country from 1984. The data reveal that the greatest increase in AIDS over time has occurred in Scotland. However, substantial decreases have occurred in that region since the mid-1990s. The trends for England and Wales are largely similar.

Of the 40,312 people who have been diagnosed with HIV infection, 16,806 have gone on to develop AIDS. Of those with AIDS, over 13,000 people have died, and 12,000 of those have been from England (Public Health Laboratory Service 2000). However, since 1984 the annual number of deaths attributed to AIDS has decreased by 70%. Again, this decline is due to the success of combination antiretroviral therapy.

RESPONSES TO HIV/AIDS

Government Efforts

The United Kingdom is one of the few countries never to have had a national policy on HIV prevention (Berridge 1996). However, an HIV and AIDS strategy was developed for England and issued for public consultation in autumn 2000 (Department of Health 2000). A parallel strategy is also being developed for Scotland, and it is anticipated that strategies for Wales and Northern Ireland will emerge over time. These strategies will make the planning, delivery, and evaluation of services for HIV prevention, treatment, and care more effective.

International experience of HIV and AIDS has led to a coherent picture of the range of ingredients necessary for successful HIV prevention and treatment (UNAIDS 1998). As well as having mechanisms for testing and treatment of patients who receive a positive diagnosis, the other factors include good public education about HIV and AIDS; focused activities for particularly, vulnerable groups and communities; access to condoms, syringes, and other injecting equipment; and good service provision for sexually transmitted infections. All of these efforts must be well coordinated and sensitive to local need.

Figure 13.3
Indexed Trends in AIDS Cases, by Country (1984 = 100)

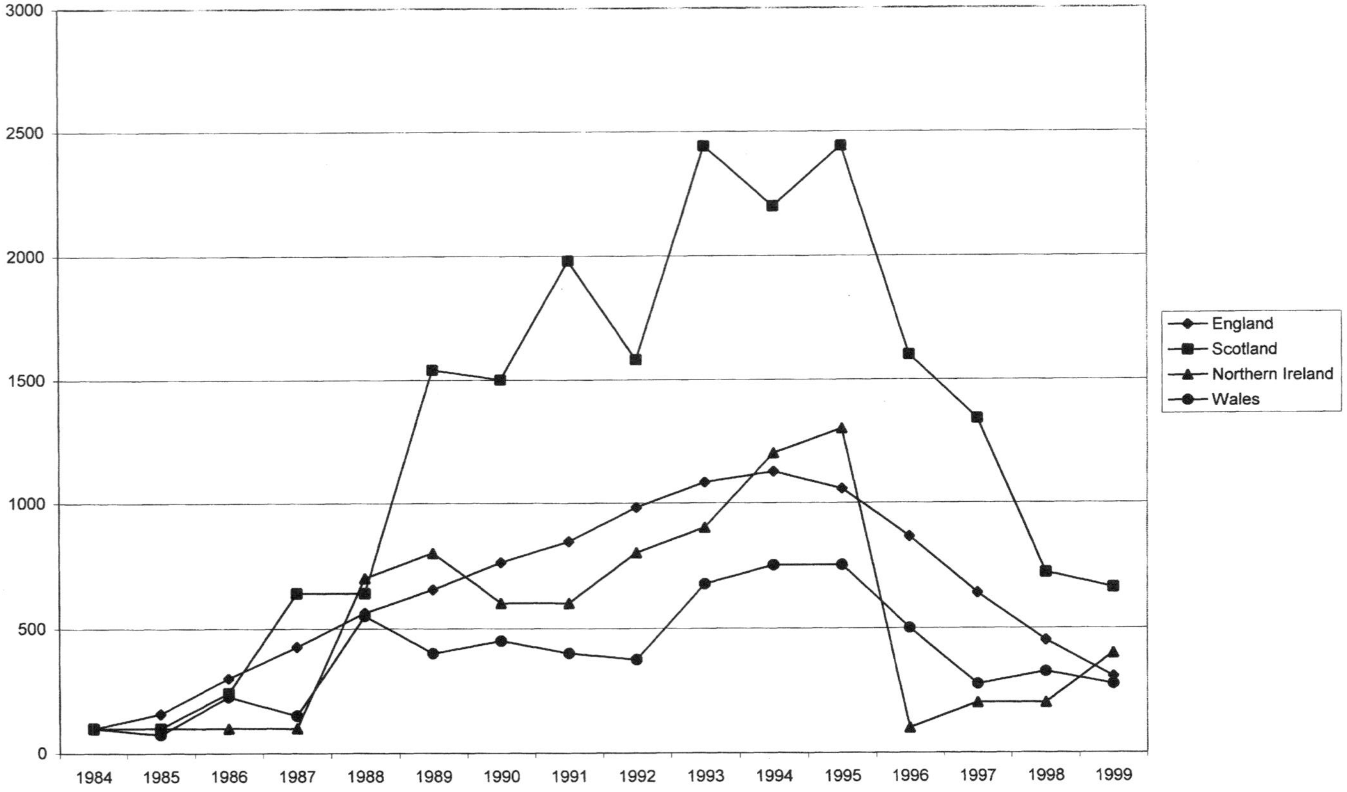

Source: Public Health Laboratory Service 2000.

Treatment and Care of People with HIV

In the early 1980s when the cause of the syndrome was unknown, the primary medical response to HIV/AIDS was to treat the immediate presenting medical problems, often unusual opportunistic infections such as Pneumocystis carinii and cytomegalovirus and rare cancers such as Karposi's sarcoma. The prognosis for those infected was extremely poor. In 1983 the virus responsible for AIDS (then called HTLV-III) was identified, and in the following year, a number of diagnostic tests were developed.

As a result of those developments the immediate clinical responsibility for diagnosis and treatment in the United Kingdom was established within genitourinary medicine (because of its presentation as a sexually transmitted disease [STD]). Other specialities including immunology, dermatology, and gastroenterology were often involved in the treatment. In Scotland, the identification of significant infection among injecting drug users (Haw and Higgins 1998; Robertson, Bucknall, and Welsby 1986) led to a different profile of clinicians being involved including those in infectious diseases, drug treatment services, and primary care. These developments in Scotland also led to a reorientation of the treatment and care of drug users both in Scotland and subsequently in the rest of the United Kingdom (Strang 1998). This new position involved wider consideration of public health issues and resulted in changes in existing treatment services as well as new HIV-specific services.

In 1988, the UK government Advisory Council on the Misuse of Drugs (ACMD) published a report on AIDS and drug misuse. The first conclusion drawn was that the transmission of HIV infection into the general population represented a greater threat to public and individual health than drug misuse. The same conclusion was reached in the McClelland Report, which was published in Scotland in the same year (Scottish Home & Health Department 1988): This concern led to the development of a network of needle and syringe exchange schemes being established across much of the United Kingdom (Stimson, Donoghoe, and Dolan 1990), often linked to outreach workers (Rhodes 1993). An important aspect of these exchanges was that they were not connected to entry into treatment. The immediate objectives of these services were to reduce needle sharing and therefore the spread of HIV. Drug treatment services also established methadone prescribing programs to encourage a shift away from the use of injectable drugs. Harm reduction became a priority for drug services. Achieving abstinence from drugs was considered to be only a long-term goal. These services have continued to operate successfully throughout much of the United Kingdom and have made a significant contribution to containment of the spread of HIV infection within drug injecting populations (Haw and Higgins 1998). The exception to this is Northern Ireland, where the relatively low prevalence of both injecting drug use and HIV infection meant that needle exchange schemes were not established. However, a substantial rise in injecting drug use in specific areas in the late 1990s has led to installation of pilot schemes in areas deemed most at risk (Northern Health and Social Services Board 2000).

During the first half of the 1980s AIDS was regarded as an incurable disease, and life expectancy following diagnosis was extremely short. As understanding of the disease increased, the treatment and prevention of opportunistic infections improved, and effective antiviral therapies were developed, life expectancy increased dramatically. The United Kingdom continues to make a contribution to the global effort in treatment advance. The use of HAART over the last three to four years has led to a dramatic reduction by about one-third in the number of people developing AIDS and a reduction by a similar proportion in the number of people dying from AIDS (Department of Health 1999). These important advances in drug treatment have led to HIV/AIDS being treated as a chronic disease. While such therapies are not completely effective, the work of the Medical Research Council trials network has ensured that new therapies continue to be supported and extended and continue to be monitored through treatment centers throughout the United Kingdom. In addition to the development of better treatments, the long-term aim is the development of a vaccine for those at risk of contracting HIV. The Medical Research Council in the United Kingdom has convened a group of the main researchers in the United Kingdom to develop a vaccine. However, it is suggested that this will not be available for 10 years (Department of Health 2000).

In the United Kingdom, HIV services are currently funded through allocations for HIV treatment and care services; HIV prevention services; and drug misuse services. As HIV in the United Kingdom as a whole has remained a primarily sexually transmitted disease, the main access point for diagnosis continues to be through genitourinary medicine. Clinical expertise in HIV is based in identified treatment centers and centers of excellence across the United Kingdom. In the case of England the concentration around the capital city of London of specialist centers has led to criticism of the accessibility of services to those with HIV infection living in other parts of the country. Such centers continue to involve clinicians from a wide range of specialties. A network of clinicians, in the form of the British HIV Association, aims to ensure that best clinical practice is developed and disseminated.

However, in addition to basic medical treatment, a range of other support services are also required to support people living with HIV and AIDS, their partners, their families, and their caregivers. These services are provided by the National Health Service (NHS), Local Authorities (LAs), and NGOs. Commissioning arrangements have evolved, particularly in those areas with a high prevalence of HIV infection, whereby in many health and local authorities there are designated officers for HIV. Joint commissioning at a regional level is the norm, and this helps ensure continuity of care between health and social services.

The Department of Health (2000) in a progress report on the development of an HIV/AIDS strategy for England identifies the main services and the interfaces between the National Health Service, LAs, and NGOs.

HIV Prevention Activity

The UK approach to prevention that developed during the 1980s and 1990s has been described as a pyramid, with national mass media campaigns targeted at the general population at the top, followed by national campaigns targeted at subgroups within the population such as black and ethnic communities, women, and tourists. Below this are targeted campaigns in special settings, for example, in prisons, schools, and the armed forces. Finally below are community-based local initiatives that are designed to reinforce the national campaigns and encourage people, particularly those in high-risk groups, to change behavior that put them at risk of contracting HIV infection (Knight and Schwarz 1992).

In 1986 the government launched its first round of newspaper advertisements with the slogan "Don't Aid AIDS." The low budget for this project was later deemed to have exacerbated rather than helped confusion surrounding AIDS. This attempt was followed by a television and leaflet campaign—"Don't Die of Ignorance"—which was run by the Department of Health and Social Security in 1986. Since then national prevention campaigns have used a variety of media including television and national and minority press and have targeted the general population, young people, gay men, and more recently, black and minority ethnic groups.

In schools, HIV prevention is addressed through sex education, which is usually taught as part of the personal and social education (PSE) curriculum. Although secondary schools are required by law to provide sex education that includes teaching about STDs and HIV, many teachers are extremely anxious about teaching about sex. Two myths seem to underpin these anxieties—the myth that parents object to teenagers being taught about sexual matters and the myth that teaching about sex encourages young people to have it (Aggleton 1999). However, research suggests that as many as 94% of parents approve of teaching sex education in school (Aggleton 1999), and a review conducted by the NHS Centre for Review and Dissemination (1997) clearly demonstrates that well-planned sex education programs do not increase sexual activity. Nevertheless, it is likely that there is wide variation in the quality of provision of sex education throughout the United Kingdom.

In the United Kingdom, community-based initiatives often involving drug treatment, sexual health services, and NGOs have been regarded as the most effective way of delivering primary HIV prevention to the high-risk groups— gay men, drug injectors, and people from black and minority ethnic groups.

The focus has been on the provision of safer sex and safer injecting messages and the distribution of condoms and injecting equipment. These efforts have involved close collaboration between health authorities/boards, local authorities, and NGOs, and joint commissioning is common.

Role of Nongovernment Organizations

There are a number of different NGOs that address HIV in the United Kingdom. The Terrence Higgins Trust was the first to be established in London in 1982. It came as a direct response to the death of a gay man from AIDS. Its initial focus was as a fund-raising body to support medical research, but this objective quickly changed to one of providing health education, support, information, and advice to people affected directly and indirectly by HIV and AIDS. Additionally the Trust now provides legal housing and welfare benefit advice and advocacy, a buddying service for gay men, and practical help with such things as decorating, cleaning, and transport support for HIV-positive prisoners. A year later, the Scottish AIDS Monitor (SAM) was set up, initially to monitor the epidemic in Scotland; but very quickly its activities expanded to include the provision of information and support services for people with HIV as well as direct input to the development of policy. Since then a range of agencies have been established. "Body Positive" began as a self-help group for people who were diagnosed with HIV in London and now has local branches across the UK. "Frontliners," a campaigning, information, and support organization runs services by and for people with AIDS.

Crusaid is the main charity fund-raising organization for HIV/AIDS. Since it was established in 1986, it has raised millions of pounds, most of which has been used to improve the quality of life and services for people living with HIV/AIDS. Early grants from Crusaid helped establish hospices in Brighton, in the southeast of England, and Edinburgh, the capital city of Scotland.

Following the proliferation of both national and local NGOs, the National AIDS Trust was established in 1987 as their coordinating body. Funded through central government the main focus of its work is on policy research and campaigning to improve the United Kingdom's HIV prevention effort.

Particularly in the 1980s, NGOs were central both to the development of government policy and to the development of services and self-help for people, caregivers, and families affected by HIV infection. Berridge (1996: 5) describes the first half of the 1980s as "a period of incoherence, of absence of knowledge, of 'groping in the dark.' . . . Informal alliances and groupings emerged . . . most notably the concordat between gay activists, public health doctors, clinicians and scientists." This ignorance led to government policy being informed from the bottom rather than the top, and organizations like the Terrence Higgins Trust were enormously influential and often had a direct line of communication to government (Berridge 1996). Although still influential, the "normalization" and "professionaliza-tion" of the field now means that NGOs make up some of the many agencies and organizations involved in the prevention, treatment, and care of HIV/ AIDS.

Changing Attitudes and Behavior

Public Attitudes toward HIV and AIDS

HIV/AIDS first came to the attention of the general public in the mid-1980s and was shaped largely by media coverage in the press and on tele-vision, which began around this time. Because of its association with the gay community, HIV/AIDS became labeled as the "gay plague." Opinion polls taken around 1986–1987 indicated that public attitudes toward gays and those with AIDS were hard-line (Berridge 1996). Similar views were held by some prominent churchmen who regarded the disease as divine retribution for unnatural acts. The links with injecting drug use also led to further attributions of personal culpability for developing HIV. These views contrasted with perceptions about hemophiliacs who had been infected through no fault of their own by the therapeutic use of contaminated blood products.

Growing understanding about the modes of transmission of HIV infec-tion led to a recognition that there was also a potential risk to the general public through sexual contact and exchange of blood products. However, although scientists had established that HIV could not be transmitted by touch, kissing, saliva, or mosquito bites, among the general public there was growing panic about how HIV/AIDS could be transmitted. Lack of knowl-edge among the general public culminated in a debate about whether churchgoers were at risk when they drank wine from the Communion cup (Berridge 1996).

In 1987, the late Princess Diana, a patron of the newly formed National AIDS Trust (NAT), opened a new AIDS ward in a London hospital, and much media attention was given to her shaking hands with an AIDS sufferer. Although there is no real way of assessing the impact of this event, it was regarded as a symbolic act that represented the beginning of the process of normalization of the disease (Berridge 1996). This change was further strengthened when the illness and deaths of popular public figures such as rock star Freddie Mercury were brought to public attention. Such high-profile deaths helped to personalize the disease, moving it away from an unspecific threat to identifying it with individuals. Television programming has also played a role in the normalization of HIV and AIDS. In addition to factual programs, the issue of HIV has also been included in the story line of leading UK soaps.

However, as a result of this normalization process, many in the United Kingdom are beginning to feel that the epidemic has ebbed away. Recent surveys of public attitudes have shown that HIV/AIDS is no longer seen as a major public health threat (Aggleton 1999). While the reduction in mortality and numbers of new infections gives grounds for this claim, there is a real danger of complacency.

Changing Behavior

The impact of individual HIV prevention initiatives is difficult to assess. However, there is some evidence of behavior change among high-risk groups. Studies have demonstrated a change in behavior among gay men that could make a difference to the transmission of HIV infection and other STDs (Gellan and Ison 1986). In addition, among some groups of drug users there has been marked reductions in both levels of sharing of injecting equipment and levels of injecting (Frischer, Goldberg, and Bloor 1992; Haw and Taylor 1994). As a result, the prevalence of drug-related HIV infection in UK cities has remained low compared to other countries (Stimson 1995). The exception is Edinburgh and Dundee, where infection rates of 19.6% (Davies et al. 1995) and 26.8% (Haw and Higgins 1998) have been reported for injecting drug users. However, the primary epidemic in both these cities appears to have occurred in 1983 and 1984, before harm reduction measures were introduced (Haw et al. 1996; Robertson, Bucknall, and Welsby 1986).

In contrast, there has been little evidence of changes in sexual behavior among the general population, either in terms of numbers of sexual partners or use of condoms (Wellings et al 1998). Indeed, data suggest that between 1998 and 1999 there was a sharp increase in cases of gonorrhea among young people (Department of Health 1999). The increase suggests that this group in particular are more likely to engage in unprotected sex. Among drug users, too, there has been little evidence of changes in sexual behavior. Indeed, a Scottish study found no difference in the sexual behavior of HIV-positive and-negative IDUs and estimated that sexual transmissions could exceed injecting transmissions by a ratio of up to 19 to 1 (Haw and Higgins 1996). Finally, among younger cohorts of gay men who are just beginning their sexual careers, there is also evidence of risk behavior (Hart 1995). A survey of gay men conducted between 1996 and 1998 also found an increase in unprotected sex among all gay men (Dodds et al. 2000).

CONCLUSION

From the early days of ignorance and national panic, HIV and AIDS have become normalized in the United Kingdom (Berridge 1996). The decreasing newsworthiness of the epidemic, treatment advance, and a decrease in activism have probably all contributed to a national reduction in the level of concern regarding HIV and AIDS. For example, recent surveys of public attitudes have shown that AIDS is no longer seen as a major public health threat (Aggleton 1999). Indeed, analysis of recent HIV and AIDS statistics presented throughout the chapter suggests that HIV and AIDS appear on the whole to be reasonably controlled at the present time. There is little evidence to suggest substantial amounts of recent HIV transmission in injecting drug users. Additionally, it appears that the level of new infections attributed to sex between men has stabilized.

However, the prevalence of HIV infection is still increasing, and people are still dying from AIDS. Additionally, patterns of transmission are shifting, with a recent increase in the spread of heterosexually transmitted HIV, especially among the younger age group and most notably in women (Department of Health 1999). Albeit at a reduced level, there is also evidence of continuing risk behavior among high-risk groups such as IDUS and homosexual men. Ironically the advent of new and more effective drug treatments has led to debate about the extent to which people's risk behavior may change if it is felt that a cure for HIV and AIDS exists (Grulich 2000). The combined effect of all these factors means that the potential for the sudden new growth of HIV in the United Kingdom remains an ever present reality.

In many ways the HIV and AIDS strategies that are being developed must attempt to address the here and now of HIV and AIDS in the United Kingdom. To be successful in achieving their goals to reduce the transmission of HIV infection and the prevalence of undiagnosed infection, it is important that action is taken in a systematic fashion. Priority must be given to raising awareness among the general population about the potential risks from HIV. This need is well demonstrated by the growth across the United Kingdom of new transmissions among the heterosexual community, particularly young people.

In this vein, HIV testing must become more accessible to all who may have been exposed to HIV. This means tailoring environments for testing to individual needs. For example, not all people will be comfortable using the traditional GUM clinics and may require more family-friendly services with HIV testing mainstreamed into other services they use. Continuation and extension of antenatal testing conducted in selected regions of the United Kingdom is important to reduce vertical transmission of HIV infection.

Additionally, there must be a sustained effort in working with those groups most susceptible to infection such as men who have sex with men, injecting drug users, men and women who have links with people in high-prevalence countries, and people already diagnosed with HIV and AIDS. For example, in Northern Ireland needle exchange schemes must be implemented in areas of high risk, and in southeast England, in particular, further prevention work within black African communities is also required, as are improvements in testing facilities and treatment. Work to promote good social and health care for people living with HIV must also be improved.

The geographical distribution of the epidemic has changed over the decade, leading to a mismatch between the location of treatment centers in relation to where people live. Efforts must be taken to ensure both equity and consistency in the care provided. Furthermore, advances in treatment mean that people with HIV are living longer and need a different range of care and support. For example, ways should be found to facilitate more innovative treatment options such as home administration of medication or from outpatient centers within local communities. The chronic nature of the disease also means that a wider range of medical and supportive services may be required. Finally and perhaps the most challenging, combating the stigma associated with HIV remains a priority. Despite the notable shift from the early days of moral panic and public outrage, from a general public perspective HIV continues to be associated with stigma and social exclusion. The new strategy will attempt to actively combat discrimination and promote service user involvement in the furtherance of this aim. The importance of such advancement is amplified by the requirements of the Human Rights Act, which came into force across the United Kingdom in October 2000 and which brings basic human rights into domestic law.

In the initial wake of the AIDS crisis, the Social Services Committee on AIDS succeeded in making it a one-nation issue. This history is why it is important that HIV and AIDS remain high on the agenda throughout the United Kingdom and that strategic policy is harmonized. It is important that this new HIV and AIDS strategy for England is promptly followed by equivalent Northern Ireland, Scottish, and Welsh documentation. At the time of this writing, Scotland had completed a draft strategy, whereas Northern Ireland and Wales both reported that it would be completed but had set no timetables.

Finally, Aggleton (1999:10) concludes that action must be taken now. He suggests that the United Kingdom faces "[a] dangerous new phase of the epidemic, one in which perceptions of the seriousness of HIV and AIDS have declined . . . but one in which there is evidence of an increase in risk related sexual behaviours." He suggests that "unless urgent action is taken many of the advances made in efforts to control the epidemic over the past decades are in danger of slipping away."

BIBLIOGRAPHY

Advisory Council on the Misuse of Drugs. 1988. *AIDS and the Misuse of Drugs Part 1. AIDS Control Act. 1987.* London: HMSO.
Aggleton, Peter. 1999. *HIV at the Cross Roads.* London: National AIDS Trust.
Berridge, Virginia. 1996. *AIDS in the UK: The Making of Policy.* Oxford: Oxford University Press.

Brown, Phylidda. 2000. "Rate of HIV Transmission among Africans in UK 'Under-estimated.' " *British Medical Journal* 320: 725.

Communicable Disease Surveillance Centre. 1983. *Communicable Diseases Report.* London: Communicable Disease Surveillance Centre, July.

Davies, A. N. Dominy, N. Peters, G. Bath, S. Burns, and A. Richardson. 1995. "HIV in Injecting Drug Users in Edinburgh: Prevalence and Correlates." *Journal of Acquired Immune Deficiency Syndromes and Human Retrovirology* 8: 399–405.

Department of Health. 1992. *Health of the Nation.* London: Author.

———. 1993. *Key Area Handbook: HIV/AIDS and Sexual Health.* London: Author.

———. 1999. *Prevalence of HIV in the United Kingdom Summary Report of the Unlinked Anonymous Steering Surveys Group.* London: Author.

———. 2000. *Developing an HIV/AIDS Strategy Progress Report.* London: Author.

Dodds, Julie, Anthony Nardone, Danielle Mercey, and Anne Johnson. 2000. "Increase in High Risk Sexual Behaviour among Homosexual Men" London 1996–8: Cross Sectional, Questionnaire Study. *British Medical Journal* 320: 1510–1511.

Frischer, Martin, David Goldberg, and Michael Bloor. 1992. "Reduction in Needle Sharing among Community Wide Samples of Injecting Drug Users." *International Journal of STD and AIDS* 3: 288–290.

Gellan, M., and C. Ison. 1986. "Declining Incidence of Gonorrhea in London: A Response to the Fear of AIDS?" *Lancet* 2: 920.

Grulich, Andrew. 2000. "HIV Risk Behaviour in Gay Men: On the Rise." *British Medical Journal* 320: 1487–1488.

Hart, Graham. 1995. "Gay Community Safer Sex Interventions." In *AIDS Drugs and Prevention*, Tim Rhodes and Richard Hartnoll, eds. London: Routledge.

Haw, Sally, and Kathryn Higgins. 1996. *Tayside Behavioral and HIV Study. Final Report to the Scottish Office Home & Health Department.* Edinburgh: Scottish Office.

———. 1998. "A Comparison of the Prevalence of HIV Infection and Injecting Risk Behaviour in Urban and Rural Samples in Scotland." *Addiction* 93: 855–863.

Haw, Sally, Kathryn Higgins, David Bell, Brian Johnston, and Allison Richardson. 1996. "Evidence of Continuing Risk of HIV Transmission among Injecting Drug Users from Dundee." *Scottish Medical Journal* 41: 3.

Haw, Sally, and Avril Taylor. 1994. "Can Prescribing Policy Influence Patterns of Drug Use and Methods of Drug Administration?" *AIDS* 7 (4): 598–600.

Knight, I., and C. Schwarz. 1992. *Preventing the HIV Spread.* London: Department of Health.

National Health Service (NHS) Centre for Review and Dissemination. 1997. "Preventing and Reducing the Adverse Effects of Unintended Teenage Pregnancies." *Effective Health Care* 3 (1): 1–9.

Northern Health and Social Services Board. 2000. Personal communication.

Public Health Laboratory Service. 1999. "1998 Surveillance of Sexually Transmitted Infections in the UK." *Eurosurveillance* 3 (6): 61–65.

———. 2000. *AIDS/HIV Quarterly Surveillance Tables* (45): 99/4.

———. 2001. *AIDS/HIV Quarterly Surveillance Tables.* (49): 00/4.

Rhodes, Tim. 1993. "Time for Community Change: What Has Outreach Got to Offer?" *Addiction* 88: 1317–1320.

Robertson, J., A. Bucknall, and P. Welsby. 1986. "Epidemic of Aids Related Virus (HTLV-III/LAV) Infection among Intravenous Drug Abusers." *British Medical Journal* 292: 527–529.

Scottish Home & Health Department. 1986. *HIV Infection in Scotland: Report of the Scottish Committee on HIV Infection and Intravenous Drug Misuse.* Edinburgh: Author.

———. 1988. *The McClelland Report.* Edinburgh: Author.

Stimson, Gerry. 1995. "Aids and Drug Injecting in the United Kingdom 1997 to 1999: The Policy Response and the Prevention of the Epidemic." *Social Science and Medicine* 41: 699–716.

Stimson, Gerry, Martin Donoghoe, and Kate Dolan. 1990. "Distributing Sterile Needles and Syringes to People Who Inject Drugs: The Syringe Exchange Experiment." In *AIDS and Drug Misuse* John Strang and Gerry Stimson, pp. 222–231. London: Routledge.

Strang, John. 1998. "AIDS and Drug Misuse in the UK—10 Years On: Achievements, Failings and New Harm Reduction Opportunities." *Drugs: Education Prevention and Policy* 5 (3): 293–304.

Taylor, Avril, Martin Frischer, Simon Green, David Goldberg, Neil McKeganey, and Laurence Gruer. 1994. "Low and Stable Prevalence of HIV among Drug Injectors in Glasgow." *International Journal of Sexually Transmitted Diseases and AIDS* 5 (2): 105–107.

UNAIDS. 1998. *Expanding the Global Response to HIV/AIDS through Focussed Action.* Geneva: Author.

Wellings, Kaye, Julia Field, Anne Johnson, and Jane Wadsworth. 1998. *Sexual Behavior in Britain in Britain. The National Survey of Sexual Attitudes and Lifestyle.* London: Penguin.

14

UNITED STATES

Dale D. Chitwood

INTRODUCTION

AIDS emerged at a time when it was believed by many that the threat of infectious disease in the United States had, for the most part, been eliminated. The first cases in the United States of what later would be known as AIDS were described by the Centers for Disease Control and Prevention (CDC) in 1981 (Centers for Disease Control and Prevention [CDC] 1981a, 1981b). Two decades have passed since these initial cases were ascertained and AIDS entered the public consciousness in the United States. HIV/ AIDS has become an enormous medical, social, and political concern. Many aspects of societal life have been affected by this epidemic. Considerable personnel and monetary resources have been allocated to combat HIV/ AIDS on multiple fronts ranging from education and behavioral intervention programs to sophisticated medical technology and research. There have been many failures in responding to the AIDS crisis but also many triumphs. While (it has been suggested that) the government was slow to recognize and adapt to the growing epidemic, public and private agencies and institutions have achieved considerable success. Basic knowledge of AIDS and HIV has advanced dramatically over the last two decades. While a cure has yet to be found, treatment advances have prolonged the life span of AIDS patients and have reduced the rate of progression from HIV to AIDS. On the social front, organizations have been formed to educate and support HIV-positive individuals and persons with AIDS (PWAs). Legislation has been enacted to provide medical assistance to PWAs and to prevent discrimination against PWAs in the workplace and other public venues.

HIV infection and AIDS continue to be enormous problems. AIDS is not curable, but it is preventable. Innovative programs have been and are being created in an attempt to change behaviors that place individuals at high risk for acquiring or transmitting HIV. There is some evidence that these programs are having an impact in retarding the spread of AIDS, a disease that has caused untold misery and suffering and has resulted in the deaths of thousands of people, most of whom were in the prime years of life.

ISSUES RELATING TO HIV AND AIDS

History

In 1981 a technician at the CDC in Atlanta, Georgia, uncovered data that reflected an unusually high number of requests for pentamidine, a drug used to treat Pneumocystis carinii pneumonia (PCP). This discovery led to a report of PCP occurring unusually in five gay men in Los Angeles, California (CDC 1981b). Shortly thereafter, an abnormally high number of Kaposi's sarcoma (KS) cases among men who have sex with men (MSM) were reported in New York (CDC 1981a).

A search began to find the cause of the increase in PCP and KS among MSM. A leading candidate for the cause was the use of nitrant inhalants, or "poppers" (Haverkos, Kopstein, and Drotman 1994). An alternative theory was that an infectious agent caused the increase in PCP and KS (CDC 1982b). In early 1982, the syndrome, which would later be known as AIDS, was referred to as Gay-Related Immune Deficiency (GRID) Syndrome, and in February of that year, the CDC reported that 251 individuals had been diagnosed with GRID, 99 of whom had died (Shilts 1987). It was soon discovered that the syndrome also was affecting men and women injecting drug users (IDUs) and hemophiliacs. GRID was no longer an appropriate description of the disease, and it was renamed acquired immuno-deficiency syndrome (AIDS).

It became apparent early in the epidemic that AIDS was transmitted through the exchange of blood and other bodily fluids. After the discovery of the virus that causes AIDS, the transmission mechanisms became clearer. Excluding the transmission of the virus through blood transfusions and the use of blood components to treat disease, the primary risk behaviors for HIV/AIDS were determined to be unsafe sex practices and the use of unsterile injection equipment.

Research studies were initiated early in the epidemic to determine the specific high-risk behaviors among gay males, IDUs, and other groups (e.g., prostitutes) thought to be at high risk for the disease. Hundreds of studies have been published on risk behaviors and related factors for the transmission of HIV, and the knowledge of these transmission factors has led to intervention programs aimed at decreasing HIV transmission among those at risk.

Since the beginning of the epidemic through the end of 1999, a total of 733,374 AIDS cases have been reported in the United States. The extent of HIV disease is unknown, but it has been estimated that there are 650,000 to 900,000 individuals with HIV infections living in the United States and that at least 40,000 new infections occur each year (CDC 1998).

AIDS and HIV Surveillance

The CDC is part of the U.S. Public Health Service and monitors reportable illnesses such as tuberculosis, hepatitis, sexually transmitted diseases (STDs), and other infectious diseases. The CDC is also assigned the task of investigating outbreaks of diseases and, in the case of a new disease entity, establishing a definition for that disease. Thus, the CDC was responsible for creating an epidemiologic definition of AIDS and collecting surveillance data for cases that met these criteria. The official definition of AIDS has evolved over the course of the epidemic. Initially, AIDS was defined as the occurrence of biopsy-proven KS and/or biopsy- or culture-proven infections at least moderately predictive of cellular immune deficiency (Jaffe, Bregman, and Selik 1983). After the discovery of the HIV retrovirus that causes AIDS and other medical advances including tests for the presence of antibodies to HIV in blood, the surveillance definition was revised in 1985. The new definition included a positive test for HIV antibodies and added several diseases to the list of indicators of AIDS for those with a positive test. For those not tested, the old criteria applied (CDC 1985). Two years later, in 1987, the surveillance case definition was expanded to include additional disease indicators (CDC 1987). In 1993 the case definition was expanded again, to include all HIV-infected persons with CD4+ t-lymphocyte counts of less than 200 cells μL or a CD4+ percentage less than 14. Pulmonary tuberculosis and invasive cervical cancer were added to the list of indicator diseases (CDC 1992).

In addition, the CDC retrospectively collected information on cases that met the definition for AIDS and that occurred prior to AIDS surveillance reporting by the states. This process identified an additional 99 cases that occurred prior to 1981 and 319 cases in addition to the original 16 cases in 1981 (see Table 14.1).

In the first years of the epidemic the monitoring of diagnosed AIDS cases provided data that reflected changes in the prevalence of HIV infection in the U.S. population. Advances in the treatment of HIV-positive individuals slowed the progression of HIV disease and led to a decrease in AIDS incidence that no longer reflected HIV prevalence. These changes made it difficult for public health agencies to monitor and plan for the HIV/AIDS

Table 14.1
AIDS Cases and Deaths by Year, Before 1981 through December 1999

Year	Cases diagnosed during interval	Deaths occurring during interval
Before 1981	99	30
1981	335	129
1982	1,201	466
1983	3,153	1,512
1984	6,360	3,518
1985	12,026	6,997
1986	19,372	12,154
1987	29,070	16,456
1988	36,064	21,189
1989	43,399	27,767
1990	49,446	31,734
1991	60,472	36,959
1992	79,477	41,480
1993	79,752	45,271
1994	72,684	49,677
1995	69,172	49,992
1996	59,832	36,930
1997	47,439	20,945
1998	38,587	16,432
1999	25,434	10,198
TOTAL	733,374	429,836

Source: CDC 2000.

epidemic. In 1997 the CDC and the Council of State and Territorial Epidemiologists (1997) recommended that all states include surveillance for HIV infection as part of their AIDS surveillance activities. Many states had implemented HIV surveillance prior to this recommendation, and by the end of 1999, 34 of the 50 states were reporting newly documented cases of HIV to the CDC (CDC 1999). The CDC now includes HIV prevalence in its semiannual reports of AIDS surveillance data. Because not all states report HIV cases, the prevalence of HIV is underestimated in the CDC semiannual reports. However, the HIV surveillance data can detect trends and provide data to better characterize populations in which HIV has been newly diagnosed (CDC 1999).

Problems unique to HIV surveillance have been identified. The AIDS surveillance program is name based but with complete confidentiality of individual names. The health care provider or institution making the AIDS diagnosis reports to the state surveillance office using the name of the patient as one aspect of the unique identifier assigned to each case. This information is then reported to the CDC using the name-based unique identifier. The reporting of HIV is more problematic; because of confidentiality concerns, some states use coded identifiers rather than individual names. These non-name-based identifiers have not proven as satisfactory as the name-based identifiers. Problems with the non-name-based identifiers include the possibility that more than one individual is assigned the same code or that one individual is assigned more than one code. In addition, codes based on constructed identifiers often were incomplete. In two states using coded identifiers from 1994 to 1996, the CDC documented that almost 50% of the reported cases had an incomplete report (CDC 1999). In addition, although anonymous testing sites exist in all states, personal identifying information is not linked to test results. Confidential testing sites do use name-based identifiers, but there has been concern that if names are reported to surveillance agencies, it might deter some individuals from being tested. With the advent of home collection kits, data on individuals who test at home are not reported. It is expected that early in the twenty-first century all 50 states will be reporting HIV cases (CDC 1999).

The first decade of the AIDS epidemic in the United States was characterized by an alarmingly high incidence of AIDS cases, with major urban areas on the East and West Coasts of the United States particularly affected. The number of AIDS cases in the United States had reached 151,079 by the end of 1989. The second decade continued this trend until 1994 when for the first time in the epidemic the number of reported AIDS cases dropped from the previous year. By the end of December 1999, 733, 374 cumulative cases of AIDS had been reported (CDC 2000).

Mortality associated with AIDS was high during most of the epidemic. Table 14.1 describes the number of AIDS cases and number of reported deaths among these cases since 1981. Of the 733,374 individuals diagnosed with AIDS, 429,836 have died. Mortality data for 1999 were incomplete, and the reported number of deaths occurring in that year may increase as additional deaths are reported to the CDC. In 1996, the number of deaths due to AIDS began to decrease (CDC 2000).

Risk Groups

The first group to be determined at high risk for AIDS was men who have sex with men. Shortly after the first cases appeared in 1981 among MSM, it was discovered that injecting drug users and persons with hemophilia also were developing the syndrome (CDC 1982c). The following year the CDC issued a report of immunodeficiency and opportunistic infections in infants under two years of age and speculated that these children possibly had AIDS (CDC 1982d). At the same time, evidence began to accumulate that individuals who had received blood transfusions were developing AIDS (CDC 1982a). The etiology of AIDS was unknown at the time, but it was becoming apparent that AIDS was transmitted through blood and other bodily fluids. Heterosexual sex was implicated in the spread of AIDS, and erroneously, early in the epidemic, Haitian immigrants were targeted as a risk group (CDC 1982b). The CDC presently reports statistics for six major risk groups among adult/adolescents. The primary groups for whom risk exposure is greatest are (1) men who have sex with men, (2) injecting drug users, (3) men who have sex with men *and* inject drugs, (4) persons with hemophilia/coagulation disorder, (5) persons who engage in heterosexual contact, and (6) persons in receipt of blood transfusion, blood components, or tissue.

Since the beginning of the epidemic until the year 2000, 724,656 adult/adolescent AIDS cases have been reported to the CDC. As presented in Table 14.2, MSM is the largest risk category, representing 47% of the total adult/adolescent AIDS cases and 56% of the cases among men. MSM have comprised the largest number of cases since the beginning of the epidemic. However, since early in the epidemic the proportion of AIDS cases attributed to MSM has steadily declined, whereas the proportion of cases attributed to IDU has steadily increased. As of the end of 1999, IDUs accounted for 25% of the reported cases. IDU is the largest risk group for women (42%) and the second largest group for men (22%). Heterosexual contact accounts for 10% of all AIDS cases. However, 40% of the cases among women resulted from heterosexual exposure, whereas only 4% of the cases among men did. Exposure through heterosexual contact has increased rapidly, particularly among women. Since 1994 more new cases among women were attributable to heterosexual contact than to IDU (CDC 2000). The major risk factor of the vast majority of women who acquire AIDS through heterosexual transmission is sex with an IDU. Among the 24,067 cases among women attributed to heterosexual contact, 19,523 (81%) reported having sex with an IDU (CDC 2000).

One of the successes in the prevention of the transmission of HIV/AIDS has been the almost total elimination of cases acquired among those with hemophilia disorder or recipients of blood transfusions or blood products. Since the ability to test blood products for the presence of antibodies to HIV became practical in 1985, measures have been adopted that have all but eliminated risk of transmission through blood and blood components.

Throughout the epidemic, blacks and Hispanics have been disproportionately affected. During the 1990s the epidemic shifted toward a decreasing proportion of cases among MSM and increasing proportion among African Americans and Hispanics. In absolute numbers, blacks have outnumbered whites in new AIDS cases and deaths since 1996, although proportionately they represent less than 15% of the total population. In 1999, the annual rate of new AIDS cases per 100,000 population was 9.0 for whites, 64.2 for African Americans, and 34.6 for Hispanics (CDC 2000). Table 14.3 presents the number of AIDS cases diagnosed among whites, African Amer-

Table 14.2
Adult/Adolescent AIDS Cases by Exposure Category and Sex, Reported through December 1999

Adult/adolescent exposure category	Males		Females		Totals	
	No.	(%)	No.	(%)	No.	(%)
Men who have sex with men	341,597	(56)	-------	-------	341,597	(47)
Injecting drug use	134,356	(22)	50,073	(42)	184,429	(25)
Men who have sex with men and inject drugs	46,582	(8)	-------	-------	46,582	(6)
Hemophilia/coagulation disorder	4,803	(1)	272	(0)	5,075	(1)
Heterosexual contact:	26,530	(4)	47,946	(40)	74,477	(10)
Sex with injecting drug user	8,696		19,523		28,219	
Sex with bisexual male	-------		3,368		3,968	
Sex with person with hemophilia	58		407		465	
Sex with transfusion recipient with HIV infection	398		581		979	
Sex with HIV-infected person, risk not specified	17,378		24,067		41,446	
Receipt of blood transfusion, blood components, or tissues	4,863	(1)	3,668	(3)	8,531	(1)
Other/risk not reported or identified	46,112	(8)	17,851	(15)	63,965	(9)
Total	**604,843**	**(100)**	**119,810**	**(100)**	**724,656**	**(100)**

Source: CDC 2000. Available on the World Wide Web at: http://www.cdc.gov/hiv/stats/hasr1102/table5.htm

Table 14.3
Adult/Adolescent AIDS Cases by Sex, Exposure Category, and Race/Ethnicity; Cumulative Data
Through December 1999

Exposure category	White, not Hispanic		Black, not Hispanic		Hispanic	
	No.	(%)	No.	(%)	No.	(%)
Men who have sex with men	216,564	(75)	74,434	(37)	45,867	(43)
Injecting drug use	26,856	(9)	68,491	(34)	38,338	(36)
Men who have sex with men and inject drugs	23,880	(8)	14,965	(8)	7,253	(7)
Hemophilia/coagulation disorder	3,725	(1)	551	(0)	424	(0)
Heterosexual contact:	5,181	(2)	15,121	(8)	5,986	(6)
Sex with injecting drug user	1,849		5,079		1,704	
Sex with person with hemophilia	29		18		10	
Sex with transfusion recipient with HIV infection	153		148		87	
Sex with HIV-infected person, risk not specified	3,150		9,876		4,185	
Receipt of blood transfusion, blood components, or tissues	3,133	(1)	1,028	(1)	574	(1)
Risk not reported or identified	11,198	(4)	24,658	(12)	9,425	(9)
Total	290,537	(100)	199,248	(100)	107,867	(100)

Female Adult/Adolescent AIDS Cases by Exposure Category and Race/Ethnicity, Reported through December 1999

Exposure category	White, not Hispanic		Black, not Hispanic		Hispanic	
	No.	(%)	No.	(%)	No.	(%)
Injecting drug use	11,074	(42)	29,059	(42)	9,613	(40)
Hemophilia/coagulation disorder	102	(0)	108	(0)	53	(0)
Heterosexual contact:	10,528	(40)	25,719	(38)	11,222	(47)
Sex with injecting drug user	4,294		9,916		5,159	
Sex with bisexual male	1,452		1,311		513	
Sex with person with hemophilia	281		80		39	
Sex with transfusion recipient with HIV infection	300		162		96	
Sex with HIV-infected person, risk not specified	4,201		14,250		5,415	
Receipt of blood transfusion, blood components, or tissues	1,789	(7)	1,230	(2)	536	(2)
Risk not reported or identified	2,805	(11)	12,413	(18)	2,407	(10)
Total	**26,298**	**(100)**	**68,529**	**(100)**	**23,831**	**(100)**

Source: CDC 2000.

icans, and Hispanics living in the United States by the associated exposure category. Among males, African Americans (34%) and Hispanics (36%) are more likely than whites (9%) to have acquired AIDS through IDU. Fewer ethnic differences are observed for females who are exposed to AIDS through IDU.

One of the tragedies of the AIDS epidemic is that it is a disease of the young. Almost two-thirds (63%) of the cases among males and 7 out of 10 cases among females were diagnosed prior to age 40 (CDC 2000). As of 31 December 1999, a total of 8,718 of the AIDS cases were classified as pediatric (i.e., were diagnosed among individuals under the age of 13). Over three-fourths of these cases (77%) were diagnosed prior to age 5, and 91% of all pediatric cases were attributed to perinatal transmission by the mother. Table 14.4 indicates the risk exposure categories for children under the age of 13 diagnosed with AIDS. Of the 7,943 cases resulting from perinatal exposure, more than one-half (57%) are associated with IDU. Perinatally acquired AIDS has declined dramatically in the 1990s as a result of the implementation of the use of zidovudine (or azidothymidine, AZT) to prevent perinatal transmission. This trend is expected to continue with the use of more aggressive therapies such as combination drugs to treat infected pregnant women.

HIV and AIDS are not distributed evenly across regions in the United States. Early in the epidemic, urban areas on the East and West Coasts of the United States were the hardest hit (Hardy et al. 1985). New York City on the East Coast has reported the highest number of AIDS cases (115,059) followed by Los Angeles (40,709) on the West Coast. The three metropolitan areas comprising the next greatest number of AIDS cases are: San Francisco, California (27,151), Miami, Florida (22,872), and Washington, D.C. (21,648).

Persons with HIV/AIDS

Much of the early hysteria and panic that resulted from incomplete knowledge of the transmission of AIDS has dissipated. In the initial stages of the epidemic, AIDS appeared to be limited to MSM and IDUs, two groups who already were marginalized by society and frequently experienced discrimination. AIDS was viewed as self-inflicted and the result of immoral and self-destructive behaviors by homosexuals and drug abusers. As long as AIDS was confined to these groups, it was easy for many persons to disregard the disease and its consequences. When it became clear that AIDS could affect the general heterosexual population, not only through sexual activities but also through receiving blood transfusions and other blood products, a "plague mentality" arose (Lamers 1988). AIDS patients and their families became "untouchables." Politicians in several states introduced legislation to segregate AIDS-infected persons from the general population.

Table 14.4
Pediatric AIDS Cases by Exposure Category and Sex, Reported through December 1999

Pediatric (<13 years old) exposure category	Males		Females		Totals	
	No.	(%)	No.	(%)	No.	(%)
Hemophilia/coagulation disorder	228	(5)	7	(0)	235	(3)
Mother with/at risk for HIV infection	3,942	(88)	4,001	(94)	7,943	(91)
Injecting drug user	1,566		1,550		3,116	
Sex with injecting drug user	740		703		1,443	
Sex with bisexual male	86		85		171	
Sex with person with hemophilia	17		15		32	
Sex with transfusion recipient with HIV infection	11		14		25	
Sex with HIV-infected person, risk not specified	574		611		1,185	
Receipt of blood transfusion, blood components, or tissues	74		79		153	
Has HIV infection, risk not specified	874		944		1,818	
Receipt of blood transfusion, blood components, or tissues	239	(5)	140	(3)	379	(4)
Risk not reported or identified	74	(2)	87	(2)	161	(2)
Total	4,483	(100)	4,235	(100)	8,718	(100)

Source: CDC 2000.

Many individuals known to have AIDS lost their jobs, their medical insurance, and the support of their families and friends.

School-age children infected with AIDS presented a particular problem. Even though epidemiologists and health authorities assured the public that AIDS was not transmitted through casual contact such as kissing, touching, or drinking from the same glass or water fountain and that children with AIDS would not infect their classmates, many parents reacted with panic, fear, and public displays of hostility (Liss 1989). Children with AIDS often were not allowed access to the classroom; various lawsuits resulted. Perhaps the most noted case is that of Ryan White who became a symbolic figure in the fight for civil rights for AIDS-infected individuals. Ryan was 13 years old when diagnosed with AIDS. He was barred from the classroom, and the matter was taken to court and resolved in White's favor. The court determined that White posed no threat to the other students. After Ryan was readmitted to school, protests occurred outside the school, and the family was subject to harassment. The White family eventually relocated to another city where Ryan was welcomed into the school and the community. Ryan White died on 8 April 1990 at the age of 18. Today, children who are HIV infected or diagnosed with AIDS routinely attend public schools with no widespread community opposition.

Much of the fear associated with HIV/AIDS has dissipated but will not disappear entirely until a cure is found. As the risk factors for HIV infection became clear and the public more educated, the hysterical reaction to HIV/AIDS-infected individuals lessened. While there is stigma attached to HIV/AIDS, antidiscrimination laws have been passed according basic civil rights to victims of the disease. The major piece of legislation that redresses discrimination against persons with AIDS or HIV disease is the Americans with Disabilities Act (ADA), which was signed into law in July 1990. This federal statute protects individuals with disabilities from discrimination in employment, housing, and public accommodations. HIV disease and AIDS meet the definition of disability in this law, and HIV-positive individuals, whether or not symptomatic, are covered under the ADA.

RESPONSES TO HIV/AIDS

Governmental Efforts to Control HIV/AIDS

The U.S. government has invested billions of dollars in HIV/AIDS research, health care, and prevention programs since the beginning of the AIDS epidemic in 1981. Federal funding for AIDS biomedical research began that same year with appropriations of several hundred thousand dollars (Kaiser Family Foundation 1998). In fiscal year 1999 (October 1998 through September 1999), the federal government spent $9.7 billion on AIDS-related programs (Kaiser Family Foundation 2000), an amount that constitutes approximately half of 1% of the total federal budget. The federal government funds HIV/AIDS programs in four general categories: (1) care and assistance, (2) research, (3) prevention, and (4) international efforts.

Care and Assistance

Programs under care and assistance are those that deliver health care services, support services, and disability assistance to persons with HIV/AIDS. Multiple governmental departments and agencies are responsible for care and assistance programs. Approximately $7 out of every $10 (71%) spent of the HIV/AIDS money is for care and assistance. Major programs in this category include Medicare (health care for those over 65), Medicaid (health care for those with low income), Supplemental Security Income (SSI), and Social Security Disability Income (SSDI). These programs receive no funds designated as HIV/AIDS money but serve many individuals who are infected with HIV. Thirty-one percent of the federal monies spent on HIV/AIDS care and assistance programs comes from funding allocated to Medicaid. In addition, individual states also contribute to Medicaid. The share of each state's Medicaid program that the state itself must pay ranges from 20% to 50%. This funding is in addition to federal monies and is not included in the estimates for federal government spending.

The Ryan White Comprehensive AIDS Resources Emergency (CARE) Act was enacted by Congress in 1990 and reauthorized in 1996 and 2000. This legislation, named in honor of Ryan White, provides emergency assistance to locales in the United States that are disproportionately affected by HIV/AIDS infections. Assistance is in the form of grants to states, local governments, and private nonprofit groups to provide a range of health and social services to people with HIV/AIDS. Approximately 19% of all funding for care and assistance is provided through the Ryan White CARE Act (Kaiser Family Foundation 1998).

Research

Research programs include a range of biomedical, epidemiological, behavioral, health services, and social science research activities. Research activities comprise approximately 19% of the federal AIDS budget. While research activities are supported by a variety of federal agencies, the vast majority of funding is funneled through the National Institutes of Health (NIH), which allocated $2 billion for AIDS-related research in the year 2000. NIH is composed of 21 individual institutes and centers, each concentrating on a particular domain of medical science. HIV/AIDS research crosses the boundaries of multiple institutes, and each of the institutes funds AIDS research programs in its particular area. Seven institutes, however, fund the bulk of HIV/AIDS research: (1) The National Institute of Allergy and Infectious Disease has the lead responsibility for the discovery and the development of interventions to treat or prevent HIV infection. (2) The

National Cancer Institute focuses its research on AIDS-related malignancies. The National Cancer Institute houses the HIV Drug Resistance Program and the NIH Vaccine Research Center, which is a joint project with the Institute of Allergy and Infectious Disease. (3) The National Institute on Drug Abuse concentrates its research on drug-related behaviors that are linked to HIV transmission and on developing intervention strategies to reduce these behaviors. (4) The National Institute of Mental Health focuses on the impact of HIV on the central nervous system and therapeutics of central nervous system involvement as well as strategies and interventions to motivate behavior change in at-risk populations. (5) The National Center for Research Resources provides critical research technologies and resources across all NIH Institutes. (6) The National Heart, Lung, and Blood Institute supports research on the pulmonary, cardiac, and hematologic complications of HIV as well as research designed to maximize the safety and adequacy of the nation's blood supply. (7) The National Institute of Child Health and Human Development supports research focused on maternal, pediatric, and adolescent HIV infection.

HIV research at the NIH is conducted through both intramural and extramural research programs. The bulk of the funding is to the extramural program, which provides grants to researchers in academic institutions across the country. The Office of AIDS Research (OAR) was created in 1988 to direct the NIH AIDS research program. The OAR develops an annual comprehensive plan and budget for NIH-supported HIV/AIDS research.

In essence, five types of research activities are supported by federal funds. Basic research studies the human immune system, the molecular structure of HIV, and ways in which the virus attacks the human body. Clinical research examines the impact of HIV on the human body, identifies medical conditions that affect people infected with HIV, and conducts clinical trials of medications to treat HIV-related disease. Epidemiologic research studies the distribution and control of HIV/AIDS, including the incidence and prevalence of HIV/AIDS, in various populations and communities. Behavioral research evaluates interventions designed to change behaviors to reduce the transmission of HIV. Health services research addresses issues such as cost, access, and outcomes of services and care.

The investment the nation has placed in HIV/AIDS research has resulted in numerous advances including:

• Verification of HIV as the causal agent of AIDS and the development of a test to detect the presence of antibodies to HIV in blood and other tissue.
• The development of drugs to treat HIV infection and advances in the treatment of several HIV-related diseases and infections.
• The use of antiretroviral drugs to reduce the risk of HIV transmission from pregnant women to the fetus.

- A doubling of the average survival time for a person living with HIV/AIDS.
- A reduction in the number of new AIDS cases in the United States most likely due to successful intervention and educational programs.
- The identification of barriers to access to care for people with HIV.

Prevention

Prevention programs are funded by grants to states and other groups for risk-reduction activities. The agency responsible for overseeing most prevention programs is the CDC, which is a component of the Department of Health and Human Services (HHS). Prevention programs include a wide range of activities including dissemination of AIDS educational materials to the general population, members of groups at high risk for HIV infection, public health practitioners, and health care professionals. In addition, the CDC funds prevention and intervention programs among high-risk groups. Approximately 8% of the federal HIV/AIDS budget is spent on prevention activities.

International Efforts

There is a range of international programs conducted mainly by the U.S. Agency for International Development. International HIV/AIDS programs account for 1.5% of the annual HIV/AIDS budget.

Nongovernmental Efforts

Since the very beginning of the AIDS epidemic the not-for-profit sector has been actively involved in support and prevention activities. Nonprofit community-based agencies sprang up in the large urban areas as early as 1982. The agencies' missions were threefold: (1) to offer support services for people living with AIDS, (2) to educate the public and health professionals about HIV, and (3) to advocate for fair and effective AIDS policies at the local, state, and federal levels. Most agencies were organized by small groups of volunteers concerned with the AIDS crisis and were oriented toward gay men. As the AIDS epidemic expanded, most agencies also expanded their services and included programs for other high-risk groups. Funded largely through private donations and volunteer workers, these agencies have performed herculean tasks and have served as the front line in the battle against AIDS.

While each agency differs somewhat in services offered and number of clients served, the AIDS Project Los Angeles (APLA) can serve as an example of the work done by these community-based organizations. APLA is the second-largest HIV/AIDS organization in the United States and serves over 8,000 individuals living with AIDS. Started in 1982 by a small group of concerned people, the agency now employs a professional staff of 175 and has a volunteer force of over 2,000 individuals. APLA can provide clients with food from its food bank, transportation services, legal services, dental care, home health care, child care, assistance in obtaining public benefits and insurance claims, mental health services, and housing assistance. In addition, the APLA offers support groups for people with HIV/AIDS and their families; an adult and child buddy program, which provides social interaction and emotional support for clients; a telephone hotline; and case management that provides assessment, planning, and referrals for clients. The agency also provides educational material concerning HIV/AIDS to the community and risk-reduction programs targeted at high-risk groups. APLA also aggressively lobbies federal, state, and local governments to enact legislation on behalf of people living with HIV disease. Agencies such as the APLA serve a vital role in the fight against HIV/AIDS.

Many creative and innovative ideas and approaches have arisen to combat HIV/AIDS in communities across the nation. Fund-raising has been accomplished by methods from "walk-a-thons" to celebrity-studded galas. Many high-profile artists and celebrities have contributed their talents to raise money for AIDS. The gay community has produced notable AIDS activists who have gained national stature.

One of the more poignant projects is the NAMES Project or the AIDS Memorial Quilt Project. Panels of quilt are created for individuals who have died of AIDS-related illnesses. The quilt is displayed in public venues and serves as both a fund-raiser and an educational tool as well as a memorial to those who have died. Presently the quilt is composed of over 42,960 panels, upon which more than 83,000 names are inscribed. If all three-feet-by-six-feet panels were laid end to end, the quilt would be 48.82 miles long; the quilt covers 773,280 square feet and weighs over 50 tons. The quilt has had more than 13 million visitors and, in the United States, has raised almost $3 million for direct services for people with AIDS. The NAMES Project now has 36 international affiliates.

Academic institutions continue to play a key role in HIV/AIDS research, education, and treatment. Medical schools and their affiliated teaching hospitals perform more than 50% of all NIH-supported research (Association of American Medical Colleges 1999). In addition, medical schools and teaching hospitals have provided a disproportionate share of AIDS care.

Private industry, particularly pharmaceutical companies and biotechnical organizations, has been active in developing new treatments and therapies for HIV-related disease. Seventy-five pharmaceutical and biotechnical companies are involved in HIV/AIDS research in the United States, and as of December 1999, 61 AIDS-related medicines have been approved for sale in the United States and 102 medications were in development (Kaiser Family Foundation 2000). The pharmaceutical companies, however, have been criticized for the high cost of HIV/AIDS treatment. Pharmaceutical companies frequently utilize the knowledge gained from NIH-supported research to assist in the development of new drugs and other biomedical products. There has been pressure on the pharmaceutical industry to discount prices to reflect the public's investment.

CONCLUSION

Much has been accomplished in the United States since the AIDS epidemic was identified in the early 1980s. Laws have been enacted to secure equality and civil rights for those living with HIV-related diseases. Major research discoveries have advanced the treatment and care of persons with HIV/AIDS, and the average life span of these individuals has increased considerably. Funding for medical treatment has been made available for those who are uninsured or do not have the means to pay. Surveillance reports indicate that the number of new AIDS cases has decreased annually in recent years.

These conclusions not withstanding, HIV/AIDS remains an enormous problem in the United States, requiring billions of dollars annually to cover costs associated with the epidemic. HIV/AIDS has caused untold human suffering and will continue to do so until a cure and a vaccine are discovered. Stigmatization of persons living with HIV-related disease persists. The United States not only must face the problems associated with AIDS from the beginning of the epidemic but must be prepared to deal with emerging problems such as the high incidence and prevalence of HIV/AIDS among minority populations.

The United States must continue to combat the health care and social consequences associated with this epidemic. The nation must participate fully with other developed nations to provide resources and expertise to address the international consequences of AIDS.

BIBLIOGRAPHY

Association of American Medical Colleges. 1999. "Maximizing the Investment: Principles to Guide the Federal-Academic Partnership in Biomedical and Health Sciences Research." Available on the World Wide Web at: http://www.aamc.org/research/dbc/maximize/contents.htm.

Centers for Disease Control and Prevention. 1981a. "Kaposi's Sarcoma and Pneumocystis Pneumonia among Homosexual Men—New York City and California." *Morbidity and Mortality Weekly Report* 30: 250–252.

———. 1981b. "Pneumocystis Pneumonia—Los Angeles." *Morbidity and Mortality Weekly Report* 30: 305–308.

———. 1982a. "Epidemiologic Notes and Reports Possible Transfusion-Associated Acquired Immune Deficiency Syndrome (AIDS)—California." *Morbidity and Mortality Weekly Report* 31: 652–654.

———. 1982b. "Opportunistic Infections and Kaposi's Sarcoma among Haitians in the United States." *Morbidity and Mortality Weekly Report* 31: 353–354, 360–361.

———. 1982c. "Update on Acquired Immune Deficiency Syndrome (AIDS) among Patients with Hemophilia A." *Morbidity and Mortality Weekly Report* 31: 644–646, 652.

———. 1982d. "Update on Acquired Immune Deficiency Syndrome (AIDS)— United States." *Morbidity and Mortality Weekly Report* 31: 507–508.

———. 1983. "Update: Acquired Immune Deficiency Syndrome (AIDS)—United States." *Morbidity and Mortality Weekly Report* 32: 688–691.

———. 1985. "Revision of the Case Definition for Acquired Immunodeficiency Syndrome for National Reporting—United States." *Morbidity and Mortality Weekly Report* 34: 373–375.

———. 1987. "Revision of CDC Surveillance Case Definition for Acquired Immunodeficiency Syndrome." *Morbidity and Mortality Weekly Report* 361(1S): 1S–15S.

———. 1992. "1993 Revised Classification System for HIV Infection and Expanded Case Definition for AIDS among Adolescents and Adults." *Morbidity and Mortality Weekly Report* 41: 1–31.

———. 1998. "Trends in the HIV and AIDS Epidemic, 1998." Available on the World Wide Web at: http://www.cdc.gov/hiv/stats/trends98.pdf.

———. 1999. "CDC Guidelines for National Human Immunodeficiency Virus Case Surveillance, Including Monitoring for Human Immunodeficiency Virus Infection and Acquired Immunodeficiency Syndrome." *Morbidity and Mortality Weekly Report* 48: 1–29.

———. 2000. *HIV/AIDS Surveillance Report, 1999, 11 (no. 2)*. Atlanta, GA: Author.

Council of State and Territorial Epidemiologists. 1997. *CSTE Position Statement ID-4: National HIV Surveillance—Addition to the National Public Health Surveillance System*. Atlanta, GA: Author.

Hardy, Ann, James R. Allen, W. Meade Morgan, and James Curran. 1985. "The Incidence Rate of Acquired Immunodeficiency Syndrome in Selected Populations." *Journal of the American Medical Association* 253: 215–220.

Haverkos, Harvey W., A.N. Kopstein, and P. Drotman. 1994. "Nitrate Inhalants: History, Epidemiology, and Possible Links to AIDS." *Environmental Health Perspectives* 102: 858–861.

Jaffe, Harold W., Dennis J. Bregman, and Richard M. Selik. 1983. "Acquired Immune Deficiency Syndrome in the United States: The First 1,000 Cases." *Journal of Infectious Diseases* 148: 339–345.

Kaiser Family Foundation. 1998. "Federal HIV/AIDS Spending: A Budget Chartbook." Available on the World Wide Web at: http://hivinsite.ucsf.edu/social/kaiser_ffamily_ffound/2098.3d3f.html.

———. 2000. "HIV/AIDS Research: Success Brings New Challenge." Capitol Hill Briefing Series on HIV/AIDS, June.

Lamers, Elizabeth P. 1988. "Public Schools Confront AIDS." In *AIDS: Principles, Practices, & Politics*, Inge B. Corless and Mary Pittman-Lindeman, eds., pp. 175–185. New York: Harper & Row.

Liss, Marsha B. 1989. "The Schooling of Children with AIDS." In *Children, Adolescents, and AIDS*, Jeffrey M. Seibert and Roberta A. Olson, eds., pp. 93–117. Lincoln: University of Nebraska Press.
Shilts, Randy. 1987. *And the Band Played On*. New York: St. Martin's Press.

INDEX

Homosexual (male) transmission: Australia and, 1, 6, 13; Africa (sub-Saharan) and, 204–5; Brazil and, 27–28; Central and Eastern Europe and, 45; China and, 75; Ireland and, 98, 99, 102, 103, 107–8; Mexico and, 153; Netherlands and, 161, 165, 167, 169–70; Poland and, 44–45; Spain and, 186, 187, 194; Switzerland and, 220, 227; United Kingdom and, 238, 240, 248, 249; United States and, 254, 257, 258
Hong Kong, 70
Hubei province, 73
Human rights, 42, 55–58, 61, 144, 205, 250, 264
Hungary, 54, 57

Immigrants, 145, 170–71, 189
India, 73
Infectious Diseases Act (IZW), 173
Injecting drug users (IDUs): Australia and, 2, 7–8; Africa (sub-Saharan) and, 205; Brazil and, 22, 25, 27, 29, 31; Ireland and, 98, 99, 102–3, 106, 107, 108–9, 111; Netherlands and, 161, 170; Spain and, 184–86, 187, 188, 189, 191–92, 193, 196; Switzerland and, 220–21, 222, 227; United Kingdom and, 238, 240, 243–44, 248, 249; United States and, 254, 257, 258. See also China; Europe, Central and Eastern
Inner Mongolia, 78
Intergovernmental Committee on AIDS (IGCA), 9
International AIDS Conference, 159
International AIDS Therapy Evaluation Center (IATEC), 166
International Conference on AIDS and STIs, 212
International Harm Reduction Development (IHRD), 59
International Monetary Fund, 17, 201
Ireland, Republic of: blood transfusions and, 99; condom use in, 106, 110; HIV testing in, 102;

homosexual (male) transmission in, 99, 102, 103; injecting drug users in, 98, 99, 102–3, 106, 107, 108–9, 111; nongovernmental organizations in, 107–8; north-south differences in, 97; prevalence rates in, 98, 102–3, 111; prevention measures in, 107–10; prison inmates in, 107; recommendations for, 111; reporting issues in, 98; risk group distribution in, 98–99; sex work in, 106; stigmatization in, 103
Irish Nationalists, 111 n.1
Irkutsk, Russia, 43
Islamic Medical Association of Uganda, 127
Italy, 220

Joint United Nations Programme on HIV/AIDS (UNAIDS): Africa (sub-Saharan) and, 202, 204; Belarus and, 43–44; Brazil and, 18; China and, 71; Europe (Central and Eastern) and, 52, 55; Haiti and, 92, 94; human rights and, 56; Kenya and, 119, 122; minority populations and, 58; Poland and, 45; Uganda and, 117, 122

Kaliningrad, 42, 43
Kaposi's sarcoma (KS), 254
Kazakhstan, 44
Kenya: age differences and, 119–20; AIDS orphans in, 125; compulsory notification in, 125; compulsory testing in, 124–25; condom use in, 129–30; denial issues in, 125; education programs in, 128; government response in, 127–29, 132; heterosexual transmission in, 119–21; information issues in, 116–17; mortality rates in, 119, 121–22; nongovernmental organizations in, 129, 131–32; premarital sex in, 120; prevalence rates in, 115, 117, 119–20, 132; prevention efforts in, 115, 125–26; sex work in, 127

ABOUT THE CONTRIBUTORS

ROBERT S. ANWYL is professor of sociology and Peter Masiko, Jr. Endowed Teaching Chair in the Department of Sociology at Miami-Dade Community College (North Campus) in Florida and has an adjunct appointment with the Comprehensive Drug Research Center at the University of Miami School of Medicine. His research interests and many publications are in the areas of epidemiology of drug abuse, AIDS, and cancer. He completed his graduate work at Florida State University.

ÁNGELA BOLEA was formerly head of the Health Information and Promotion Service at the Government Department for Health in Prisons in Spain. Since 1995 she has headed the AIDS prevention branch in the Secretariat of the National Plan on AIDS at the Ministry of Health. She coordinates mass media campaigns, courses, and workshops related to the prevention of HIV/STD (sexually transmitted disease) transmission as well as the Spanish Ministry of Health financing of nongovernmental organizations who work on AIDS.

JESÚS CASTILLA is head of the HIV/AIDS Surveillance Unit at the National Center for Epidemiology and adviser for the National Plan on AIDS at the Spanish Ministry of Health. He coordinates the HIV/AIDS epidemiological surveillance systems, including the AIDS surveillance registry. He is a researcher in collaborative studies in the field of HIV/AIDS and analyzes transmission, natural history, and estimates of HIV incidence and prevalence.

ROBERTO CASTRO is a full-time researcher at the Regional Center for Multidisciplinary Research of the National University of Mexico in Cuernavaca, Mexico, where he is the coordinator of the research program "Health, Violence, and Society." He has recently conducted social research on family and AIDS, violence against pregnant women, abortion and social networks, abuse against women in the health services during delivery, and violent men. His most recent book is *Life in Adversity: The Meaning of Health and Reproduction among the Poor* (2000).

DALE D. CHITWOOD is professor of medical sociology and chairperson of the Department of Sociology at the University of Miami where he holds secondary appointments in the Departments of Epidemiology & Public Health and Psychiatry & Behavioral Sciences. He has conducted research on drug abuse for the past 25 years and since 1986 has been studying the relationship between HIV/AIDS and illicit drug use. Dr. Chitwood has published extensively in the areas of drug misuse, HIV/AIDS, and health services research among drug users. Currently he is principal investigator of a National Institute on Drug Abuse–funded grant that is assessing the effectiveness of behavioral interventions in reducing HIV risk behavior and preventing persons who sniff heroin from progressing to injection drug use.

MARY COMERFORD is a senior research associate in the Department of Sociology at the University of Miami. She has been working in the field of substance abuse and HIV/AIDS for the past 15 years. She has traveled to Haiti frequently for the past 10 years, where she has served as a volunteer with several organizations.

LUIS DE LA FUENTE is an epidemiologist in the Secretariat of the National Plan on AIDS and the National Center for Epidemiology in Spain. He has worked in the substance abuse field since 1988, first with the National Plan on Drugs and since 1998 with the National Plan on AIDS. His research focuses currently on the epidemiology of health-related problems in drug users, mainly HIV infection, overdose, and mental health.

DOUGLAS FELDMAN is an anthropologist and research associate professor and director of the AIDS Social Research Program in the Department of Psychiatry and Behavioral Sciences at the University of Miami School of Medicine. He is the editor of four volumes on HIV/AIDS, most recently *The AIDS Crisis: A Documentary History* (1998). He has conducted AIDS social research in the United States, Zambia, Rwanda, Uganda, and Senegal and received the Kimball Award in Public and Applied Anthropology in 1996.

KAREN GIFFIN is a professor and researcher at the National School for Public Health of the Oswaldo Cruz Foundation, Brazilian Health Ministry (ENSP/FIOCRUZ), in Rio de Janeiro. She entered the area of public health through development of community-based proposals for women's and children's health. Her research and publications have focused on gender and health, with emphasis on reproductive health.

SUSAN GOODE is a research assistant at the Australian Institute of Criminology, with a background in geography. Her primary interests are drugs and crime, and she is currently completing a monograph on the relationship between drugs and criminal careers among incarcerated property offenders.

JEAN-PAUL C. GRUND specializes in the study of the relationship between humans and intoxicants and is director of research at DV8 Research, Training and Development. He recently completed a study of drug use among the Roma population of Central and Eastern Europe and is conducting two multisite evaluation studies of needle exchange programs in Russia and Eastern Europe. At The Lindesmith Center, Open Society Institute, he founded the International Harm Reduction Development program, which fosters the development of practical harm reduction programs in Central Eastern Europe and Russia.

SALLY HAW is a research specialist (substance misuse) for the Health Education Board for Scotland. Much of her work has focused on the epidemiology of problem drug use and HIV infection in Scotland. In the early 1990s she developed a methodology for recruiting community samples of drug users in order to estimate the prevalence of HIV infection in injecting drug users. Most recently she has been involved in the development of a research strategy to support the Scottish Drug Misuse Strategy and was adviser to Scottish parliamentary inquiry into the relationship between drug misuse and deprivation.

KATHRYN HIGGINS is a research fellow at the Centre for Child Care Research, Queens University, Belfast, Northern Ireland. Her research interests and publications lie in the field of drug use, particularly injecting use and associated health risk behaviors, adolescent substance use, and methodological issues relating to the study of hidden populations. She is currently co-investigator on the Belfast Youth Development Study, a longitudinal cohort study of adolescent drug use.

HELEN JACKSON was the director of SAfAIDS, Southern Africa AIDS Information Dissemination Service, a regional nongovernmental organization based in Zimbabwe that provides information and advisory services on HIV/AIDS and development to a wide multisectoral constituency. She is currently with the United Nations Population Fund (UNFPA) country support team for Southern Africa. She has extensive experience with HIV/AIDS programming, research, and policy in southern Africa and beyond. Prior to establishing SAfAIDS, she was a lecturer and then director of research at the School of Social Work, University of Zimbabwe.

JOHANNES C. JAGER is a theoretical biologist by training and currently deputy head of the Department for Health Services Research (CZO) at the National Institute of Public Health and the Environment (RIVM) in Bilthoven, the Netherlands. For many years he has coordinated European multinational projects, for example, the Concerted Action of the European Communities on Multinational AIDS Scenarios (MAS). He directs the Department's project Cost-Effectiveness of Interventions in Care and Prevention in Chronic and Infectious Diseases. His present research concerns general methodology, scenario analysis, and economic evaluation applied to public health and health care.

SHENGHAN LAI is an associate research professor of epidemiology at the Johns Hopkins School of Hygiene and Public Health. His research areas include cancer, HIV, and drug abuse. In the last four years, Dr. Lai has published more than 40 papers.

TIM LEE is deputy director at the International HIV/AIDS Alliance, a nongovernmental organization (NGO) specializing in supporting community action on AIDS in developing countries. Prior to this appointment, he was based in Zimbabwe for three years, working for local and regional AIDS NGOs. Before joining the NGO sector, he was lecturer in social policy at the University of Bath, United Kingdom, for eight years.

RENÉ LEYVA is a full-time researcher in the Division of Community Health and Social Wellfare, within the National Institute of Public Health, in Cuernavaca, Mexico. He is currently conducting social research on drug consumption in private pharmacies and participates in a project on migration and AIDS in Central America, a study from which his most recent published articles have been taken.

WIEN C.M. LIMBURG is an information specialist at the Department for Health Services Research (CZO) at the National Institute of Public Health and the Environment (RIVM) in Bilthoven, the Netherlands. She is involved in various research projects concerning public health and health care. Her present activities focus on hepatitis C in intravenous drug users in the European Union and care profiles of chronically ill people.

TONI MAKKAI is deputy-director of research at the Australian Institute of Criminology. She has written widely on drugs and crime and compliance and regulation. She has also held teaching and research positions in the United Kingdom and at the Australian National University, Australia. Her latest work involves monitoring illicit drug use among police detainees and evaluating the impact of drug courts in Australia.

CLYDE B. MCCOY is director of the Comprehensive Drug Research Center and Health Services Research Center, a federally funded center designated by the National Institute on Drug Abuse. He is also professor and chair of the Department of Epidemiology and Public Health at the University of Miami School of Medicine. Dr. McCoy has had continuous federal funding for his research for more than 25 years and has served as principal investigator or coprincipal investigator on numerous studies. He currently is conducting both national and international research projects. His research interests include epidemiology, drug use, demography, HIV/AIDS prevention among drug users, and cancer prevention. He has more than 200 publications in these areas.

KAREN MCELRATH is a reader in sociology at Queen's University, Belfast, Northern Ireland. Prior to that appointment she worked in the Department of Sociology at the University of Miami. She completed the first in-depth study of injecting drug users (IDUs) in Northern Ireland, and her current research interests focus on the relationship between drug policies and risk behaviors among IDUs as well as drug use in political conflict. She was co-investigator of the first project to examine the lifestyles of Ecstasy users in Northern Ireland.

LISA R. METSCH is assistant professor of epidemiology and public health at the University of Miami School of Medicine. Dr. Metsch's funded research and publications focus on behavioral interventions in substance abuse and HIV. She is the recipient of a research scientist development award from the National Institute on Drug Abuse and the principal investigator on grants funded by the Centers for Disease Control and Prevention and the Robert Wood Johnson Foundation.

ELIZABETH PISANI trained as a medical demographer at the London School of Hygiene and Tropical Medicine. She has worked extensively on the surveillance of HIV and the behaviors associated with transmission of the virus for the Joint United Nations Programme on HIV/AIDS (UNAIDS), the World Health Organization, and other groups. She is the principal author of regular UNAIDS reports on the epidemiology of HIV and is currently based in Nairobi, Kenya.

THOMAS STEFFEN has worked at the Institute for Addiction Research in Zurich. Prior to that appointment, he worked as a physician and scientific assistant at the University of Basel, where his work focused mainly on social pediatry, environmental medicine, and evaluation research in the addiction sector (tobacco and illegal drugs). His current research interests include social medicine research projects in the illegal drugs sector, especially heroin-supported treatment, and general evaluation research.

MÓNICA SUÁREZ is a civil servant in the Secretariat of the National Plan on AIDS at the Ministry of Health and responsible for HIV prevention among injecting drug users. She has worked in the substance abuse field since 1990, both with the United Nations and with Spanish organizations.

Her research focuses currently on HIV/STI (sexually transmitted infection)–related sexual risk behaviors. She is a member of the Spanish subcommittee on AIDS Prevention and the committee on guidelines for needle exchange programs in prisons.

LETÍCIA LEGAY VERMELHO is an associate professor and researcher at the Federal University of Rio de Janeiro in the Nucleus for Studies of Collective Health (NESC/UFRJ). She has acted as adviser to the Brazilian Health Ministry's AIDS program. Her current research focuses on the areas of violence as a cause of death, and AIDS.

XUE-REN WANG is a professor of statistics and is well published, with over 50 peer-reviewed publications and six books. In November 1995, Professor Wang, as the president of Yunnan University, set up the Comprehensive Drug Research Center of Yunnan University, which was approved by the Provincial Government.